The Complete Guide to Ketogenic Diet for Women Over 50

Useful Tips and 470 Delectable Recipes
30 Days Keto Meal Plan to Shed Weight, Heal Your Body, and Regain Confidence

Sandra Grant

2022

POMEGRANATE MOLASSES ROASTED CHUCK 96
SPICY MINCED LAMB WITH PEAS AND TOMATO SAUCE 97
ROASTED LAMB SHANKS WITH VEGETABLES 97
CLASSIC MEATLOAF STUFFED WITH MOZZARELLA 97
BARACOA-STYLE SHREDDED BEEF 98
BEEF SHAWARMA WITH TAHINI SAUCE 98
AVOCADO BEEF CHILI WITH COCONUT YOGURT 99
SPARE RIBS WITH CURRY SAUCE 99
RED PEPPER FLAKES BEEF RIBS WITH RICE 99
SIMPLE CORNED BEEF 100
BEEF BOURGUIGNON 100
ASIAN BEEF CURRY 100
BORDEAUX POT ROAST 100
BEEF HOT POT 101
BEEF AND PASTA CASSEROLE 101
KOREAN HOT BEEF SALAD 101
CHINESE BEEF AND BROCCOLI 101
BRISKET AND CABBAGE HODGEPODGE 102
MERLOT LAMB SHANKS 102
ROSEMARY LAMB RIBS 102
MEDITERRANEAN LAMB 102
CREAMY LAMB CURRY 103
LAMB AND VEGETABLE HOT POT 103
MOROCCAN LAMB 103
LAMB RAGOUT 104
LAMB AND BARLEY BOWLS 104
MEXICAN STYLE LAMB 104
GOAT AND TOMATO POT 104
CORNED BEEF WITH VEGETABLE 105
SPICY TACO MEAT 105
BEEF BEAN RICE 105
BEEF STROGANOFF 105
CHILE LIME STEAK FAJITAS 106
KETO BEEF AND BROCCOLI 106
MEATLOAF RECIPE 106
MOROCCAN MEATBALLS 107
LOW CARB BEEF BOLOGNESE SAUCE 107
KETO LAMB CHOPS ON THE GRILL 107
KETO LAMB CURRY 108
ROSEMARY DIJON ROASTED LAMB CHOPS 108
KETO LAMB KOFTAS 108
GREEK LAMB AND CABBAGE BOWLS 108
LAMB MEATBALLS WITH MINT GREMOLATA 109
LAMB CASSOULET WITH BEANS 109
ITALIAN RICE CASSEROLE 109
SWISS CHEESE BEEF ZUCCHINI CASSEROLE 110
CHILI VERDE WITH POTATOES 110
SIMPLE & CLASSIC GOULASH 110
BEEF AND BROCCOLI STIR-FRY 110
CHEDDAR-STUFFED BURGERS WITH ZUCCHINI 111
BEEF AND BROCCOLI STIR-FRY 111
HEARTY BEEF AND BACON CASSEROLE 111
SLOW COOKER BEEF BOURGUIGNON 111
PEPPER GRILLED RIBEYE WITH ASPARAGUS 112
STEAK KEBABS WITH PEPPERS AND ONIONS 112
SEARED LAMB CHOPS WITH ASPARAGUS 112

LAMB CHOPS WITH KALAMATA TAPENADE 112
ROSEMARY-GARLIC LAMB RACKS 113
LAMB LEG WITH SUN-DRIED TOMATO PESTO 113
SIRLOIN WITH BLUE CHEESE COMPOUND BUTTER 113
GARLIC-BRAISED SHORT RIBS 113
BACON-WRAPPED BEEF TENDERLOIN 114
CHEESEBURGER CASSEROLE 114
ITALIAN BEEF BURGERS 114

PORK AND HAM 115

HAM AND PROVOLONE SANDWICH 116
SPRING SALAD WITH SHAVED PARMESAN 116
THREE MEAT AND CHEESE SANDWICH 116
HAM, EGG, AND CHEESE SANDWICH 116
CHOPPED KALE SALAD WITH BACON DRESSING 117
CREAMY HONEY & MUSTARD PORK RIBS 117
TENDER AND JUICY SHREDDED PORK 117
KETO PROSCIUTTO SPINACH SALAD 117
BRIGHT SALSA PORK CHOPS 117
LOADED CAULIFLOWER 118
PAN-SEARED PORK TENDERLOIN MEDALLIONS 118
COCONUT PORK CURRY 118
THE BEST BAKED GARLIC PORK TENDERLOIN 118
PORK SKEWERS WITH CHIMICHURRI 119
APRICOT GLAZED PORK 119
EASY BBQ HAM 119
CHEESY SCALLOPED POTATOES WITH HAM 119
SALAD WITH BROCCOLI, CAULIFLOWER AND BACON 119
ASPARAGUS WRAPPED IN PROSCIUTTO 120
BRATWURSTS AND SAUERKRAUT 120
ROSEMARY ROASTED PORK WITH CAULIFLOWER 120
SAUSAGE STUFFED BELL PEPPERS 120
CHEDDAR, SAUSAGE, AND MUSHROOM CASSEROLE 121
CAULIFLOWER CRUST MEAT LOVER'S PIZZA 121
BACON-WRAPPED PORK TENDERLOIN WITH CAULIFLOWER 121
ROASTED PORK LOIN WITH GRAINY MUSTARD SAUCE 121

FISH AND SEAFOOD 123

QUICK & EASY KETO TUNA FISH SALAD 124
SIMPLE TUNA SALAD ON LETTUCE 124
FRIED TUNA AVOCADO BALLS 124
THAI COCONUT SHRIMP SOUP 124
SHRIMP AVOCADO SALAD 124
CAPRESE TUNA SALAD STUFFED TOMATOES 125
SPICY KIMCHI AHI POKE 125
PROSCIUTTO BLACKBERRY SHRIMP 125
SPICY SHRIMP TACO LETTUCE WRAPS 125
KETO SHRIMP THAI SALAD 126
SHRIMP AND NORI ROLLS 126
CRISPY FISH STICKS WITH CAPER DILL SAUCE 126
CREAMY SHRIMP AND MUSHROOM SKILLET 126
BUTTERED COD IN SKILLET 127
AVOCADO LIME SALMON 127
BROCCOLI AND SHRIMP SAUTÉED IN BUTTER 127
KETO CALAMARI 127
CALAMARI STUFFED WITH PANCETTA AND VEGETABLES 128
LOW CARB ALMOND CRUSTED COD 128

Introduction

Age is never an excuse to let go of yourself. *Why?* you ask. Because I can proudly say that I am a 53-year-old woman who is living her life to the fullest. I am in the best (and the hottest) shape that I have ever been in my entire life. People often ask me how I can look so fit despite my age. And my reply is, "Keto. You have to go against the grain." Puns aside, the keto diet has changed my whole life. I don't crave snacks every 30 minutes. My skin is glowing like I have drenched myself in the most expensive highlighter. Weight loss has never been so effortless and joyful, and with the keto diet, I have lost twenty pounds in two months!

Unbelievable right? But that is the magic of ketosis, where the body burns fat instead of glucose as energy. So, the body becomes a fat-burning machine that breaks down fat into ketone bodies that are used as fuel for the entire body. The diet works by using a meal consisting of high fat, low carb, and moderate protein ratio, also known as "keto" or "ketogenic."

This book is a holy grail for middle-aged women who want to know everything there is to become more fit and live a nutritional life packed with energy and lots of ketos.

One aging factor for middle-aged women is when their menstrual cycle stops; this is called menopause. It usually occurs after women hit the age of 50. As menopause occurs, it brings forth many problems, such as weight gain and irregular sleep schedules. In addition, your bones will weaken, putting you at a higher risk for osteoporosis. It happens due to the low estrogen levels and the decrease in the growth hormone. These are both essential in bone remodeling.

Hormones play a vital role in determining where and how much fat will be stored throughout the body. After menopause, most fat starts to get stored in the belly, causing increased belly fat. The right diet can help control fat storage, increasing overall health in women. The ketogenic diet is one of the best options for women going through this stage of menopause while staying healthy. I am living, breathing proof that this diet works wonders for women aged 50 years and above. I have been following it for the past two years. The hardest step to any diet is taking the first step ahead and thoroughly researching the technicalities that you can easily read in the upcoming chapters of this book.

When you first start the keto diet, it's important to know if and when you're in ketosis when you first start eating low-carb. Not only is it a great confidence booster, but testing also lets you know that you're doing things right, or wrong, and whether you need to make any changes.

An easy test is to sniff for "keto-breath." After a few days, you might notice a taste that's somewhat fruity and a bit sour or even metallic. The reason for this? When your body is in ketosis, it creates the ketone bodies: acetone, acetoacetate, and beta-hydroxybutyrate. Acetone in particular is excreted through your urine and breath, which causes "keto-breath." This change in the smell of your breath and the taste in your mouth usually diminishes after a few weeks.

A more accurate way to tell is by using ketone urine test strips. They're fairly inexpensive and can instantly check the ketone levels in your urine. You can find them in packs of 100 for under $10 online or at most pharmacies. Try to take the test a few hours after you wake up in the morning, because being dehydrated after a night's sleep can cause a false positive.

The most accurate test involves a blood ketone meter. This type of test is a bit pricier at around $40 for the meter and up to $5 per test strip. The upside is it's much more accurate because it tests your blood directly. For nutritional ketosis, your reading should be between 0.5 and 5.0 millimeters.

Long term, it's not necessary to continuously check on your ketone levels. Within a few weeks, you'll know if you're eating right, and it becomes very easy to stay in ketosis.

Living in Ratios

Just like the USDA's Food Pyramid, the keto diet is built on ratios. It's important to get the right balance of macronutrients so your body has the energy it needs and you're not missing any essential fat or protein in your diet.

Macronutrients are what foods are made of. They are fat, protein and carbohydrates. Each type of macronutrient provides a certain amount of energy (calories) per gram consumed.

- Fat provides about 9 calories per gram

- Protein provides about 4 calories per gram

- Carbohydrates provide about 4 calories per gram

On the keto diet, 65 to 75 percent of the calories you consume should come from fat. About 20 to 25 percent should come from protein, and the remaining 5 percent or so from carbohydrates.

Here are the same numbers broken down into an average 2000-calorie daily diet by grams and percentages:

Keep in mind that 2000 calories is just an example—the number of calories you consume daily should be tailored to your body, activity levels, and goals.

The number of calories you should eat depends on a few factors, including:

- Current lean body weight (total body weight minus body fat)

- Daily activity levels (do you work in an office, wait tables, compete as a professional athlete?)

- Workout regimen? If so:

o The types of workouts (weight lifting, cardio, or both)

o   Hours per week of each type

- Goal:

o   Lose weight
o   Maintain weight
o   Gain muscle

There are many ketogenic-based macro calculators available online, such as tasteaholics.com/keto-calculator and ketogains.com/ketogains-calculator. You can also find plenty of others through a quick Google search for "keto calculator." You'll be able to easily and quickly plug in your numbers and get an immediate estimation of your body's caloric needs.
One of the great things about the keto diet is that it's not necessary to track each and every number to hit your goals. Yet if you want to track, it's a great way to speed up your progress, and tracking will give you a visual reminder to stay on course every day.

Necessary Nutrients

It's crucial to drink plenty of water when beginning the keto diet. You may even notice that you're visiting the bathroom more often, and that's normal!
This happens because you're cutting out a lot of processed foods and have started eating more whole, natural foods instead. Processed foods have a lot of added sodium, and the sudden change in diet causes a sudden drop in sodium intake.
Additionally, the reduction in carbs reduces insulin levels, which in turn tells your kidneys to release excess stored sodium. Between the reduction in sodium intake and flushing of excess stored sodium, the body begins to excrete much more water than usual, and you end up low on sodium and other electrolytes.
When this happens, you may experience symptoms such as fatigue, headaches, coughing, sniffles, irritability, and/or nausea.
This state is generally known as the "keto flu." It's very important to know that this is not the actual influenza virus. It's called the keto flu only due to the similarity in symptoms, but it's neither contagious nor a real virus.
Many who experience these symptoms believe the keto diet made them sick and immediately go back to eating carbs. But the keto flu phase actually means your body is withdrawing from sugar, high carbs, and processed foods, and is readjusting so it can use fat as its fuel. The keto flu usually lasts just a few days while the body readjusts. You can abate its symptoms by adding more sodium and electrolytes to your diet.

Getting Ready to Go Keto

Now that you understand the benefits and science behind the ketogenic diet, you're ready to get started. In the following chapters, you'll get all the information you need to succeed with your keto diet, including what to buy and what to avoid,full recipes, and how to exercise to maximize your health.

CHAPTER 1

GO KETO IN FIVE STEPS

YOU NOW KNOW THE SCIENCE behind the keto diet and why it works. In this chapter, you'll learn how to get started and maximize success. Here's a quick and easy step-by-step guide to use as you begin, and to refer to any time throughout your journey, for support and guidance.

Step 1: Clean Out Your Pantry

Out with the old, in with the new. Having tempting, unhealthy foods in your home is one of the biggest contributors to failure when starting any diet. To succeed, you need to minimize any triggers to maximize your chances. Unless you have the iron will of Arnold Schwarzenegger, you should not keep addictive foods like bread, desserts, and other non–keto friendly snacks around.

If you don't live alone, be sure to discuss and warn your housemates, whether they're significant others, family, or roommates. If some items must be kept (if they're simply not yours to throw out), try to agree on a special location to keep them out of sight. This will also help anyone you share your living space with understand that you are serious about starting your diet, and will lead to a better experience for you at home overall (people love to tempt anyone on a diet at first, but it will get old and they'll tire quickly).

STARCHES AND GRAINS

Get rid of all cereal, pasta, rice, potatoes, corn, oats, quinoa, flour, bread, bagels, wraps, rolls, and croissants.

SUGARY FOODS AND DRINKS

Get rid of all refined sugar, fountain drinks, fruit juices, milk, desserts, pastries, milk chocolate, candy bars, etc.

LEGUMES

Get rid of beans, peas, and lentils. They are dense with carbs. A 1-cup serving of beans alone contains more than three times the amount of carbs you want to consume in a day.

PROCESSED POLYUNSATURATED FATS AND OILS

Get rid of all vegetable oils and most seed oils, including sunflower, safflower, canola, soybean, grapeseed, and corn oil. Also eliminate trans fats like shortening and margarine—anything that says "hydrogenated" or "partially hydrogenated." Olive oil, extra virgin olive oil, avocado oil, and coconut oil are the keto-friendly oils you want on hand.

FRUITS

Get rid of fruits that are high in carbs, including bananas, dates, grapes, mangos, and apples. Be sure to get rid of any dried fruits like raisins as well. Dried fruit contains as much sugar as regular fruit but more concentrated, making it easy to eat a lot of sugar in a small serving. For comparison, a cup of raisins has over 100 grams of carbs while a cup of grapes has only 15 grams of carbs.

Yes, you're "getting rid" of unwanted foods in your pantry, but these foods can feed many others. Please, don't throw them away! Find a local food bank or homeless youth shelter to donate them to.

Your pantry will seem empty after the cleanout. That's because products meant for longer-term storage are usually high in carbs and full of unhealthy additives and preservatives. You'll fill your refrigerator shortly (Step 2) with healthy, natural foods.

FINDING SUPPORT

Sticking to your diet in the beginning can prove difficult when close friends and family aren't eating the same as you. Even worse, they are eating all the things you're trying not to eat. Every person is different, and you likely know who will support you and who will not. For those who support you, explain that you're avoiding carbs (and which foods include carbs) and request politely that they not offer you anything when you're eating together.

Telling the naysayers that you've quit eating grains and sugar will usually suffice. The terms keto and low-carb will usually spark a debate or argument with certain people because they've been told their whole lives to eat carbs and low-fat products. Try to avoid using those terms when explaining your diet goals. Avoid direct debates by recommending they read about the benefits of being in ketosis and the health benefits of eating a low-carb diet.

Step 2: Go Shopping

It's time to restock your pantry, refrigerator, and freezer with delicious, keto-friendly foods that will help you lose weight, become healthy, and feel great!

THE BASICS

- With these basics on hand, you'll always be ready to prepare healthy, delicious, and keto-friendly meals and snacks.

- Water, coffee, and tea

- All spices and herbs

- Sweeteners, including stevia and erythritol

- Lemon or lime juice

- Low-carb condiments like mayonnaise, mustard, pesto, and sriracha

- Broths (chicken, beef, bone)

- Pickled and fermented foods like pickles, kimchi, and sauerkraut

- Nuts and seeds, including macadamia nuts, pecans, almonds, walnuts, hazelnuts, pine nuts, flaxseed, chia seeds, and pumpkin seeds.

MEATS

Any type of meat is fine for the keto diet, including chicken, beef, lamb, pork, turkey, game, etc. It's preferable to use grass-fed and/or organic meats if they're available and possible for your budget. You can and should eat the fat on the meat and skin on the chicken.
All wild-caught fish and seafood slide into the keto diet nicely. Try to avoid farmed fish.
Go crazy with the eggs! Use organic eggs from free-range chickens, if possible.

VEGGIES

You can eat all nonstarchy veggies, including broccoli, asparagus, mushrooms, cucumbers, lettuce, onions, peppers, tomatoes, garlic (in small quantities—each clove contains about 1 gram of carbs), Brussels sprouts, zucchini, eggplant, olives, zucchini, yellow squash, and cauliflower.
Avoid all types of potatoes, yams and sweet potatoes, corn, and legumes like beans, lentils, and peas.

ABOUT THOSE SWEETENERS ...

The sweeteners may sound strange if you haven't heard of them before. They both come from natural sources and are safe to use in any quantity.
Stevia is extracted from the leaves of a plant called Stevia rebaudiana. Stevia has zero calories and contains some beneficial micronutrients like magnesium, potassium, and zinc. It's readily available in liquid or powder form online and in most supermarkets. It's much sweeter than sugar, so containers are usually very small—you won't need nearly as much.
Erythritol is a sugar alcohol that is low in calories, about 70 percent as sweet as sugar, and can be found naturally in some fruits and vegetables. Sugar alcohols are indigestible by the human body, so erythritol cannot raise your blood sugar or insulin levels. Several studies have proven it to be safe. Sugar alcohols can sometimes cause temporary digestive discomfort, but out of the few available sugar alcohols like xylitol, maltitol, and sorbitol, erythritol is considered to be the most forgiving and best for everyday use.

FRUITS

You can eat a small amount of berries every day, such as strawberries, raspberries, blackberries, and blueberries. Lemon and lime juices are great for adding flavor to your meals. Avocados are also low in carbs and full of healthy fat.
Avoid other fruits, as they're loaded with sugar. A single banana can contain around 25 grams of net carbs.

DAIRY

Eat full-fat dairy like butter, sour cream, heavy (whipping) cream, cheese, cream cheese, and unsweetened yogurt. Although not technically dairy, unsweetened almond and coconut milks are great as well.
Avoid milk and skim milk, as well as sweetened yogurt, as it contains a lot of sugar. Avoid any flavored, low-fat, or fat-free dairy products.

FATS AND OILS

Avocado oil, olive oil, butter, lard, and bacon fat are great for cooking and consuming. Avocado oil has a high smoke point (it does not burn or smoke until it reaches 520°F), which is ideal for searing meats and frying in a wok. Make sure to avoid oils labeled "blend"; they commonly contain small amounts of the healthy oil and large amounts of unhealthy oils.

Step 3: Set Up Your Kitchen

Preparing delicious recipes is one of the best parts of the keto diet, and it's quite easy if you have the right tools. The following tools will make cooking simpler and faster. Each one is worth investing in, especially for the busy cook.

FOOD SCALE

When you're trying to hit your caloric and macronutrient goals, a kitchen food scale is a necessary appliance. You can measure any solid or liquid food, and get the perfect amount every time. Used in combination with an app like MyFitnessPal, you'll have all the data you need to hit your goals sooner. Food scales can be found online for $10 to $20.

FOOD PROCESSOR

Food processors are critical to your arsenal. They are ideal for blending certain foods or processing foods together into sauces and shakes. Blenders don't cut it, powerwise, for many foods, especially tough vegetables like cauliflower.
One great food processor/blender is NutriBullet. The containers you blend in come with lids or drink spouts so you can take them to go or use them as storage. They're also easy to clean, making the whole system extremely convenient. They typically sell for about $80 online.

SPIRALIZER

Spiralizers make vegetables into noodles or ribbons within seconds. They make cooking a lot faster and easier—noodles have much more surface area and take a fraction of the time to cook. For example, a spiralizer turns a zucchini into zoodles, and with some Alfredo or marinara sauce, you can't tell you aren't eating noodles. Spiralizers cost around $30 and can be found in large retail stores and online.

ELECTRIC HAND MIXER

If you've ever had to beat an egg white by hand until you get stiff peaks, then you know just how difficult it is. Electric hand mixers save your arm muscles and massive amounts of time, especially when mixing heavy ingredients. You can find a decent one online for $10 to $20.

CAST IRON PANS

They've been used for centuries and were one of the first modern cooking devices. Cast iron skillets don't wear out and are healthier to use (no chemical treatment of any kind), retain heat very well, and can be moved between the stove and oven. They are simple to clean up—just wash them out with a scrub sponge without soap, dry them off, and then rub them with cooking oil. This prevents rust and encourages the buildup of "seasoning," a natural nonstick surface. Many cast iron pans come preseasoned, and this method preserves the coating. You can find them in many retail stores and online for $10 to $80, depending on the brand and size; Lodge is a popular brand, still made in the United States.

KNIFE SHARPENING STONE

Most of prep time is spent on cutting. You'll see your cutting speed skyrocket with a sharp knife set. It's also a pleasure to use sharp knives. Aim to sharpen your knives every week or so to keep them in good shape (professional chefs sharpen their knives before every use). Sharpening stones cost under $10 and can be ordered online.

KETO-FRIENDLY ALTERNATIVES

You'd be surprised just how many carbs are in common everyday foods. Below is a chart of common foods and their keto-friendly alternatives that you can enjoy at any time.

Note: Net carbs are the total carbs minus dietary fiber (soluble and insoluble) and sugar alcohols. Fiber and sugar alcohols are not counted toward net carbs because the human body cannot digest and break them down into glucose, so they do not spike blood sugar.

NICE-TO-HAVE EQUIPMENT

The kitchen section of any store can be a wonderland. There are so many intriguing gadgets. It's also nice (although not necessary) to have these other tools on hand if you can't resist the lure:

INSTANT COOKING THERMOMETER Cooking steak and chicken is much easier when you can easily prod the meat and find out whether it's at the level of doneness that you're shooting for. These can usually be found for $10 to $20 in most retail stores or online.

MEASURING SPOON SET Get the right amount of an ingredient quickly. These sets can go from $5 to $10 in any supermarket, store, or online.

TONGS Tongs reduce splatter when working quickly (compared to using a fork or spatula to flip something in a hot pan). It's best to get tongs with nylon heads so you don't scratch any of your pots or pans. You can get a pair online or in retail stores for $10 to $15.

Step 5: Exercise

As you start your diet and the pounds fall off, think about how to lose more weight or get healthier to feel even better. This is a great time to become more active through exercise.

Increase the amount you exercise relative to what you do now. If you don't exercise at all, start taking short walks or slow jogs, or a combination of both, for 15 minutes every other day. If you already go to the gym or lift weights, add an extra exercise or start doing cardio. It doesn't matter what level you're at, try to do a little more than you're doing now. That's all it takes to become healthier. Exercise is incremental, and every increment is a boost to weight loss and feeling better.

If you have the time, try taking a class or doing an activity that involves moving, like a step class or dancing, or start playing a sport like basketball. It doesn't have to be competitive, nor do you need to be good or have any previous experience. Such activities are an easy way to get on your feet, and you can learn a new skill in the process.

Staying fit through regular physical activity has been proven to reduce blood pressure and cholesterol levels as well as reduce risk for various heart diseases and type 2 diabetes. In combination with the keto diet, your health will improve dramatically, and so will your energy levels.

Any exercise, even if it's 15 minutes a week, is better than no exercise. Don't worry about how much you do in the beginning. Just start doing something and you'll build from there naturally.

EASY EXERCISE SEQUENCES

Here are a few easy exercise sequences if you're just starting out. Once every other day is enough in the beginning. If possible, try doing these with a friend or significant other for support and accountability. If you can't do some of them, that's absolutely all right! Simply focus on the ones you can do.

CARDIOVASCULAR ACTIVITY Any aerobic activity, like walking, running, or bicycling, for 15 to 30 minutes, twice a week or more.

STRENGTH CONDITIONING One set of exercises (for at least 10 repetitions, or it's too easy) targeting each of the major muscle groups: chest, shoulders, back, abs, and legs.

- Push-ups or assisted push-ups

- Pull-ups or chin-ups

- Crunches

- Squats

Chapter 2: Keto Diet 101 and Its Amazing Benefits

This book discusses how the keto diet benefits women 50 years of age and above. Of course, the biggest health concern that most women face is menopause. It is one of the most impactful health concerns that may increase problems such as weight gain, mood swings, bone weakness, etc. It is about how the keto diet is effortless to follow; unlike other diets, ketosis is a lifestyle. It might seem unbelievable since I have only been following this diet for the past two years. But trust me, as I have researched how lifelong health is affected due to many factors, especially blood sugar.

After following this diet, I have experienced positive changes in my overall health and energy. It is by far the most rewarding and effortless approach I have come across through lots of research. The two years I have spent exploring this ketogenic eating style have brought me closer to a life filled with happiness and health. It is evolutionary indeed!

Using a food-loving approach, this book will satisfy all the needs necessary for the lifelong health we all dream of. This includes calories reductions, saturated fats boost, control of blood sugar, boosted cell health, and so much more.

It doesn't just include a handful of recipes in a meal plan but also an introduction to ketosis. It includes things I wish I had known before I started this diet. For example, I never knew what 75% fat, 15% protein, and 10% carbs looked like on a plate and their effect on our body. But don't worry because that is what I'm going to help you with!

Problems Faced by Women After 50

Before we jump into ketosis and its benefits, we first have to learn about the problems that women face. The first step to every solution is recognizing your problems before jumping to any conclusion.

In women, the reproductive system is the only system that starts working at the ages of seven or eight and ceases to work around 60 to 65. So no matter how hard it might seem, every woman has to go through this phase in her life. The reverse phase is often called menopause. This period often takes ten years or more to completely stop, but the process stops the childbearing function first, then the menstrual function.

This entire process of the reverse reproductive system is divided into four-stage periods:

- Pre-menopausal period: 45 until the onset of menopause
- Peri-menopausal period: 44–45 years of age
- Menopause: last menstrual period around 50
- Postmenopausal period (the last stage): begins after menopause at approximately 65–69

The program for the development and aging of an organism is individual. If we were to divide the percent of a woman's life, then 33 percent would be dedicated to this period, for the arrival for which they are completely unarmed.

Besides age-related changes in the reproductive system, there are also some climacteric changes that occur during life. The lack of estrogen can lead to the development of osteoporosis, hormonal cardiopathy, depression, and psychoses related to age. The second female hormone, which is connected to targeted organs, will get affected, causing diseases such as uterine fibroids, breast tumors, etc. The correct relationship between all the elements and hormones is crucial during the menstrual cycle.

In addition, the damage accumulated as a result of past illnesses, stressful situations, and the peculiarities of a modern lifestyle is of concern. Exposure to high frequency or ultraviolet rays also manifests any existing pathology.

The growing deficiency of female sex hormones might also lead to a decrease in the body's adaptive capabilities. Female hormones affect all organs, including our central nervous system, blood vessels, heart bones, urinary system, etc.

The symptoms of the climacteric syndrome may include hot flashes (burning sensations) to the face, upper body accompanied by sweating, dizziness, and rapid heartbeat. These could lead to sleep deprivation along with weakness, fatigue, and irritation.

Metabolic disorders such as atherosclerosis and osteoporosis may occur five or more years after menopause, leading to the likelihood of diseases like hypertension, myocardial infarction, and bone fractures. Earlier menopause may also result in early metabolic disturbance due to the disappearance of the protective effect of estrogen on bones, hearts, and blood vessels.

Today, a low-carb ketogenic diet can help to compensate for the ongoing hormonal changes and eliminate the symptoms of the climatic period, accompanied by complete rest and engagement in enjoyable activities and hobbies

Benefits Of the Ketogenic Diet for Women

According to my research, the ketogenic diet can have several benefits, especially for women going through menopause.

Helps Improve Blood Sugar Levels
During menopause, insulin levels may drop, which causes a rise in blood sugar levels. Insulin is a hormone that is responsible for transporting sugar from the blood to the cells. Some studies showed that a ketogenic diet with a reduced intake of carbs could help lower your insulin levels. In addition, women who have insulin resistance are more likely to have hot flashes, and keto diets help get rid of them.

Prevention Of Obesity
The most common associated system of menopause is sudden weight gain. It occurs due to hormonal changes and a slower metabolism. Some women might also face a decrease in their height with weight gain that increases body mass (BMI). The keto diet is the opposite of low-fat diets that can actually cause weight gain.

Suppression Of Hunger
Another symptom of menopause for many women is an increase in appetite. If started at the right time during menopause, the ketogenic diet can help regulate the appetite.

This book will help you learn about the best ketogenic foods involved in this diet that will help you balance hormone levels and relieve symptoms of any unpleasant condition.

Other Important Benefits of the Ketogenic Diet

Arthritis and Benefits of Ketogenic Diets

How Do You Define Arthritis?

Arthritis is the inflammation of your joints, and the most commonly found types are osteoarthritis and rheumatoid arthritis.

Osteoarthritis is the cause of the degeneration of joints over time. It causes wearing and tearing conditions in the joints.

Rheumatoid arthritis causes a burning and painful sensation in the joints, so for this type, the body is attacking the joints; as a result, you will feel pain and inflammation.

The most common symptoms of this disease are low mobility, joint pain, and swelling. People also report redness of the skin. A study showed that almost 25% of people would face arthritis once in their lives. Another study showed that the prevalence of osteoarthritis doubled and rheumatoid arthritis almost halved.

Diet Of Arthritis

Your lifestyle can influence the severity and symptoms of arthritis in addition to your environment and genetic history.

Being obese or overweight can increase your risk of developing arthritis by 3–400%. It is no surprise that any diet that includes processed foods and desserts increases inflammation and blood sugar levels, which increases the risk of arthritis symptoms. While following a diet (especially the ketogenic diet) can help healthily control body weight, foods with antioxidants, polyphenols, and probiotics can help balance the body's overall health, reducing the symptoms of arthritis.

Omega 3 Fatty Acids

Foods that contain omega-3, especially fatty fish, are perfect for reducing joint pain, swelling, and inflammation. You can consume whole foods (sardines, tuna, oysters, squid, etc.) and also combine various additives like krill oil in your meals.

Virgin Olive Oil

Scientists believe that people in the Mediterranean region have lower levels of arthritis because of the high consumption of olive oil in their meals.

Another study showed that Greeks ate large amounts of vegetables cooked in extra virgin olive oil, reducing their risk of arthritis.

It can be a little tricky when using olive oil in your meals because it tends to contain inflammatory compounds when cooked on high heat. That's why I would advise you to either cook it on low heat or, better yet, drizzle it on your food after cooking. It will make it taste even better!

Boney Beef Broth

Collagen is a unique type of protein that makes up the cartilage. Arthritis is a disease that affects the cartilage by either inflaming or damaging it. Collagen has a high concentration of the amino acids glycine and proline and makes up about 27% of your body.

The use of collagen protein directly affects the body's damaged tissues and helps repair them. The best way to consume daily collagen is by boiling beef bone broth. You can use it in your ramen or any other dish that requires broth. Psst! Look up some delicious Korean hot-pot recipes online; they are always my go-to!

Garlic
Haven't we all heard about how garlic helps keep vampires away? Just kidding! But seriously, it is one of the most-used ingredients in many recipes because it contains anti-inflammatory properties that help reduce joint pain and even lower the risk of arthritis.

Turmeric
Turmeric is a holy grail ingredient used in many recipes, especially in India, Pakistan, and other South Asian countries. It's also used as an anti-bacterial agent for any bone fractures or swelling of the joints. It is said that if you warm some turmeric powder with oil and a bit of salt, layering it on the affected area, the skin will then absorb all the goodness of the turmeric, causing the wound to heal faster.
You can use powdered turmeric or even fresh turmeric and brew some tea, or you could even use it in your meals as a spice; it will add some color and enhance the flavor of your dish.

Green Tea
Any person hoping to lose weight should try green tea before anything else! It has been said that it boosts your metabolism and contains many antioxidants that can help with the inflammation and pain due to arthritis. In addition, a random clinical trial found that patients who added green tea to their diet along with medications found it to be more effective in reducing pain and other arthritis symptoms.

Leafy Greens
Fresh greens, like cabbage, are a superfood for those who are looking for a good diet. It's a versatile ingredient that you can use in smoothies or even in salads and other dishes.
Cabbage contains anti-inflammatory compounds known as sulforaphane and diindolylmethane. Greens like kale contain 93 milligrams of vitamin C and a good 7,812 IU of vitamin A in every 100-gram serving, which can do wonders for those who have arthritis. Conversely, a lack of vitamins C and A can increase your risk of arthritis.

Keto Helps with Gout

A commonly found type of arthritis, known as gout, is a sudden and painful inflammation of the joints, mainly the thumb. The pain and inflammation are caused by increased uric acid levels in the blood. Perhaps surprisingly, the keto diet is the best solution for gout.
A diet low in carbohydrates and calories is the best choice for treating gout. However, carbohydrates should be limited enough to increase ketone production. The main source should be plant foods and dairy products for protein and limit meat and fish consumption.
Proper maintenance of hydration and electrolyte levels is also very crucial. Following a keto diet that allows you to maintain ketosis and lose excess fat may include the following ratio:
- 5.5 or fewer servings of meat
- One or fewer servings of seafood
- Get protein from high-fat dairy food and plant-based keto foods
- Extra consumption of water and electrolytes like sodium and potassium

Ketosis Diet and Fatty Liver Disease

Also known as liver steatosis, fatty liver disease usually occurs when more than 5% of the liver's hepatocytes are composed of triglycerides and is usually the result of the overconsumption of alcohol. Still, there are cases in which people drank very little or none at all.

It affects about 25% of the western countries' population; according to some researchers, it can be fixed with preventable measures while also altering your lifestyle.

Ingredients To Help with Liver Steatosis

Green Tea

Rich in catechins, green tea can help reduce liver fat, liver enzymes, and inflammation, according to a 12-week controlled study, by consuming green tea with at least 1 gram of catechins or more.

Monounsaturated Fat

Food high in monounsaturated fats can have protective effects on liver health. One study on overweight adults found that a diet high in monounsaturated fats helps in significant reductions in liver fat levels, no matter how much physical activity they did.

What's the best source for such good fats? My favorite is avocado, olives, olive oil, peanuts, and almonds. You can combine them and make yourself a delicious and healthy fatty salad!

Whey Protein

An antioxidant named glutathione is produced by the body to help neutralize and protect cells. Whey protein may help people with fatty liver disease because it may increase the body's glutathione levels. In a study, some people who consumed 20 grams of whey protein a day for 12 weeks showed a significant increase in their glutathione levels and decreased stress and liver fat markers.

Fatty Fish

Rich in Omega-3 polyunsaturated fatty acids, oily and fatty fish have powerful anti-inflammatory properties.

In a detailed review of ten controlled studies, omega-3s were shown to reduce liver fat and other fatty liver disease inflammatory markers.

The best sources of fish are anchovies, mackerel, and herring (which can make for a perfect dinner, in my opinion!). Slightly grilled fish lightly seasoned with a side of greens is perfect after a day of exhaustion and stress.

Polyphenols

Foods with polyphenols are high in antioxidants that belong to a group of compounds known as phytochemicals, which are found in plants. Catechins found in greens are one of 4,000 other types present in different foods. These include coffee (my favorite!), berries, tomatoes, and spices like turmeric and cinnamon. According to many pieces of research, these are beneficial for people who are suffering from fatty liver disease.

Probiotics

Imbalance in gut bacteria can also be a cause of fatty liver disease. A study conducted in 2017 showed that probiotics are beneficial in reduced liver fat and enzymes. Some recommendations might include fermented foods such as Greek yogurt and kimchi, which contain natural probiotics that will help support your gut health and improve your overall health.

Collagen Benefits Of the Keto Diet

Over 25% of body weight is accounted for with collagen protein. It has at least 16 types present in the human body. Collagen contains three amino acids: proline, glycine, and hydroxyproline. Ninety percent of the types are I, II, and III. Type I is mainly found in skin, bones, and tissue fluids. Type II is found in cartilage, and the third type is found in skin, muscles, and blood vessels.

A dietary supplement like collagen hydrolyzate increases collagen levels in the human body. It contains broken pieces of amino acids called collagen peptides that help the supplement dissolve in the liquids present in the body. After absorption, these peptides travel through the bloodstream and help repair the damaged tissues. Gelatin is a mixture of collagen peptides that contains antioxidant, antihypertensive, and cholesterol-lowering properties.

Benefits Of Collagen in The Keto Diet

Anti-Aging Therapy
Collagen is known for its miracle anti-aging properties. Unfortunately, with age, our body starts reducing the collagen levels, which causes fine lines and wrinkles on our skin. Adding collagen-friendly food or supplements to our diet can help keep our appearance fresher and younger.

Reduces Cellulite
Collagen peptides used as an oral supplement can do wonders for the cellulite present on our thighs. In addition, it can help reduce the cellulite and waviness of the skin in overweight women.

Improves Bone Health
Collagen is responsible for about 25% of our body weight, which includes the cartilage of our bones. Using food rich in collagen can help those who have arthritis by increasing hydroxyproline levels, an amino acid present in collagen. It reduces joint pain and inflammation. In addition, it aids wound healing and helps strengthen the bones.

Supports Nitrogen Balance
With age, we tend to reduce protein intake in our diet, leading to nitrogen imbalances and unnecessary weight loss. According to a study, the supplement containing collagen helped maintain the nitrogen levels of nine healthy older women. At the same time, they complained that whey protein supplements caused them to lose weight in an extraordinary manner that affected their overall health.

Prevent Hair Loss
Hair loss is something many women have to deal with, especially after menopause, because of hormonal changes and mood swings. Research shows that type XVII collagen can help prevent early hair loss, graying, and thinning.

Products that contain collagen include fish, berries, vegetables, bone broth, and grass-fed meats (chicken, lamb, beef, etc.)

Ketogenic Diet And Alzheimer's Disease

The leading cause of dementia—and the most common neurodegenerative disease—is known as Alzheimer's and is found in many older women. It is a progressive disease that has yet to be treated.

How Can Ketones Help Fight Alzheimer's?

Reduces Oxidative Stress
Oxidative stress ketones can cause plaque formation in the brain. Compared to sugar, it generates much lower stress levels in the brain.

Provides Neuroprotective Properties
Antioxidants present in the ketones can help protect the brain from damage.

Increases Mitochondrial Production
Ketones have a trigger effect in the generation of new mitochondria and improve the pathways of older ones. However, low regenerative properties can typically occur due to age as our brain cells become sluggish.

Regulates the Glutamatergic Neurotransmitter System
The body learns to use ketones as fuel and increases the GABA levels significantly. The constant trigger of glutamatergic neurotransmitters can help increase the speed of degeneration; with the increase of GABA neurotransmitters, it decreases the damage to the brain

Along with benefits to the brain, ketones can have additional benefits to the body, such as a decrease in sugar levels, reducing the glucose used by the brain and the problems caused by glucose metabolism.

Decreased Insulin Levels
The ketogenic diet helps reduce insulin levels making the brain cells sensitive to insulin and increasing the energy levels caused by insulin.

Autophagy Activation
Because of the carbohydrate restriction, a process known as autophagy is activated, which is a cell cleansing process essential for maintaining healthy cells and improving their functioning in the body.

Other Ways to Protect Your Brain and Potentially Reverse Alzheimer's

Aside from the ketogenic diet and ketone supplements, there are many other ways to improve brain health. Keep reading to find out!

Eating Whole Foods
Cutting out sugars and carbs from your diet can help reduce the speed of brain aging. Avoid processed foods, alcohol, and omega-6 fatty acids and replace them with low-carb nuts, meats, avocado, and high-quality oils.

Eating More Vegetables
Veggies produce a transcription factor responsible for activating the process of detoxification and protecting the brain from oxidative stress.

Eating Omega-3 Fatty Acids
Eat foods like fish or fish oil supplements daily to reduce inflammation. Usually, one to three grams per day is the recommended dose.

Drinking Caffeine
Daily consumption of caffeine may protect your brain against any cognitive impairment. In a study, mice were fed caffeine, which suppressed the buildup of beta-amyloid plaque in the brain.

Consuming Curcumin
It can help prevent plaque buildup, remove the plaque, and hopefully improve brain health. It is also known to reduce cholesterol levels and remove iron and copper from the brain.

Consume Vitamin B
Vitamin B is *so* essential for brain health! It can improve cognition and prevent plaque formation in the brain, especially vitamins B3 and B1.

Physical Activity
Exercising daily and being more physically active has been shown to slow brain diseases and improve overall cognitive and physical performance.

Getting Sufficient Sleep
Sleep is something we tend to ignore, so getting a good recommended eight hours of sleep is crucial as it can contribute to cognitive dysfunction. Lack of sleep has proven to slow down brain functioning, making you prone to getting infected with brain-related diseases.

Learn To Relieve Stress
Another bad thing that can affect brain functioning and reduce sensitivity to insulin and memory loss is chronic stress. Using techniques like meditation and yoga can help calm your anxiety and stress; also, using breathing techniques can be very helpful in providing sufficient oxygen to the brain.

Brain Exercise

Using different methods of exercise that help stimulate the brain can potentially protect it from damage. Just like weight lifting, trying new things that the brain has yet to do can help the brain develop new synaptic connections and improve its functioning. Challenging your brain can work as muscle growth, helping the brain stay fit and healthy and protecting it from unnecessary decline.

The Ketogenic Diet Helps Reduce Belly Fat

Also known as visceral fat, belly fat can put you at risk of several serious diseases such as type 2 diabetes, cardiovascular disease, and certain types of cancer. In addition, recent research suggests that the amount of fat present in a certain body part can affect your health more than where it is present in the body.

Subcutaneous fat: A fatty tissue layer just below the skin's surface anywhere on your body. It is normal to have in your body and is not that bad, even if it is excessive.

Visceral fat: Als known as abdominal fat, it may form in the stomach cavity and around the stomach, liver, and intestines. Increasing the level of inflammation could lead to health problems, which is why it's also known as the "heart-attack fat."

Ectopic fat: Fat that occurs in abnormal organs of the body and can be extremely harmful to your health. It may affect areas like the liver, health, and muscles.

A difference in fat distribution can be why some overweight people are "healthier" while others who are not overweight may have health problems due to more heart-attack fat.

An easier way to assess how much visceral fat you have is by measuring the size of your waist. The larger your waist circumference, the more visceral fat you have.

Ways the Keto Diet Burns Belly Fat

In a ketogenic diet, you lower your carb and sugar intake, which improves your insulin sensitivity. Hence, the body learns to burn fat as a primary energy source. As a result, people who have become keto-adapted can burn fat almost ten times faster than others.

Due to the absence of carbs, keto forces the body to burn fat as fuel both during exercise and at rest. On other diets that concentrate on carbs more, the body burns fat only during fasting (including sleep) and exercise. But a keto diet helps you burn fat 24/7.

Ketones help reduce food craving and hunger, resulting in stable and long-term weight loss without counting calories! Great, right?

Effectiveness Of Keto Through Research

An analysis of 13 studies from 2013 involving 1,415 subjects found that the keto diet resulted in longer-lasting weight loss and improved overall health compared to a low-fat diet. In addition, a 2012 study compared low-calorie diets to low-carb diets by using a patient with type 2 diabetes, who found that the keto diet resulted in a more significant reduction in body weight, waist circumference, and insulin resistance than a low-calorie diet.

A review of 12 studies of the keto diet in overweight adults in 2020 found that the average weight loss was between 10 to 15.6 kg and the average decrease in the waist by 12.5 cm. In addition, the results of the keto subjects were stable throughout the follow-up period of up to two years, and 92.5% of them were able to stick to the diet.

Keto Diet Can Help with Acne

A group of researchers examined the potential benefits of a ketogenic diet for acne treatment. It helps with acne in three ways:

Firstly, as we've already talked about earlier, the keto diet helps regulate insulin levels, which can help with acne. Secondly, it helps with inflammation by reducing the redness of acne. Thirdly, it can help regulate the sebum levels and prevent the pores from clogging, which is the main cause of acne. Based on these three ways, it was proved that acne patients could follow the ketogenic diet to help improve their skin health and potentially improve their acne to some extent. There have been cases where people followed the keto diet to lose weight but ended up with completely cleared-up skin. Can't complain about that!

However, there have been cases where people have started suffering from even severe acne and inflammation problems after following the keto diet. This could mean that acne is not caused by carbs but by something else.

The Link Between Acne and Dairy

When facing severe acne, we have often heard that you should avoid dairy food as it helps increase the insulin and IGF-I levels, which may be the main cause of acne besides carbs. Like milk and whey-based products, dairy products can stimulate higher insulin and IGF-1 levels. In addition, some researchers have reported that hormones present in milk can help stimulate the acne-causing germs in your body. And whey protein is said to create a potent insulin response that can further accelerate any acne issues.

How the Ketogenic Diet Potentially Worsens Acne

It could be due to the intake of dairy and whey protein products; therefore, you can start by cutting down on such products. Common keto-friendly dairy products (such as yogurt and cream) contain hormones that stimulate acne breakouts. Also, other foods like cheese and butter may harm your skin health because it contains some active hormones. You can use plant-based dairy products like coconut milk and coconut cream to reduce your dairy intake. However, some people don't like the strong flavor of coconut in recipes made from it. Therefore, it could prove a safer choice for those suffering from acne. You can use dairy-free cheese, also known as vegan cheese, which is low in fat.

Other Ways to Improve Skin Health and Reduce Acne

Limiting your carb and dairy intake can definitely make a big impact on your skin's health, but after a while, that also stops working as well. Keeping that in mind, you could switch to other suggestions, like eating fatty fish several times a week. As we talked about, omega-3 is an anti-inflammatory agent that may help improve skin health. This could include sardines, anchovies, salmon, and mackerel.

Consume low-calorie vegetables as a side with every meal. Leafy greens are known to promote hormone regulation and improve skin health, plus they're tasty.

Drinking green tea, which is full of antioxidants, can help significantly reduce acne. And trust me, green tea leaves aren't just for drinking! You can use the leftover soaked leaves to make an awesome skin mask to help soothe that redness away.

Exercising daily can help increase your insulin sensitivity and improve the condition of your skin. You can start by taking short walks of about 10 to 15 minutes and gradually increase them if you like.

Keto Helps With Polycystic Ovary Syndrome

It is a condition in which the ovaries produce an abnormal amount of male sex hormone (androgen), and small cysts are formed in the ovaries. It can also be known as infertility. Almost 70% of fertility problems are caused by it. Only a few women know of PCOS and its symptoms despite it being the most common hormonal problem in women.

Common symptoms include irregular periods, weight gain/loss, infertility, problems with conceiving a child, acne, male pattern baldness, fatigue, and hirsutism (hair growth in abnormal areas).

What Causes Polycystic Ovary Syndrome?

Understanding the nature of the disease may help us better understand its cause. Women with PCOS are at risk of insulin resistance, obesity, diabetes, hypertension, glucose intolerance, and dyslipidemia. These could be due to inappropriate lifestyles. We live in a world of an abundance of food such as cookies, chips, cakes, and so on. This combination of excess calories and insulin resistance can easily cause any chronic disease.

How Insulin Resistance Causes PCOS

As we previously talked about, the symptoms of PCOS include higher insulin levels and resistance. It causes the ovaries to produce more androgen (male sex hormones). It also decreases the sex hormone present in a female body. With increasing androgen and a decrease in sex hormones, free testosterone can move in the blood and interact with cells which can cause chest and facial hair growth, fatigue, mood swings, and other PCOS symptoms.

Diet for PCOS

In a study on five overweight women consuming a keto diet for 24 weeks, the results showed an average weight loss of 12%, decreased free testosterone by 22%, and a decrease in insulin levels by 54%. Also, two women who were suffering from infertility became pregnant!

However, there is one important caveat. Restricting carbohydrates during a ketone diet can increase stress levels and promote insulin resistance. This is why it's important to follow a ketogenic diet with little variation.

A New and Improved Diet for PCOS

Following guidelines when it comes to a diet plan is essential. Restricting carbs can cause stress for some women who follow the keto diet and potentially reverse the results.

Limiting Carbohydrates

The recommended dose for beginners is less than 35 grams of carbs per day. At the start, it's safe to try reducing your daily carb intake to 5–10 grams per day; that will help gradually increase your ketone levels and your ability to burn fat. It is important to take things slowly at first and gradually increase to have your body get used to the new diet.

Vegetables That Are High in Fiber

Greens like broccoli, spinach, and kale can help reduce inflammation and fight insulin levels. Adding them as a side for every meal is the best decision.

The Right Amount of Protein

Adding more calories if you find your body fat to be an unhealthily low percentage can help maintain the weight and save you from any harmful side effects it may cause. But if you are overweight, you might need to be a little calorie deficit to help promote weight loss.

By following these guidelines, you'll be able to lower your insulin levels, balance your hormones, and reverse many PCOS symptoms. However, things like stress and inactivity can still limit your results. For best results, combine a healthy lifestyle with a ketogenic diet.

Exercising With the Ketogenic Diet

Exercise has always proved to help aid any diet plan. To keep the body healthy, we need to move. Doing any kind of physical activity such as weight training, aerobics, yoga, and meditation can help improve your globulin levels and decrease the number of male sex hormones in your body.

The Keto Diet Helps Improve Blood Pressure

According to a study from 2007, a ketogenic diet is a solution for the rise in blood pressure that has been the cause of 12.8% of deaths around the world. Comparing women who followed a low-calorie diet with those who followed a low-carb diet showed that those who followed a low-calorie ketogenic diet reduced high blood pressure symptoms. It doesn't mean that you can replace blood pressure medication with a ketogenic diet. Instead, remove some carbohydrates from your daily meal plan and see the results for yourself!

The recommendation for those interested in lowering their blood pressure would be to consume 50 grams or less of carbohydrates per day. But it is important to check it with your doctor or dietitian before you make big changes to your diet on your own.

Chapter 3: Problems with the Keto Diet and Ways to Overcome Them

Common Side Effects While on a Ketogenic Diet

As I have said before, the keto diet is not a cure for all diseases, and it might have side effects like any other diet. However, the smart thing to do would be to learn how to cope with the side effects so you'll be able to get the most out of the diet. It's the first few months that'll be hard; once your body gets used to the diet, it's a smooth sail ahead. Now I will tell you what problems women on a low-carb diet can face.

Keto Diet and Its Effects on Uric Acid Levels

Because of the severe restriction of carbohydrate intake, the keto diet has the lowest glycemic index compared to any other diet. A short-term study proved that it only lasts the first few weeks because the body is getting used to changing the energy-providing mechanism. The uric acid levels usually return to their original levels or even become lower with time. The rise in uric acid levels is normal in the early stages of the ketosis diet due to the breakdown of the protein for energy. The need for sugar in the body will decrease with the uric acid and protein breakdown.

Overall, it may appear that during the first two weeks, a keto diet may increase the risk of gout while potentially reducing the risk as the body burns more ketones for energy. Many people had different effects from the ketogenic diet. Some said that it cured their gout, while others said that they started noticing gout symptoms after starting the diet, which can be due to many reasons like an increase in the consumption of meat and fish.

Constipation During the Keto Diet

Gut problems may arise when you switch to a new diet. It is mainly due to the change in food, and your body needs time to get accustomed to goin without foods that you've always been eating; we call it the *adaption phase*. A ketogenic diet can have a dramatic impact on your eating habits, especially if you're someone like me who loves food containing a high rate of carbohydrates. It is a temporary phase that your body may go through to get used to not eating the foods you consume every day. However, you need to be very careful if you feel discomfort when using the toilet. Reach out to your dietitian or doctor right away as it could be due to other things as well.

Keto-friendly foods are very nutritious but smaller in volume; therefore, you may generate less waste, which is obvious. Also, the keto diet doesn't require fiber, and your body is used to consuming a high amount of fiber every day. Therefore, you need to walk every other day; this is just a normal sign that your body is used to a new way of life. If you cannot use the toilet for more than three days and are in pain, then you may do several things that could help you feel better. Some effective remedies for constipation that are low in carbs are:

Drink Plenty Of Water
Dehydration is directly related to your gut health, so making sure to stay hydrated is important when following a low-carb diet. Water is also a detoxifying agent; it helps wash out all the bad acids in your body, helping you melt the fat and feel refreshed.

Consume Enough Electrolytes
Electrolytes present in sodium or potassium are very important for your body. The lack of electrolytes could lead to headaches, dizziness, and overall weakness. A cause of constipation can also be due to not having enough sodium or potassium in your body. You can get your daily dose of around 2,000–4,000 grams from foods like avocado, salmon, chicken breast, and broccoli—instead of supplements, as they could be dangerous for your health while on a diet.

Take Magnesium Supplements
Magnesium is a mild laxative that can help you with indigestion and provides good relief from constipation. In addition, it has a calming effect on your nervous system as sometimes constipation can be activated due to stress.

Getting Adequate Fiber from Leafy Greens
Fiber is found in all plant foods. Green vegetables are particularly a good source of low-carb fiber supplements. Some of the best vegetables you can include in your meals during the keto diet are spinach, celery, avocado, zucchini, asparagus, mushroom, and cauliflower. The regular consumption of vegetables helps balance your diet by adding the necessary vitamins and minerals to it and helping alleviate constipation.

Drinking Hot Drinks on An Empty Stomach
Consuming warm drinks like coffee, tea, or even honey dissolved in water on an empty stomach can boost your metabolism and help wash out any "leftover" waste in your stomach. I have been trying that ever since I started the diet, and it has helped me a lot with my constipation as well as the unnecessary bloating. It also adds a boost to your day, making you feel fresh like a flower in bloom. No wonder the Chinese have hot vending machines; you can rarely find any cold drinks in China.

Try MCT Oil
Oil made up of medium-chain triglyceride fats mostly extracted from coconut oil helps with many digestive problems, such as constipation and stomach pain, which you are likely to experience when following a ketogenic diet. Apart from curing digestive problems, it has other benefits like improving energy, lowering cholesterol, and improving brain functioning and memory.
You can easily use MCT oil to make a delicious cup of keto coffee. Simply mix one or two teaspoons with one or two tablespoons of butter and 340 grams of coffee. It's been my favorite way to make coffee ever since I started the keto diet. You can start by using small amounts of the oil and gradually increase; just make sure to check your symptoms in case you are intolerant to it.

Brittle Nails

Your nails might start to exfoliate or get prone to breaking while you're on a keto diet. Don't panic; I have been through it myself. You can use the following tips to help improve your nail health.

Consume Vitamin A
Keto-friendly foods like eggs, spinach, and milk high in vitamin A can help with your nails' growth and positively affect bones, teeth, and tissue.

Increase Zinc Levels
A lack of zinc can easily slow down the growth of your nails as well as cause them to change color. Zinc is essential as it stimulates cell growth and division, which affects your skin, hair, and nails. Foods like cashews, flax seeds, spinach, and soybeans are high in zinc and keto-friendly.

Biotin Consumption
We've all heard about the wonder of biotin for our hair and nail health. You can get a supplement prescribed by your dietitian or use foods that contain vitamin H like lettuce, walnuts, and raspberries.

Add Folic Acid (Vitamin B9) To Your Diet
Folic acid isn't just limited to when you're pregnant, but it is essential for women of all ages. It helps moisturize and nourish your nails and hair. In addition, food such as beets, avocados, and eggs are full of vitamin B9.

Sleep Problems with the Keto Diet

There could be several reasons you face sleep problems during the keto diet that are not related to the diet. These could include:
Hormonal changes, caffeine or other stimulants, stress, anxiety or depression, and alcohol or drug addiction. However, suppose the above reasons aren't causing you a lack of sleep. In that case, there might be some lifestyle changes that cause insomnia during a keto diet.

Late-Night Eating

Sometimes we get used to eating right when we're about to go to bed, which can keep us up all night. It is recommended not to eat anything four hours before going to bed. This gives you enough energy to last through the night without getting hungry because we don't lose that much energy while we sleep.

Electrolyte Imbalance
Monitor your electrolyte intake before and during the ketosis diet. It is very important as a lack of certain electrolytes, especially magnesium, can cause insomnia symptoms. Consuming supplements with a perfect magnesium balance can help improve your sleep quality, relax your muscles, and remove any leg cramps you might face during the night. Suppose you prefer not to take any supplements and want to rely wholey on food. In that case, you might use bone broth, which is perfect for replenishing electrolytes.

Having Blue Lights Around You

We all live in a world full of gadgets. Can we even survive a day without our phones? A study proved that using blue light-emitting gadgets around you when sleeping can affect your sleeping pattern, making you prone to insomnia. So I would recommend that you switch off your phone half an hour before going to bed and maybe read a few pages of that book you've always wanted to read!

Exercising Before Bed

Since we are so busy during the day, we often think it's better to exercise at night. However, since working out wakes up your entire body and increases the Adeline in your body, it might be difficult for you to fall asleep. Try to exercise during the day; if you can use the early morning to exercise, it will do wonders for your body. You can even switch to yoga before bed, which will help relax your muscles and improve your sleep quality.

Drinking Caffeine Before Bed

Caffeine makes our blood rush, causing our body and brain to wake up. It may stay in your body for up to six hours after consumption. I would advise you to drink coffee only in the mornings and switch to green tea in the afternoon, as it helps calm your nerves.

During ketosis, your body will switch to new macros and redefine how it functions. This can affect sleep patterns as well. Other reasons might also be causing poor sleep.

Additional Energy

An additional surge of energy due to the intake of healthy fats is normal during ketosis. This additional energy may keep you awake and more alert than you usually are.

Stress Regarding Intermittent Fasting

The intermittent fasting that comes as a part of the keto diet pushes the body's limits by inducing a glucose-deficient state to start ketosis within the body. This glucose deprivation can cause an increase in stress hormones in women, cause irritability, and as a result, disturb your sleep cycle.

Electrolyte Imbalance

Low levels of electrolytes (such as magnesium) can cause you to become restless and have a night of disturbed sleep. Lack of electrolytes can also cause your muscles to cramp and affect sleep quality.

Keto Flu

When you remove carbs from your diet and replace them with fat as your body's main energy source, it can give you the "keto flu." It can induce insomnia as well. The symptoms of the keto flu include:

- Stomachache
- Difficulty in concentration
- Nausea
- Vertigo
- Irritability
- Heart palpitations
- Cravings for desserts
- Irregular bowel movement

Keto flu isn't very different than the regular stomach flu. However, the symptoms usually ease within three days, along with any ensuing insomnia.

Diarrhea and the Keto Diet

Diarrhea symptoms usually occur alongside keto flu, and some of you lucky ones might not even have to experience the nasty keto flu at all. However, diarrhea is not necessarily aligned with keto flu. It will, however, disappear in about two weeks. Just like how we discussed constipation during the early stages of the diet, diarrhea can also be caused due to a drastic change in eating. Our stomach is getting used to not having tons of glucose and carbs in it and using fat for energy sources.

Possible Causes of Diarrhea on the Keto Diet

Bile
Since your body fat increases during the keto diet, it starts producing more bile used by the body to break down fats that lubricate your colon and potentially lead to diarrhea. By reducing added fats from butter and coconut oil, you can switch to natural fats such as avocado, meats, and nuts. Once your body adapts, you can gradually add other sources of fat.

Too Much Magnesium
Excessive magnesium can cause digestive problems. Those who follow a low-carb diet might face electrolyte imbalance. Many people try adding more vitamins and minerals to their diet, leading to diarrhea and other digestive problems. It is important to monitor your electrolyte intake and stop taking any supplements that might contain magnesium. Switch to using foods that have magnesium in them, like bone broth. Try sticking to 3,000 mg of magnesium per day.

Food Intolerance
Sometimes when we switch to eating foods that we are not used to, our body has trouble digesting them. The best way to notice this symptom is when you start noticing chunks of fecal matter when using the toilet. It's easy to figure out what food caused this by eating only one type of vegetable per meal.

How to Deal with Symptoms of Keto Diarrhea

While figuring out what causes your diarrhea, you can follow some steps that might help relieve symptoms.
Start by adding more leafy greens into your diet, which are low in carbs. Fiber is important for digestive health and regular stools. It helps reduce the symptoms of diarrhea. Maintain a healthy balance of gut bacteria by adding probiotics to your diet. They carry many health benefits besides digestive health. You need to maintain a decent balance of good bacteria in your gut to help fight the harmful bacteria that may cause your digestive problems. You may use probiotics as powdered supplements, the best choice for dealing with diarrhea. Drink plenty of water to help eliminate any extra electrolytes present inside your body. As we discussed, the earlier increase of magnesium may cause digestive issues.

Increase In Urination

During ketosis, the body urinates more because while depleting your body's glycogen stores, the body releases three to four grams of water per gram of glycogen. This increased water release increases the urge to urinate more frequently, even at night. This frequent disturbance hinders a peaceful, full night's sleep. However, this problem goes away as soon as your body burns through its glycogen stores.

Color and Smell of Urine on the Keto Diet

While on the keto diet, your urine might become different in color and smell. Frequent urination is a sure sign of ketosis because the body releases a lot of water while dissolving its glycogen stores. This water is excreted through urination.

During ketosis, your body will produce sweat or even fruity-smelling urine. This is due to the ketones that leech through the blood and into the urine, changing their smell and appearance.

I have discussed the different colors of urine while on the keto diet and their meanings here.

- **Clear urine:** Clear urine is a sign of excess water intake. This is a sign that you should be drinking lesser water, but only until the urine becomes light yellow.
- **Dark yellow urine:** Dark-colored urine means you are not drinking enough water and need to increase your water intake. Remember that you will feel thirsty only after your body is dehydrated, so don't wait to feel thirsty. Be sure to ration the water out; drink a glass of water every two hours or so.
- **Fatty urine:** When the body reaches ketosis, many waste products stored in the body's fat start to get released into the bloodstream and then excreted through urine in the form of acetoacetate. This will cause the urine to become greasy and fatty. It would help if you took this as a signal that your body has reached ketosis.
- **Foamy urine:** People mistake foamy toilet water for foamy urine. When the urine is under excessive pressure, it will often be excreted with a lot of pressure and cause bubbles in the toilet bowl. Unless it is cloudy or hurts while urinating, there's nothing to worry about. However, cloudy or painful urine may indicate a urinary tract infection that will require immediate medical attention.

Frequent Heart Palpitations

During the first few weeks of keto, heart palpitations are normal due to a lack of salt and water in the body. As a result, the heart needs to work double to pump the blood with reduced fluid.

Dehydration

The body can very quickly get dehydrated during ketosis. The main way to solve this is to increase your water intake and ensure that it carries electrolytes, especially sodium. Heart palpitations result from dehydration and should subside within a week or so. But if they don't, be sure to consult your doctor.

To find out if you are dehydrated, check the color of your urine. Dark yellow-colored urine means dehydration, and a brownish color means severe dehydration.

Signs and Symptoms of Dehydration

The most distinguishing signs of dehydration are:

- Heart palpitations
- Irregular breathing
- Brain fogginess
- Slight dizziness
- Fatigue and lethargy
- Chest pain
- Muscle cramps

Treatment

The most effective and reliable cure for this condition is to drink plenty of water. Also, make sure you have enough sodium (salt) in your diet. If that doesn't help, then heart palpitations can trigger stress hormones. However, it's usually a temporary condition that should go away on its own within a week.

If the rapid heartbeat is episodic and instantly passes, this does not pose a serious threat. But if the symptoms recur, be sure to consult a doctor!

Keto Cramps

When the body is low on hydration and electrolytes, it can develop many deficiencies of necessary vitamins and minerals. This can result in severe cramping of muscles and disturbed sleep as well as hindered exercise.

Minerals

Cramps can be caused due to a deficiency of minerals as well. The four key minerals that you should be ingesting are discussed in the following sections.

Sodium

Decreased salt levels in the body can cause kidney dysfunction and force the body to use potassium, which is necessary for other muscular functions such as the heart. To curb a sodium deficiency, make sure you consume 3,000 to 5,000 milligrams of sodium per day.

Potassium

As discussed above, potassium is important for muscular and nerve functions. Therefore, make sure you consume between 3,000 and 4,000 milligrams of potassium per day.

Magnesium

Most people do not get enough magnesium per day, even though they only need 400 milligrams daily. However, it is a well-known fact that the keto diet does not usually result in magnesium deficiency in the body.

Vitamin E

If your mineral intake is normal, try taking vitamin E supplements to curb muscular cramps.
Here is a recipe to make your own electrolyte drink:
Ingredients
- Purified water or herbal tea (decaffeinated): 5 glasses
- Lemon or lime juice: 1/2 cup
- Pink Himalayan salt: 1/4 teaspoon or to taste
- Powdered magnesium supplement: 2 tablespoons
- Potassium chloride powder: 1/2 teaspoon

- Sweetener (erythritol or liquid stevia): to taste

Mix all ingredients in a two-liter bottle or jug and enjoy.

Headaches On Keto

There are several reasons you might have headaches during the keto diet. However, there is no need to worry as it might be due to the positive changes in your body.

Dehydration
Due to the new carb-free lifestyle, your body might be able to urinate more than it used to. This is one of the main reasons you face dehydration, leading to dizziness and heaviness in the brain, causing you a headache.

Sodium Deficiency
Because of carb restriction, people who follow a ketogenic diet face a decrease in insulin levels, decreasing absorption, and sodium deficiency. This can be solved by consuming at least a ½ teaspoon of table salt per day.

Sugar Withdrawal
Sugary drinks mostly cause dehydration and sodium deficiency. But, a sudden decrease in sugar intake can also cause headaches.

Caffeine Withdrawal
During keto, people stop consuming coffee and soy drinks, resulting in headaches.

Sensitivity to Histamines
Suppose we rule out dehydration, sodium, sugar, and caffeine as potential sources of headaches. In that case, you may be suffering from histamine intolerance.

Foods High in Histamines
Foods like pickles, sauerkraut, old cheeses, dried meats, shellfish, and nuts can be removed if your headache still doesn't stop.

Ways to Get Rid of Headaches During the Keto Diet

Five remedies that may help with immediate relief of headaches include:
1. **Drinking warm water with salt in it**. Try mixing a simple solution of half a teaspoon of table salt dissolved in a 680 ml glass of warm water and drink it. As discussed earlier, this will help the headache if it's due to dehydration or sodium deficiency.
2. **Drink bone broth.** You can drink broth made from beef bone or chicken to get sodium in your body as well. Remember to drink it warm.
3. **Drink vegetable broth.** Simply boil two cups of water, then add them to a broth made of vegetables and mix well.
4. **Drinking chicken broth with additional salt.** Add a full teaspoon of salt to two cups of chicken broth (low in carbohydrates), then microwave it for one minute; this can help relieve the headache.
5. **Drink caffeine**. Caffeine is the safest way of getting rid of headaches. The best way is to make coffee with butter and salt. I know it sounds weird but trust me, it tastes better than it sounds. All you have to do is add two tablespoons of butter or coconut oil and half a teaspoon of salt into your regular coffee and enjoy!

Keto Rash

At the beginning of the keto diet, developing an itchy rash all over your body is quite normal. This is called a "keto rash." Some reasons for the keto rash that have been discovered are:

- Your body produces ketones during ketosis that can cause inflammation around the blood vessels and take the form of rashes.
- A low-carb diet and excessive fasting will push the body into ketosis and cause a rash.
- You might be allergic to one or many keto foods.
- Your body might be going through deficiencies in various nutrients that have been excluded from your diet, and these deficiencies might result in rashes.

How to Treat a Keto Rash

There is a high chance that your body will adjust to ketosis and get used to ketone production, and the rashes will disappear independently. However, if they don't, try one of these remedies:

- ***Eat more carbs.*** Experiment by increasing your carb intake or taking a gentler path to ketosis with a higher carb proportion than most people. Find the optimal balance of carbs in your diet over time that will reduce the appearance of rashes without compromising the state of ketosis.
- ***Try identifying if you have any allergies.*** You might be developing a rash due to being allergic to any keto foods. The most common allergens in keto diets are dairy, bollocks, fish, tree nuts, and peanuts. Try removing each of the keto foods from your diet for a few weeks at a time and check if the rash decreases in intensity. If it doesn't, add the food back and remove another one. If the rash subsides or becomes better, move on to the next food item.
- ***Take vitamin and mineral supplements***. Consult your doctor and start supplements to curb any nutrient deficiency your body might be going through. Minerals you should be focusing on are calcium, magnesium, sodium, and potassium. Vitamins D, A, and omega-3 are important for fat dissolution. Various bile salts such as deoxycholic, chenodeoxycholic, and lithocholic acids encourage liver function and digestion of lipids.

How to Prevent Rashes

The following recommendations can help reduce the appearance of rashes, in general:

- ***Avoid sweating***. Take a few days off from the gym or reduce the intensity of workouts. Be sure to shower after every workout
- ***Avoid friction***. To alleviate the rash, avoid rubbing the affected area in any way possible. This includes wearing fitted clothes, exfoliation, rigorous wiping, scratching, using Band-Aids, and sleeping on the affected area. Lotion or rash cream can also help soothe the skin and reduce friction.

Loss of Hair On the Keto Diet

Some people report an increase in hair loss when they shift to a keto lifestyle and attribute it to the diet. So, they end up quitting the diet rather than actually diagnosing the issue behind the hair loss. So far, no studies suggest a relationship between hair loss and ketosis. On the contrary, people often report better hair growth and quality due to the low-carb intake. Therefore, if you are on a keto diet and experiencing a sudden increase in hair loss, it might be due to one of the following factors:

- *Biotin deficiency*. According to a 2013 study, hair loss on keto can be explained by biotin deficiency. The study explains that biotin is a water-soluble vitamin responsible for acting as a cofactor for several enzymes. The study went on to say that Japan has a children's version of a low-carb diet called the ketone formula, but it doesn't contain enough biotin. Biotin deficiency in infants can cause skin rashes, cramps, developmental delays, poor muscle tone, and hair loss. Fortunately, biotin deficiency is easily treated with supplements.

- *Telogen effluvium*. Another reason why people experience hair loss, especially when they first start a keto diet, is because their hair goes into shock. According to the American Osteopathic College of Dermatology, some systemic shocks occur when you first go on a ketogenic diet. This happens when about 70% of the hair on the scalp falls out within two months and immediately—in large quantities. Medically speaking, this type of hair loss is described as telogen effluvium. In other words, your body may be shocked at first, but once it adapts to the new diet, your hair needs to adjust. The worst thing you can do in this situation is to give up keto and go back to a high-carb diet.

- *Thyroid problems or autoimmune diseases*. In some cases, hair loss has nothing to do with the keto diet and can be caused by thyroid problems or autoimmune diseases. For example, hypothyroidism or hyperthyroidism can cause changes in hormone levels, which can cause hair loss. In addition, alopecia is an autoimmune condition characterized by hair loss. Although the cause is unknown, research shows that it is associated with hyperthyroidism.

- *Iron deficiency*. The hair can be affected by iron deficiency, so you need to take a blood test to determine if you have a deficiency of vitamins or minerals. In most cases, an iron and vitamin B supplement can help provide the nutrients you need for your hair growth.

- *Protein or calorie deficits*. Hair loss can also be associated with a lack of protein or eating too few calories. While keto isn't exactly a high-protein diet, it's enough. You can adjust your protein intake to see if hair loss can be stopped. However, keep in mind that excessive amounts of protein can knock you out of ketosis, so keep a close eye on your macros.

- **Stress and little sleep**. Keep in mind that a timeline regarding when hair loss occurs is of great importance. If you start experiencing hair loss within one to three months of starting the diet, don't worry. Your hair loss is most likely temporary, and it won't last very long. On the other hand, suppose you have been on a keto diet for at least six months or longer, and you're suddenly having trouble. In that case, you need to adjust your eating and lifestyle habits to ensure you're not depriving yourself of nutrients, sleep well (at least seven to eight hours a night), and fight stress through meditation, yoga, or daily outdoor activities.

How to Stop Hair Loss

Here are some remedies that can help in the natural growth of hair.

- **Peppermint oil**. According to research, peppermint essential oil promotes hair growth by stimulating the scalp and does not contain any harmful side effects.

- **Collagen**. According to a study conducted by a team of researchers in Japan, a lack of collagen can cause poor stem cell performance. The publication stated that a deficiency of type XVII collagen, which is located near the hair follicle and stem cells under the scalp, is the cause of hair loss.

- **Caffeine**. This is good news for coffee lovers. According to a 2014 study, caffeine helps hair grow faster by reducing the effects of DHT on the scalp. Among the sources of caffeine are green tea, black tea, and coffee. Green tea is particularly beneficial for hair growth as it has been shown to boost your metabolism, boosting the growth rate of new hair. One study found that a compound in green tea known as epigallocatechin-3-gallate, or EGCG, promoted hair follicle growth and stimulated dermal papilla cells, causing hair to grow much faster. Green tea is also high in antioxidant polyphenols, which can help your hair grow as it protects cells from oxidative damage and stress. In addition, antioxidants help slow down the aging process, thus affecting the hair. In addition, green tea contains a lot of antioxidants, such as panthenol, which is often used in shampoos, helping you grow strong hair.

- **Pumpkin seeds**. Pumpkin seeds contain a lot of zinc. Studies show that their deficiency is often associated with hypothyroidism and hair loss. Also, pumpkin seeds contain vitamin E, which has an anti-inflammatory effect on the scalp. Keep in mind that although pumpkin seeds contain a large amount of fat, they also include a lot of carbohydrates, so be careful how much you consume.

- **Palmetto**. Studies show that saw palmetto extract allows you to maintain testosterone balance, promoting hair growth. One study found that men and women who used palmetto extract lotion as a shampoo for three months had a 35% increase in hair density.

- **Ginkgo biloba**. This is a herb often associated with helping in hair regrowth. It strengthens the hair roots and prevents thinning. It's also great for stimulating blood flow, which helps nourish your hair.

- **Probiotics**. Probiotics help restore the balance of good bacteria in your body and get rid of bad things, including any bacteria on your head that prevent your hair from growing.
- **Apple cider vinegar**. Some research suggests that apple cider vinegar can help stimulate hair growth because it improves blood flow to the scalp and gives hair more nutrients, and it also contains natural antibacterial properties, so you can use it to fight dandruff.

Constipation On a Keto Diet

When you switch to a new diet, there are often some problems with the intestines. After all, your body has gotten used to the other food, and now it needs time to adjust.

A ketogenic diet can be a pretty drastic change in your eating habits, especially if you're used to high-carb foods, so it's no surprise that you may experience various problems—specifically, temporary constipation.

You need to clarify right away if the regularity of your bowel movements has changed or if you do not experience pain or discomfort when visiting the toilet. This may be completely normal, and you do not need to do anything.

Keto foods are very nutritious, so they are smaller in volume. Therefore, it is natural that you will produce less waste. A well-designed ketogenic diet plan doesn't need fiber. Still, depending on what you've eaten before, your gut may have gotten used to higher amounts of fiber.

So, if you are used to regular stools once or twice a day but now need to walk every other day without experiencing bloating, pain, hard stools, etc., it's just a normal sign that your body is getting used to a new lifestyle.

Normal bowel activity is considered between three times a day and three times a week, so if you are in this range and have no other symptoms, just let your body enter a new rhythm.

However, if you experience discomfort and can't go to the bathroom for more than three days, or if you experience pain, there are a few things you can do.

Here are the most effective remedies for constipation on a low-carb and ketogenic diet.

- *Make sure you drink plenty of water.* Dehydration can have a direct effect on your gut, so you need to make sure you're drinking enough fluids.

- *Make sure you are getting enough sodium and potassium*. Insufficient amounts of sodium or potassium in the body can lead to weakness, dizziness, headaches, high blood pressure, and constipation. Your daily sodium intake should be between 2,000 and 4,000 grams. If you're particularly active and sweating, you may need even more. The recommended amount of potassium you should consume daily is 4,700 mg; however, it is best to get it from real foods such as avocados, broccoli, salmon, chicken breast, and the like, as supplements can be dangerous.

- *Take magnesium supplements*. Magnesium is another element that is needed during the keto diet. In addition, it acts as a mild laxative. It can help with indigestion and is a good relief for constipation. In addition to aiding in defecation, magnesium has a calming effect on the nervous system, as stress can exacerbate constipation.

- *Eat enough fiber (from green vegetables).* You can find fiber in all plant foods. Green vegetables are a particularly good source, as they are low in net carbs and will help you get other essential micronutrients. Some of the best fiber-loaded vegetables for the keto diet are spinach, celery, avocado, asparagus, cabbage, bok choy, arugula, zucchini, mushrooms, and cauliflower. These vegetables contain essential minerals and vitamins that would maintain the balance of your diet and help with regular stools.

- *Drink a cup of hot coffee or tea (or plain water) on an empty stomach*. If you suffer from constipation for a few days and begin to experience unpleasant side effects, such as bloating, coffee or tea on an empty stomach may help. In addition, drinking hot liquid causes slight contractions in the intestines, so if you are not a fan of coffee or tea, you can just drink hot water—it will also help with digestion, reduce stress levels, and help with dehydration.

- ***Try MCT oil***. MCT oil consists of medium-chain triglyceride (MCT) fats, which in most cases are extracted from coconut oil. As many keto dieters say, MCT oil can help with digestive problems such as constipation and stomach pain. MCT also has several other benefits, such as improved energy levels, lowering cholesterol levels, and improved brain function and memory. When you first try MCT oil, take a small amount first and slowly build up to higher doses, as some people are intolerant to it.

Three Female Keto Problems – And How to Solve Them

Despite having countless benefits, the keto diet can pose some unique challenges for women. You will find three major stumbling blocks that women on the ketogenic diet face listed below and what they can do to overcome them.

Problem 1: The Keto Plateau – No Weight Gain Or Loss Is Happening

Ensure that at least 60% of your diet is full of high-quality fats, which you can find in foods such as avocado, olive oil, grass-fed beef, coconut oil, eggs, and clarified butter (ghee).

Using MCT coconut oil can help increase ketone production in the body and speed up ketosis. This will give your body more ketones to burn as fuel. MCT oil is also known for reducing food cravings and increasing energy levels, which will also increase your metabolism. You can use this easily throughout the day by simply drizzling it over your salad or mixing it in your coffee or smoothie.

As discussed earlier, intermittent fasting helps boost the ketone-burning process and reduces your caloric intake. This is a perfect way to speed up your weight loss. You can simply follow it by skipping breakfast and having a cup of keto coffee rich in MCT oil that will help boost the fat burning mechanism

Also, try using a food tracker. Tracking your food or calorie intake can help you maintain your body's proper balance.

Problem 2: Hormonal Imbalance

Hormones may cause many problems for women, especially as they get older. Fibroids, heavy periods, and endometriosis are signs that the body is producing too much estrogen.

Keeping a check on your body fat can help improve estrogen production. Hormones can cause problems, especially those trying to cut their body fat. The optimal fat amount in a female body should be 22–29, which is the perfect fat percentage that helps the hormones feel good.

Don't strive for an ideal weight. Talk to your doctor and do some research on what the ideal is for *you*. By stressing hard about reaching that ideal weight, we cause our hormones to react badly to present fat and cause an imbalance. A ketogenic diet is ideal as it is compatible with your hormones. It is better to synchronize your diet with your period cycle by increasing the protein intake from day 1 to day 5. From days 6 to 11, aim for very low carbs and moderate protein intake in your meals. From days 12 to 16, choose keto foods like avocado, broccoli, garlic, and parsley. At the end of your cycle, on days 17 to 28, increase your carbs once or twice with vegetables.

Problem 3: Not Enough Exercise

The keto diet is a low-carb diet, which means that you are limiting your carbohydrates too much, which can affect hormones and your exercise.

30-Day Keto Diet Weight Loss Meal Plan

1. The purpose of this plan is to show you what types of keto foods you can eat, ways you can prepare your foods, what a typical keto meal looks like, and recipes.

2. How to use this plan:

3. Each day will be between 1,500-1,700 calories (designed for weight loss).

4. Make sure you know your daily macros (how much fat, protein, carbs, and calories you need to achieve your goal).

5. Each recipe has anywhere between 2-10 servings, so be sure to prepare according to your macros and personal needs. For example, if you only cook for yourself, you might want to make 1 serving at a time, or make as many servings as you want and keep the leftover for the next days.

6. This meal plan is designed for one person. If you would like to use them for multiple people, simply multiply the ingredient uantities by the total number of people.

7. Be flexible. We don't know your personal goal, your budget, your cooking skills, what your favorite foods are, or what foods you don't like to eat, so we cannot personalize the meal plan just for you. This plan is just to give you ideas of what to cook for breakfasts, lunches, and dinners. So please feel free to adjust and personalize it to make it work for you.

8. Feel free to replace any of the recipes or ingredients with your personal choices and adjust the ingredient amounts to fit your macros and situation.

If you follow a very strict keto diet, make sure to personalize this meal plan to make it work for you.

	Breakfast	Lunch	Dinner
DAY 1	COCONUT MILK PANCAKES	COCONUT CHICKEN TENDERS	KETO SHRIMP THAI SALAD
DAY 2	AVOCADO OMELETTE	MEXICAN MEATZA	CRISPY FISH STICKS WITH CAPER DILL SAUCE
DAY 3	KETO BREAKFAST DAIRY-FREE SMOOTHIE BOWL	CHICKEN WITH SPINACH AND FETA	CREAMY SHRIMP AND MUSHROOM SKILLET
DAY 4	EASY SHAKSHUKA	CREAMY HONEY & MUS-TARD PORK RIBS	THAI GREEN CURRY
DAY 5	FARMER CHEESE PANCAKES	CHICKEN EGG SALAD WRAPS	KETO MASHED GARLIC TURNIPS
DAY 6	MATCHA BREAKFAST BOWL	BLUE CHEESE BACON BURGERS	CHICKEN LIVER PTE
DAY 7	BROCCOLI QUICHE CUPS	GROUND BEEF AND CABBAGE STIR-FRY	BUTTERED COD IN SKILLET
DAY 8	DENVER OMELET SALAD	COCONUT CHICKEN TENDERS	ZUCCHINI PIZZA BOATS
DAY 9	BROCCOLI & CHEESE OMELET	BAKED CHICKEN NUGGETS AND FRESH SALAD	SESAME TOFU WITH EGGPLANT

DAY 10	AVOCADO BACON AND EGGS	FRIED TUNA AVOCADO BALLS	THAI BEEF SALAD
DAY 11	PEANUT BUTTER GRANOLA	KALE CAESAR SALAD WITH CHICKEN	CAPRESE MEATBALLS
DAY 12	CHORIZO BREAKFAST BAKE	CHICKEN ENCHILADA SOUP	BROCCOLI AND SHRIMP SAUTÉED IN BUTTER
DAY 13	LEMON POPPY RICOTTA PANCAKES	SHRIMP AVOCADO SALAD	CRISPY CHIPOTLE CHICKEN THIGHS
DAY 14	SWEET BLUEBERRY COCONUT PORRIDGE	CHICKEN ENCHILADA BOWL	AVOCADO LIME SALMON
DAY 15	EGG STRATA WITH BLUEBERRIES AND CINNAMON	SPINACH MOZZARELLA STUFFED BURGERS	CALAMARI STUFFED WITH PANCETTA AND VEGETABLES
DAY 16	SOUTHWESTERN OMELET	MEXICAN MEATZA	KETO CALAMARI
DAY 17	PEPPERONI, HAM & CHEDDAR STROMBOLI	CHICKEN PHILLY CHEESESTEAK	LOADED CAULIFLOWER
DAY 18	VEGETABLE TART	SPICY SHRIMP TACO LETTUCE WRAPS	EASY CASHEW CHICKEN

DAY 19	ZUCCHINI EGG CUPS	CHICKEN QUESADILLA	MEXICAN FISH STEW
DAY 20	KETO CROQUE MADAME	MEATBALLS IN TOMATO SAUCE	LOW CARB ALMOND CRUSTED COD
DAY 21	KETO PROTEIN BREAKFAST SCRAMBLE	RIBS IN WHITE SAUCE	MEXICAN FISH STEW
DAY 22	3-INGREDIENT PESTO ZOODLE BOWL	CHICKEN WINGETTES WITH CILANTRO DIP	GRILLED SALMON WITH AVOCADO SALSA
DAY 23	CHOCOLATE PROTEIN PANCAKES	BEEF STEW	CREAMY KETO FISH CASSEROLE
DAY 24	POACHED EGG AND BACON SALAD	TURKEY TACO BOWLS	(INSTANT POT) COCONUT CURRY MUSSELS WITH ZUCCHINI NOODLES
DAY 25	SPINACH PANCAKES	JALAPENO CHICKEN	KETO ASIAN STEAK SALAD
DAY 26	GRIDDLED HALLOUMI AND WATERMELON SALAD	CLASSIC MEATLOAF STUFFED WITH MOZZARELLA	PORK SKEWERS WITH CHIMICHURRI
DAY 27	TURKISH-STYLE BREAKFAST RECIPE	BARACOA-STYLE SHREDDED BEEF	LEMON KALAMATA OLIVE SALMON

DAY 28	POACHED EGGS MYTILENE	TURKEY LASAGNA WITH RICOTTA	SEAFOOD MEDLEY STEW
DAY 29	KETO BREAKFAST SANDWICH	CREAMY LAMB CURRY	CRUNCHY ALMOND TUNA
DAY 30	ROASTED RADISH AND HERBED RICOTTA OMELET	TENDER AND JUICY SHREDDED PORK	CARAMELISED TILAPIA

RECIPES

BREAKFAST

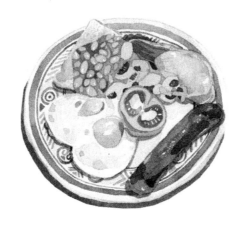

Coconut Milk Pancakes

Nutrition: Cal 442;Fat 35g;Carb 15g;Protein 16,2g
Serving 4; Cook time 15min

Dry Ingredients

6 tablespoons coconut flour
4 tablespoons granulated sweetener
1 teaspoon baking powder

Wet Ingredients

•6 tablespoons unsweetened coconut milk
•4 large eggs
•2 teaspoons vanilla extract

Instructions

1. In a mixing bowl add all of the dry ingredients.
2. In a separate bowl mix together coconut milk, eggs, and vanilla extract. Be sure to shake can before opening.
3. Preheat skillet or pan on medium heat for cooking and add coconut oil or butter.
4. Combine dry and wet and beat well with a whisk until batter is smooth and free of lumps.
5. Add to pan and cook each side evenly. If cooking too fast, pull off heat and lower temperature. Pancakes should be fluffy and not runny on the inside but golden brown on the outside.

Keto Breakfast Casserole

Nutrition: Cal 200;Fat 15g;Carb 4g;Protein 13 g
Serving 10; Cook time 70min

Ingredients

• Drizzle of oil
• ½ cup onion
• 1 tablespoon garlic, minced
• 1 pound breakfast sausage
• 12 eggs
• ½ cup almond milk
• 2 teaspoons mustard powder
• 1 teaspoon oregano
• ¼ teaspoon salt
• Pepper, to taste
• 1½ cups broccoli florets
• 1 zucchini, diced
• 1 red bell pepper, diced (or 3–4 cups veggies of choice)

Instructions

1. Preheat oven to 375°F (190°C).
2. In a skillet over medium heat, add a drizzle of oil and sauté onion and garlic.
3. Once transparent, add sausage and cook until browned, 7–10 minutes.
4. Add to a 13×9-inch casserole or baking dish and set aside.
5. In a large bowl, whisk together eggs, milk of choice, and seasonings. Stir in chopped veggies.
6. Pour mixture over sausage.
7. Bake until firm and cooked through, 30–40 minutes.
8. Allow to cool slightly before slicing into squares, serving, and enjoying!

9. Store leftovers in the fridge for up to 5 days, and reheat individual portions in the microwave.

Avocado Omelette

Nutrition: Cal 310;Fat 23g;Carb 11g;Protein 16 g
Serving 2; Cook time 5min

Ingredients

3 eggs, lightly beaten
3 tablespoons almond milk
Nonstick cooking spray, as needed
1/2 cup tofu cheese
1 tablespoon sliced green onion
1/4 cup chopped red bell pepper
1 ripe, fresh California avocado; seeded, peeled, and cubed

Instructions

1. Mix eggs and milk.
2. Spray a large skillet with nonstick cooking spray and heat over medium low heat. Pour egg mixture into skillet. Cook eggs until top is almost set.
3. Sprinkle with cheese and green onion. Cook, about 2 minutes.
4. Top with red pepper and avocado, fold over, and serve immediately.

Keto Breakfast Dairy-Free Smoothie Bowl

Nutrition: Cal 642;Fat 45g;Carb 10g;Protein 22,2g
Serving 3; Cook time 10min

Ingredients

• 1 ½ cups (350 ml) full-fat coconut milk
• 1 cup (110 g) frozen raspberries
• ¼ cup (60 ml) MCT oil or melted coconut oil, or ¼ cup (40 g) unflavored MCT oil powder
• ¼ cup (40 g) collagen peptides or protein powder
• 2 tablespoons chia seeds
• 1 tablespoon apple cider vinegar
• 1 teaspoon vanilla extract
• 1 tablespoon erythritol, or 4 drops liquid stevia

Instructions

1. Place all the pudding ingredients in a blender or food processor and blend until smooth. Serve in bowls with your favorite toppings, if desired.

Crispy Keto Corned Beef & Radish Hash

Nutrition: Cal 252;Fat 16g;Carb 1,5g;Protein 23g
Serving 2; Cook time 10min

Ingredients

• 2 tablespoons olive oil
• 1/2 cup diced onions
• 2 cups radishes, diced to about 1/2 inch
• 1 teaspoon kosher salt
• 1/2 teaspoon ground black pepper
• 1 teaspoon dried oregano (Mexican if you have it)
• 1/2 teaspoon garlic powder
• 2 twelve-ounce cans corned beef or 2 cups finely chopped corned beef, packed

Instructions

1. Heat the olive oil in a large saute pan and add the onions, radishes, salt, and pepper.
2. Saute the onions and radishes on medium heat for 5 minutes or until softened.
3. Add the oregano, garlic powder, and corned beef to the pan and stir well until combined.
4. Cook over low to medium heat, stirring occasionally for 10 minutes or until the radishes are soft and starting to brown.
5. Press the mixture into the bottom of the pan and cook on high heat for 2–3 minutes or until the bottom is crisp and brown.
6. Serve hot.

Coconut Flour Porridge
Nutrition: Cal 345;Fat 28,5g;Carb 11g;Protein 13 g
Serving 1; Cook time 7min

Ingredients
- 2 tablespoons coconut flour
- 2 tablespoons golden flax meal
- 3/4 cup water
- Pinch of salt
- 1 large egg, beaten
- 2 teaspoons butter or ghee
- 1 tablespoon heavy cream or coconut milk
- 1 tablespoon low-carb brown sugar (or your favorite sweetener)

Instructions
1. Measure the first four ingredients into a small pot over medium heat and stir. When it begins to simmer, turn it down to medium-low and whisk until it begins to thicken.
2. Remove the coconut flour porridge from heat and add the beaten egg, a half at a time, while whisking continuously. Place back on the heat and continue to whisk until the porridge thickens.Remove from the heat and continue to whisk for about 30 seconds before adding the butter, cream, and sweetener.
3. Garnish with your favorite toppings (4 grams net carbs).

Easy Shakshuka
Nutrition: Cal 216;Fat 12,8g;Carb 16,6g;Protein 112
Serving 6; Cook time 35min

Ingredients
- 2 tablespoons olive oil
- 1 large yellow onion, chopped
- 1 large red bell pepper or roasted red bell pepper, chopped
- 1/4 teaspoon fine sea salt
- 3 cloves garlic, pressed or minced
- 2 tablespoons tomato paste
- 1 teaspoon ground cumin
- 1/2 teaspoon smoked paprika
- 1/4 teaspoon red pepper flakes (reduce or omit if sensitive to spice)
- 1 large can (28 ounces) crushed tomatoes, preferably fire-roasted
- 2 tablespoons chopped fresh cilantro or flat-leaf parsley, plus addition cilantro or parsley leaves for garnish
- Freshly ground black pepper, to taste
- 5 to 6 large eggs

Instructions
1. Preheat the oven to 375°F. Warm the oil in a large, oven-safe skillet (preferably stainless steel) over medium heat. Once shimmering, add the onion, bell pepper, and salt. Cook, stirring often, until the onions are tender and turning translucent, about 4 to 6 minutes.
2. Add the garlic, tomato paste, cumin, paprika, and red pepper flakes. Cook, stirring constantly, until nice and fragrant, 1 to 2 minutes.
3. Pour in the crushed tomatoes with their juices and add the cilantro. Stir, and let the mixture come to a simmer. Reduce the heat as necessary to maintain a gentle simmer and cook for 5 minutes to give the flavors time to meld.
4. Turn off the heat. Taste (careful, it's hot!), and add salt and pepper as necessary. Use the back of a spoon to make a well near the perimeter and crack the egg directly into it. Gently spoon a bit of the tomato mixture over the whites to help contain the egg. Repeat with the remaining 4 to 5 eggs, depending on how many you can fit. Sprinkle a little salt and pepper over the eggs.
5. Carefully transfer the skillet to the oven (it's heavy) and bake for 8 to 12 minutes, checking often once you reach 8 minutes. They're done when the egg whites are an opaque white and the yolks have risen a bit but are still soft. They should still jiggle in the centers when you shimmy the pan (keep in mind that they'll continue cooking after you pull the dish out of the oven).

Steak and Eggs
Nutrition: Cal 210;Fat 36g;Carb 3g;Protein 44g
Serving 1; Cook time 15min

Ingredients
- 1 tablespoon butter
- 3 eggs
- 4 ounces sirloin
- 1/4 avocado
- Salt
- Pepper

Instructions
1. Melt your butter in a pan and fry 2–3 eggs until the whites are set and yolk is to desired doneness. Season with salt and pepper.
2. In another pan, cook your sirloin (or favorite cut of steak) until desired doneness. Then slice into bite-sized strips and season with salt and pepper.
3. Slice up some avocado and serve together!

Farmer Cheese Pancakes
Nutrition: Cal 200;Fat 12g;Carb 2,5g;Protein 18g
Serving 5; Cook time 20min

Ingredients
- 1 lb Farmer Cheese
- 1 cup coconut flour

- •2 eggs
- •Pinch of salt, to taste (optional)
- •1 tsp Stevia, to taste (optional)

Instructions

1. Mix farmer cheese, coconut flour, salt, and 2 eggs. Mixture should be like paste texture.
2. Form pancakes into round shape. Dust it just a bit with coconut flour.
3. Fry till both sides are golden brown.

French Omelet

Nutrition: Cal 186;Fat 9g;Carb 4g;Protein 22 g
Serving 2; Cook time 10min

Ingredients

- •2 large eggs
- •4 large egg whites
- •1/4 cup fat-free milk
- •1/8 teaspoon salt
- •1/8 teaspoon pepper
- •1/4 cup cubed fully cooked ham
- •1 tablespoon chopped onion
- •1 tablespoon chopped green pepper
- •1/4 cup shredded reduced-fat cheddar cheese

Instructions

1. Whisk together first five ingredients.
2. Place a 10-in. skillet coated with cooking spray over medium heat. Pour in egg mixture. Mixture should set immediately at edges. As eggs set, push cooked portions toward the center, letting uncooked eggs flow underneath.
3. When eggs are thickened and no liquid egg remains, top one half with remaining ingredients. Fold omelet in half. Cut in half to serve.

Corned Beef and Radish Hash

Nutrition: Cal 252;Fat 16g;Carb 2g;Protein 23 g
Serving 4; Cook time 20min

Ingredients

- •1 tablespoon olive oil
- •1/4 cup diced onions
- •1 cup radishes, diced to about 1/4 inch
- •1/2 teaspoon kosher salt
- •1/4 teaspoon ground black pepper
- •1/2 teaspoon dried oregano (Mexican if you have it)
- •1/4 teaspoon garlic powder
- •1 - 12 ounce can corned beef or 1 cup finely chopped corned beef, packed

Instructions

1. Heat the olive oil in a large saute pan and add the onions, radishes, salt, and pepper.
2. Saute the onions and radishes on medium heat for 5 minutes or until softened.
3. Add the oregano, garlic powder, and corned beef to the pan and stir well until combined.
4. Cook over low to medium heat, stirring occasionally for 10 minutes or until the radishes are soft and starting to brown.
5. Press the mixture into the bottom of the pan and cook on high heat for 2-3 minutes or until the bottom is crisp and brown.

Matcha Breakfast Bowl

Nutrition: Cal 150;Fat 10g;Carb 5g;Protein 13g
Serving 1; Cook time 10min

Ingredients

Matcha Chia Bowl

- •1 cup plant-based milk such as coconut, almond, or macadamia
- •2 tablespoons chia seeds
- •1-2 teaspoons matcha to taste (we use 2 teaspoons)
- •Vanilla stevia drops or preferred sweetener, to taste
- •Pinch of pink Himalayan salt

For the Smooth Version (optional)

- •1/4-1/2 avocado, to taste
- •Mint extract or fresh mint leaves

Serving Suggestions (optional)

- •Shredded coconut, lightly toasted
- •Almonds, lightly toasted
- •Fresh strawberries

Instructions

1. Mix chia seeds with your chosen milk, matcha, sweetener, and salt. Cover and refrigerate overnight. For the milk, I like to mix 1-2 tablespoons of full-fat coconut milk (the canned stuff) with 1 cup of water.
2. Add more liquid as needed to reach desired consistency (optional). Sweeten to taste and serve with toppings of choice.
3. To make the smooth version, simply blend in a high-speed blender. You can add some avocado for added creaminess, mint leaves (or extract) for a fresh touch, and a handful of ice.
4. Chia pudding (without the avocado) can be kept refrigerated in an airtight container for up to a week (it's ideal for meal prepping!)

Southwestern Omelet

Nutrition: Cal 390;Fat 31g;Carb 7g;Protein 22g
Serving 4; Cook time 10min

Ingredients

- •1/2 cup chopped onion
- •1 jalapeno pepper, minced
- •1 tablespoon canola oil
- •6 large eggs, lightly beaten
- •6 bacon strips, cooked and crumbled
- •1 small tomato, chopped
- •1 ripe avocado, cut into 1-inch slices
- •1 cup shredded Monterey Jack cheese, divided
- •Salt and pepper, to taste
- •Salsa (optional)

Instructions

1. In a large skillet, saute onion and jalapeno in oil until tender; remove with a slotted spoon and set aside. Pour eggs into the same skillet; cover and cook over low heat for 3-4 minutes.
2. Sprinkle with the onion mixture, bacon, tomato, avocado, and 1/2 cup cheese. Season with salt and pepper.
3. Fold omelet in half over filling. Cover and cook for 3-4 minutes or until eggs are set. Sprinkle with remaining cheese. Serve with salsa if desired.

Pulled Pork Hash
Nutrition: Cal 354;Fat 22g;Carb 8g;Protein 21g
Serving 2; Cook time 20min

Ingredients
•2 tablespoons FOC (fat of choice, I use lard)
•1 turnip, diced (115 g)
•1/2 teaspoon paprika
•1/4 teaspoon salt
•1/4 teaspoon garlic powder
•1/4 teaspoon black pepper
•3 Brussels sprouts, halved (50 g)
•1 cup chopped lacinato kale, about 2 leaves (45 g)
•2 tablespoons diced red onion (30 g)
•3 ounces pulled pork
•2 eggs

Instructions
1.Heat the oil in a large cast iron skillet over medium-high heat. Add the diced turnip and the spices to the skillet. Cook 5 minutes, stirring occasionally.
2.Add the remaining vegetables to the skillet and cook another 2-3 minutes until they start to soften. Add in the pork and cook 2 minutes.
3.Make 2 divots in the hash and crack in two eggs. Cover and cook 3-5 minutes, just until the whites are set.

Ham & Feta Omelet
Nutrition: Cal 290;Fat 20g;Carb 5g;Protein 21 g
Serving 2; Cook time 15min

Ingredients
•4 large eggs
•1 green onion, chopped
•1 tablespoon 2% milk
•1/4 teaspoon dried basil
•1/4 teaspoon dried oregano
•Dash of garlic powder
•Dash of salt
•Dash of pepper
•1 tablespoon butter
•1/4 cup crumbled feta cheese
•3 slices deli ham, chopped
•1 plum tomato, chopped
•2 teaspoons balsamic vinaigrette

Instructions
1.In a small bowl, whisk eggs, green onion, milk, and seasonings until blended. In a large nonstick skillet, heat butter over medium-high heat. Pour in egg mixture. Mixture should set immediately at edge.
2.As eggs set, push cooked portions toward the center, letting uncooked eggs flow underneath. When eggs are thickened and no liquid egg remains, top one side with cheese and ham.
3.Fold omelet in half; cut into two portions. Slide onto plates; top with tomato. Drizzle with vinaigrette before serving.

Ham Steaks with Gruyere, Bacon & Mushrooms
Nutrition: Cal 352;Fat 22g;Carb 5g;Protein 34 g
Serving 14; Cook time 15min

Ingredients
•2 tablespoons butter

•1/2 pound sliced fresh mushrooms
•1 shallot, finely chopped
•2 garlic cloves, minced
•1/8 teaspoon coarsely ground pepper
•1 fully cooked boneless ham steak (about 1 pound), cut into four pieces
•1 cup shredded Gruyere cheese
•4 bacon strips, cooked and crumbled
•1 tablespoon minced fresh parsley (optional)

Instructions
1.In a large nonstick skillet, heat butter over medium-high heat. Add mushrooms and shallot; cook and stir 4-6 minutes or until tender. Add garlic and pepper; cook 1 minute longer. Remove from pan; keep warm. Wipe skillet clean.
2.In same skillet, cook ham over medium heat 3 minutes. Turn; sprinkle with cheese and bacon. Cook, covered, 2-4 minutes longer or until cheese is melted and ham is heated through. Serve with mushroom mixture. If desired, sprinkle with parsley.

Broccoli Quiche Cups
Nutrition: Cal 291;Fat 24g;Carb 4g;Protein 17 g
Serving 12; Cook time 20min

Ingredients
•1 cup chopped fresh broccoli
•1 cup pepper jack cheese
•6 large eggs, lightly beaten
•3/4 cup heavy whipping cream
•1/2 cup bacon bits
•1 shallot, minced
•1/4 teaspoon salt
•1/4 teaspoon pepper

Instructions
1.Preheat oven to 350°. Divide broccoli and cheese among 12 greased muffin cups.
2.Whisk together remaining ingredients; pour into cups. Bake until set, 15-20 minutes.

Broccoli & Cheese Omelet
Nutrition: Cal 230;Fat 17g;Carb 5g;Protein 15g
Serving 4; Cook time 15min

Ingredients
•2-1/2 cups fresh broccoli florets
•6 large eggs
•1/4 cup 2% milk
•1/2 teaspoon salt
•1/4 teaspoon pepper
•1/3 cup grated Romano cheese
•1/3 cup sliced pitted Greek olives
•1 tablespoon olive oil
•Shaved Romano cheese and minced fresh parsley

Instructions
1.Preheat broiler. In a large saucepan, place steamer basket over 1 inch of water. Place broccoli in basket. Bring water to a boil. Reduce heat to a simmer; steam, covered, 4-6 minutes or until crisp-tender.

2. In a large bowl, whisk eggs, milk, salt, and pepper. Stir in cooked broccoli, grated cheese, and olives. In a 10-inch ovenproof skillet, heat oil over medium heat; pour in egg mixture. Cook, uncovered, 4-6 minutes or until nearly set.
3. Broil 3-4 inches from heat 2-4 minutes or until eggs are completely set. Let stand 5 minutes. Cut into wedges. Sprinkle with shaved cheese and parsley

Denver Omelet Salad
Nutrition: Cal 230;Fat 14g;Carb 7g;Protein 17 g
Serving 4; Cook time 10min

Ingredients
- 8 cups fresh baby spinach
- 1 cup chopped tomatoes
- 2 tablespoons olive oil, divided
- 1-1/2 cups chopped fully cooked ham
- 1 small onion, chopped
- 1 small green pepper, chopped
- 4 large eggs
- Salt and pepper, to taste

Instructions
1. Arrange spinach and tomatoes on a platter; set aside. In a large skillet, heat 1 tablespoon olive oil over medium-high heat. Add ham, onion, and green pepper; saute until ham is heated through and vegetables are tender, 5-7 minutes. Spoon over spinach and tomatoes.
2. In same skillet, heat remaining olive oil over medium heat. Break eggs one at a time into a small cup, then gently slide into skillet.
3. Immediately reduce heat to low; season with salt and pepper. To prepare sunny-side-up eggs, cover pan and cook until whites are completely set and yolks thicken but are not hard. Top salad with fried eggs.

Turkey Breakfast Sausage
Nutrition: Cal 85;Fat 5g;Carb 2g;Protein 10g
Serving 8; Cook time 10min

Ingredients
- 1 pound lean ground turkey
- 3/4 teaspoon salt
- 1/2 teaspoon rubbed sage
- 1/2 teaspoon pepper
- 1/4 teaspoon ground ginger

Instructions
1. Crumble turkey into a large bowl. Add the salt, sage, pepper, and ginger. Shape into eight 2-inch patties.
2. In a nonstick skillet coated with cooking spray, cook patties over medium heat for 4-6 minutes on each side or until a thermometer reads 165° and juices run clear.

. Avocado Bacon and Eggs
Nutrition: Cal 125;Fat 9g;Carb 2g;Protein 8g
Serving 2; Cook time 15min

Ingredients
- 1 medium avocado
- 2 eggs
- 1 piece bacon, cooked and crumbled
- 1 tablespoon low-fat cheese

- Pinch of salt

Instructions
1. Preheat oven to 425°F.
2. Begin by cutting the avocado in half and removing the pit.
3. With a spoon, scoop out some of the avocado so it's a tad bigger than your egg and yolk. Place in a muffin pan to keep the avocado stable while cooking.
4. Crack your egg and add it to the inside of your avocado. Sprinkle a little cheese on top with a pinch of salt. Top with cooked bacon.
5. Cook for 14-16 minutes. Serve warm.

Peanut Butter Granola
Nutrition:Cal 338;Fat 30g;Carb 9g;Protein 10 g
Serving 12; Cook time 30min

Ingredients
- 1 1/2 cups almonds
- 1 1/2 cups pecans
- 1 cup shredded coconut or almond flour
- 1/4 cup sunflower seeds
- 1/3 cup Swerve sweetener
- 1/3 cup vanilla whey protein powder OR collagen protein powder
- 1/3 cup peanut butter
- 1/4 cup butter
- 1/4 cup water

Instructions
1. Preheat oven to 300°F and line a large rimmed baking sheet with parchment paper.
2. In a food processor, process almonds and pecans until they resemble coarse crumbs with some larger pieces. Transfer to a large bowl and stir in shredded coconut, sunflower seeds, sweetener, and vanilla protein powder.
3. In a microwave-safe bowl, melt the peanut butter and butter together.
4. Pour melted peanut butter mixture over nut mixture and stir well, tossing lightly. Stir in water. Mixture will clump together.
5. Spread mixture evenly on prepared baking sheet and bake 30 minutes, stirring halfway through. Remove and let cool completely

. Avocado Bacon and Eggs
Nutrition: Cal 125;Fat 9g;Carb 2g;Protein 8g
Serving 2; Cook time 15min

Ingredients
- 1 medium avocado
- 2 eggs
- 1 piece bacon, cooked and crumbled
- 1 tablespoon low-fat cheese
- Pinch of salt

Instructions
1. Preheat oven to 425°F.
2. Begin by cutting the avocado in half and removing the pit.
3. With a spoon, scoop out some of the avocado so it's a tad bigger than your egg and yolk. Place in a muffin pan to keep the avocado stable while cooking.

4. Crack your egg and add it to the inside of your avocado. Sprinkle a little cheese on top with a pinch of salt. Top with cooked bacon.
5. Cook for 14-16 minutes. Serve warm.

Spinach-Mushroom Scrambled Eggs
Nutrition: Cal 200;Fat 11g;Carb 2g;Protein 14g
Serving 2; Cook time 10min

Ingredients
- 2 large eggs
- 2 large egg whites
- 1/8 teaspoon salt
- 1/8 teaspoon pepper
- 1 teaspoon butter
- 1/2 cup thinly sliced fresh mushrooms
- 1/2 cup fresh baby spinach, chopped
- 2 tablespoons shredded provolone cheese

Instructions
1. In a small bowl, whisk eggs, egg whites, salt, and pepper until blended. In a small nonstick skillet, heat butter over medium-high heat.
2. Add mushrooms; cook and stir 3-4 minutes or until tender. Add spinach; cook and stir until wilted. Reduce heat to medium.
3. Add egg mixture; cook and stir just until eggs are thickened and no liquid egg remains. Stir in cheese.

Eggs Florentine Casserole
Nutrition: Cal 271;Fat 20g;Carb 7g;Protein 17 g
Serving 12; Cook time 30min

Ingredients
- 1 pound bulk pork sausage
- 2 tablespoons butter
- 1 large onion, chopped
- 1 cup sliced fresh mushrooms
- 1 package (10 ounces) frozen chopped spinach, thawed and squeezed dry
- 12 large eggs
- 2 cups 2% milk
- 1 cup shredded Swiss cheese
- 1 cup shredded sharp cheddar cheese
- 1/4 teaspoon paprika

Instructions
1. Preheat oven to 350°. In a large skillet, cook sausage over medium heat 6-8 minutes or until no longer pink, breaking into crumbles; drain and transfer to a greased 13 x 9-inch baking dish.
2. In same skillet, heat butter over medium-high heat. Add onion and mushrooms; cook and stir 3-5 minutes, or until tender. Stir in spinach. Spoon vegetable mixture over sausage.
3. In a large bowl, whisk eggs and milk until blended; pour egg mixture over vegetables. Sprinkle with cheeses and paprika. Bake, uncovered, 30-35 minutes or until the center is set and a thermometer inserted in center reads 165°. Let stand 10 minutes before serving.

Taco Breakfast Skillet
Nutrition: Cal 523;Fat 44g;Carb 9g;Protein 22g
Serving 6; Cook time 45min

Ingredients
- 1 pound ground beef
- 4 tablespoons taco seasoning
- 2/3 cup water
- 10 large eggs
- 1 1/2 cups shredded sharp cheddar cheese, divided
- 1/4 cup heavy cream
- 1 roma tomato, diced
- 1 medium avocado, peeled, pitted, and cubed
- 1/4 cup sliced black olives
- 2 green onions, sliced
- 1/4 cup sour cream
- 1/4 cup salsa
- 1 jalapeno, sliced (optional)
- 2 tablespoons torn fresh cilantro (optional)

Instructions
1. Brown the ground beef in a large skillet over medium-high heat. drain the excess fat.
2. To the skillet, stir in the taco seasoning and water. Reduce the heat to low and let simmer until the sauce has thickened and coats the meat. About 5 minutes. Remove half of the seasoned beef from the skillet and set aside.
3. Crack the eggs into a large mixing bowl and whisk. Add 1 cup of the cheddar cheese and the heavy cream to the eggs and whisk to combine.
4. Preheat the oven to 375°F.
5. Pour the egg mixture over top of the meat retained in the skillet and stir to mix the meat into the eggs. Bake for 30 minutes, or until the egg bake is cooked all the way through and fluffy.
6. Top with remaining ground beef, the remaining ½ cup of cheddar cheese, tomato, avocado, olives, green onion, sour cream, and salsa.
7. Garnish with jalapeno and cilantro, if using

Keto Cacao Coconut Granola
Nutrition: Cal 112;Fat 6g;Carb 7g;Protein 7g
Serving 3; Cook time 30min

Ingredients
- 1/2 cup chopped raw pecans
- 1/2 cup flax seeds
- 1/2 cup superfine blanched almond flour
- 1/2 cup unsweetened dried coconut
- 1/4 cup cacao nibs
- 1/4 cup chopped raw walnuts
- 1/4 cup sesame seeds
- 1/4 cup sugar-free vanilla-flavored protein powder
- 3 tablespoons granulated erythritol
- 1 teaspoon ground cinnamon
- 1/8 teaspoon kosher salt
- 1/3 cup coconut oil
- 1 large egg white, beaten

Instructions
1. Preheat the oven to 300°F.
2. Line a 15x10-inch sheet pan with parchment paper.
3. Stir all of the ingredients until the mixture is crumbly and holds together in small clumps.
4. Spread out on the parchment-lined pan.

5. Bake for approximately 30 minutes or until golden brown and fragrant (oven times may vary).
6. Let the granola cool completely in the pan before removing.
7. Store in an airtight container in the refrigerator for up to 2 weeks.

Chorizo breakfast bake
Nutrition:Cal 212;Fat 11g;Carb 11g;Protein 9g
Serving 4; Cook time 50min

Ingredients
- 2 tablespoon olive oil
- 1 red bell pepper
- 1 yellow bell pepper
- 200 grams (7 ounces) chorizo sausage
- 6 large eggs
- 2 large red onion (cut into wedges)
- 2 cloves garlic (minced)
- ½ cup coconut milk
- Salt and pepper

Instructions
1. Preheat the oven to 425 degrees Fahrenheit (220 degrees Celsius).
2. Cut the bell peppers in half, remove the seeds and stem and place the halves on a baking tray. Drizzle with 1 tbsp olive oil and put in the oven to roast for 20 minutes. After 10 minutes of baking, place the red onion wedges on the tray, drizzle with a splash of olive oil and return to the oven to cook for another 10 minutes. The peppers are done when they are soft and have a slightly charred skin. When the peppers are done, place them on a cutting board and place a bowl overtop to trap the steam. Leave them to rest for 5 minutes (this will make it easier to peel off the skin).
3. In a cast iron skillet heat 1 tbsp olive oil on medium high heat. Stir in the minced garlic and cook for 20 seconds until fragrant and then add in the chopped chorizo and cook for 5 minutes until the chorizo is cooked through and then remove from the heat.
4. While the chorizo is cooking peel the skin off of the roasted bell peppers. Cut the peeled peppers into thin strips.
5. In a bowl whisk together the eggs, coconut milk, paprika, cayenne, salt and pepper.
6. Add the sliced peppers and red onion to the cast iron skillet and pour the egg mixture overtop. Transfer to the oven to bake for 20-25 minutes until the egg has set and the top of the frittata is firm to the touch. Serve sprinkled with chopped parsley.

Baked Eggs in Avocado
Nutrition: Cal 125;Fat 10g;Carb 3g;Protein 8g
Serving 2; Cook time 15min

Ingredients
- 1 medium avocado
- 2 tablespoons lime juice
- 2 large eggs
- Salt and pepper
- 2 tablespoons shredded cheddar cheese

Instructions

1. Preheat the oven to 450°F and cut the avocado in half.
2. Scoop out some of the flesh from the middle of each avocado half.
3. Place the avocado halves upright in a baking dish and brush with lime juice.
4. Crack an egg into each and season with salt and pepper.
5. Bake for 10 minutes, then sprinkle with cheese.
6. Let the eggs bake for another 2 to 3 minutes until the cheese is melted. Serve hot.

Breakfast Egg Muffins Filled with Sausage Gravy
Nutrition: Cal 607;Fat 46g;Carb 6g;Protein 42 g
Serving 6; Cook time 35min

Ingredients
For the muffins:
- 12 large eggs
- Sea salt
- Black pepper
- 1 pound thin shaved deli ham
- 4 ounces shredded mozzarella cheese
- 4 ounces grated parmesan cheese
- Low-carb sausage gravy   For the gravy:
- 1/2 ground pork sausage
- 8 ounces softened cream cheese
- 3/4 cups beef broth
- Sea salt
Black pepper

Instructions
1. Prepare the eggs and gravy.
2. Whisk eggs together with salt and pepper to taste.
3. Cook the sausage over medium heat until thoroughly cooked through.
4. Add in the cream cheese and the broth and stirring constantly, cook until the mixture comes to a soft simmer and thickens.
5. Then reduce the heat to medium-low, still stirring constantly and simmer for 2 more minutes.
6. Season to taste with salt and pepper.
7. Set mixture aside.
8. Preheat oven to 325°F.

Assemble the muffins:
1. Place two pieces of ham in the bottom of each muffin cup, careful to overlap and try and cover the whole surface.
2. Evenly divide sausage gravy between each muffin.
3. Pour eggs into each muffin, dividing the mixture evenly.
4. Top each muffin with equal parts of the two types of cheeses.
5. Bake for approximately 30-40 minutes or until muffin is firm and cheese is melted.

Lemon Poppy Ricotta Pancakes
Nutrition: Cal 370;Fat 26g;Carb 6,5g;Protein 29 g
Serving 2; Cook time 20min

Ingredients
- 1 large lemon, juiced and zested
- 6 ounces whole milk ricotta
- 3 large eggs
- 10 to 12 drops liquid stevia
- ¼ cup almond flour

- 1 scoop egg white protein powder
- 1 tablespoon poppy seeds
- ¾ teaspoons baking powder
- ¼ cup powdered erythritol
- 1 tablespoon heavy cream

Instructions
1. Combine the ricotta, eggs, and liquid stevia in a food processor with half the lemon juice and the lemon zest—blend well, then pour into a bowl.
2. Whisk in the almond flour, protein powder, poppy seeds, baking powder, and a pinch of salt.
3. Heat a large nonstick pan over medium heat.
4. Spoon the batter into the pan, using about ¼ cup per pancake.
5. Cook the pancakes until bubbles form on the surface of the batter, then flip them.
6. Let the pancakes cook until the bottom is browned, then remove to a plate.
7. Repeat with the remaining batter.
8. Whisk together the heavy cream, powdered erythritol, and reserved lemon juice and zest.
9. Serve the pancakes hot, drizzled with the lemon glaze.

Egg Strata with Blueberries and Cinnamon
Nutrition: Cal 188;Fat 15g;Carb 4g;Protein 8g
Serving 4; Cook time 20min

Ingredients
- 6 large eggs
- 2 tbsp softened butter
- 1 tsp vanilla
- 1/2 cup blueberries (or 1/4 cup, depending upon taste)
- 1/2 tsp cinnamon (you could probably double this if you like cinnamon)
- 1 tbsp coconut oil

Instructions
1. Preheat oven to 375°F.
2. In an 8" - 9" cast iron skillet (or any oven-proof skillet), heat coconut oil over medium heat.
3. In a medium bowl beat eggs, butter, cinnamon, and vanilla together with a hand mixer until combined and fluffy (about 1-2 minutes).
4. Pour egg mixture into heated pan and allow bottom to cook slightly (about 2 minutes). Gently drop blueberries into egg mixture and place pan in oven. Cook for 15-20 or until cooked through and browned on top (but not burned).
5. Remove from oven and allow to cool slightly.

Sweet Blueberry Coconut Porridge
Nutrition: Cal 390;Fat 22g;Carb 12g;Protein 10 g
Serving 2; Cook time 15min

Ingredients
- 1 cup unsweetened almond milk
- ¼ cup canned coconut milk
- ¼ cup coconut flour
- ¼ cup ground flaxseed
- 1 teaspoon ground cinnamon
- ¼ teaspoon ground nutmeg
- Pinch salt
- 60 grams fresh blueberries

- ¼ cup shaved coconut

Instructions
1. Warm the almond milk and coconut milk in a saucepan over low heat.
2. Whisk in the coconut flour, flaxseed, cinnamon, nutmeg, and salt.
3. Turn up the heat and cook until the mixture bubbles.
4. Stir in the sweetener and vanilla extract, then cook until thickened to the desired level.
5. Spoon into two bowls and top with blueberries and shaved coconut.

Low-Carb Breakfast Quiche
Nutrition: Cal 450;Fat 36g;Carb 6g;Protein 24g
Serving 4; Cook time 55min

Ingredients
- 1 lb ground Italian sausage
- 1.5 cups shredded cheddar cheese
- 8 large eggs
- 1 tbsp ranch seasoning
- 1 cup sour cream

Instructions
1. Preheat oven to 350°F.
2. In an oven-safe skillet, brown ground sausage and drain the grease.
3. In a large bowl, whisk together egg, sour cream, and ranch seasoning. You may want to use a hand mixer.
4. Mix in cheddar cheese.
5. Pour egg mixture into pan and stir until everything is fully blended.
6. Cover with foil and bake for 30 minutes.
7. Remove foil and bake for another 25 minutes or until golden brown.

Fat-Busting Vanilla Protein Smoothie
Nutrition: Cal 540;Fat 46g;Carb 8g;Protein 25 g
Serving 2; Cook time 5min

Ingredients
- 11 scoop (20g) vanilla egg white protein powder
- ½ cup heavy cream
- ¼ cup vanilla almond milk
- 4 ice cubes
- 1 tablespoon coconut oil
- 1 tablespoon powdered erythritol
- ½ teaspoon vanilla extract
- ¼ cup whipped cream

Instructions
1. Combine all of the ingredients, except the whipped cream, in a blender.
2. Blend on high speed for 30 to 60 seconds until smooth.
3. Pour into a glass and top with whipped cream.

Savory Ham and Cheese Waffles
Nutrition: Cal 575;Fat 45g;Carb 5g;Protein 35g
Serving 2, Cook time 25min

Ingredients
- 4 large eggs, divided
- 2 scoops (40 g) egg white protein powder
- 1 teaspoon baking powder
- 1/3 cup melted butter

- •½ teaspoon salt
- •1 ounce diced ham
- •¼ cup shredded cheddar cheese

Instructions

1. Separate two of the eggs and set the other two aside.
2. Beat 2 of the egg yolks with the protein powder, baking powder, butter, and salt in a mixing bowl.
3. Fold in the chopped ham and grated cheddar cheese.
4. Whisk the egg whites in a separate bowl with a pinch of salt until stiff peaks form.
5. Fold the beaten egg whites into the egg yolk mixture in two batches.
6. Grease a preheated waffle maker then spoon ¼ cup of the batter into it and close it.
7. Cook until the waffle is golden brown, about 3 to 4 minutes, then remove.
8. Reheat the waffle iron and repeat with the remaining batter.
9. Meanwhile, heat the oil in a skillet and fry the eggs with salt and pepper.
10. Serve the waffles hot, topped with a fried egg.

Avocado Smoothie with Coconut Milk
Nutrition: Cal 283;Fat 25g;Carb 14g;Protein 3,2 g
Serving 15; Cook time 5min

Ingredients

- •1 cup coconut milk, unsweetened
- •1 tsp ginger, fresh and grounded
- •1/2 avocado
- •5 leaves spinach
- •1 tsp lime juice (optional)
- •1 tsp Stevia (optional)
- •1 tsp chia seeds

Instructions

1. Wash your ginger and spinach thoroughly.
2. Peel the ginger and avocado. Slice them into pieces.
3. Using a blender, mix all of the ingredients (except chia seeds and stevia) for a minute to obtain a smooth and uniform mixture. Optionally, pour some water and lime juice into the blender to produce the desired thickness.
4. Include some ice cubes and the sweetener into the mix just to flavor it up. Transfer to a glass and garnish with a teaspoon of chia seeds on top. Serve immediately.

Coconut Flour Pancakes
Nutrition: Cal 274;Fat 23g;Carb 8g;Protein 8g
Serving 2; Cook time 20min

Ingredients
Main Ingredients:

- •2 tbsp coconut flour
- •2 eggs
- •½ tbsp So Nourished Erythritol or a dash of stevia extract
- •¼ tsp baking powder
- •2 tbsp sour cream
- •2 tbsp melted butter
- •½ tsp vanilla extract

For the topping:

- •50 g strawberries
- •1 tbsp shredded coconut
- •1 tbsp almond slices
- •1 tbsp maple syrup (optional)

Instructions

1. Put the eggs, sour cream, 1 ½ tbsp. of melted butter (you'll need the rest for frying the pancakes), vanilla extract, and mix well.
2. Add the coconut flour, baking powder, erythritol to the mixture and mix again. Let the mixture sit for about 15 minutes. If the mixture is too thick, add a little bit of water (20-30 ml) and mix again until the consistency is right.
3. In a pan on medium heat, add butter in and fry the pancakes in butter. The number of pancakes you make will depend on the size you want. We made 6 pancakes with this recipe.

Southwestern Omelet
Nutrition: Cal 390;Fat 31g;Carb 7g;Protein 22g
Serving 4; Cook time 10min

Ingredients

- •1/2 cup chopped onion
- •1 jalapeno pepper, minced
- •1 tablespoon canola oil
- •6 large eggs, lightly beaten
- •6 bacon strips, cooked and crumbled
- •1 small tomato, chopped
- •1 ripe avocado, cut into 1-inch slices
- •1 cup shredded Monterey Jack cheese, divided
- •Salt and pepper, to taste
- •Salsa (optional)

Instructions

1. In a large skillet, saute onion and jalapeno in oil until tender; remove with a slotted spoon and set aside. Pour eggs into the same skillet; cover and cook over low heat for 3-4 minutes.
2. Sprinkle with the onion mixture, bacon, tomato, avocado, and 1/2 cup cheese. Season with salt and pepper.
3. Fold omelet in half over filling. Cover and cook for 3-4 minutes or until eggs are set.
4. Sprinkle with remaining cheese. Serve with salsa if desired.

Easy Cloud Buns
Nutrition: Cal 50;Fat 5g;Carb 1g;Protein 2.5 g
Serving 10; Cook time 40 min

Ingredients

3 large eggs, separated
1/8 teaspoon cream of tartar
3 ounces cream cheese, chopped

Instructions

1. Preheat the oven to 300°F and line a baking sheet with parchment.
2. Beat the egg whites until foamy then beat in the cream of tartar until the whites are shiny and opaque with soft peaks.

3. In a separate bowl, beat the cream cheese and egg yolks until well combined then fold in the egg white mixture.
4. Spoon the batter onto the baking sheet in ¼-cup circles about 2 inches apart.
5. Bake for 30 minutes until the buns are firm to the touch.

Pepperoni, Ham & Cheddar Stromboli
Nutrition: Cal 525;Fat 37g;Carb 16g;Protein 32 g
Serving 3; Cook time 40min

Ingredients
- 1 ¼ cups shredded mozzarella cheese
- ¼ cup almond flour
- 3 tablespoons coconut flour
- 1 teaspoon dried Italian seasoning
- Salt and pepper
- 1 large egg, whisked
- 6 ounces sliced deli ham
- 2 ounces sliced pepperoni
- 4 ounces sliced cheddar cheese
- 1 tablespoon melted butter
- 6 cups fresh salad greens

Instructions
1. Preheat the oven to 400°F and line a baking sheet with parchment.
2. Melt the mozzarella cheese in a microwave-safe bowl until it can be stirred smooth.
3. In a separate bowl, stir together the almond flour, coconut flour, and dried Italian seasoning.
4. Pour the melted cheese into the flour mixture and mix it with some salt and pepper.
5. Add the egg and work it into a dough then put it onto a piece of parchment.
6. Lay a piece of parchment on top and roll the dough out into an oval.
7. Use a knife to cut diagonal slits along the edges, leaving the middle 4 inches untouched.
8. Layer the ham and cheese slices in the middle of the dough then fold the strips over the top.
9. Brush the top with butter, then bake for 15 to 20 minutes until the dough is browned. Slice the Stromboli and serve with a small salad.

Eggs and Asparagus Breakfast Bites
Nutrition: Cal 426;Fat 35g;Carb 6g;Protein 20 g
Serving 2; Cook time 25 min

Ingredients
- 4 medium eggs
- 100 g asparagus, fresh or canned
- 1 tbsp butter, melted
- ¼ tsp baking powder
- 1 tbsp coconut flour
- 80 g cream cheese
- 40 g shredded cheddar cheese
- Salt, to taste

Instructions
1. For fresh asparagus, chop them into about 2-cm long pieces. Pan fry for around 5 minutes in melted butter. For canned asparagus, simply chop them into pieces. Reserve.

2. Combine the rest of the ingredients in a bowl. Stir well to mix together. Put aside for 10 minutes.
3. Brush a decent amount of oil in the baking molds. Place some pieces of asparagus in the molds then add the combined mixture you reserved earlier. Avoid filling up to the brim.
4. Place in the oven set at 350°F for 20 minutes, checking occasionally if the bites are cooked thoroughly.
5. Serve on a plate and enjoy.

Avocado Breakfast Muffins
Nutrition: Cal 250;Fat 19g;Carb 2,5g;Protein 17g
Serving 20; Cook time 30min

Ingredients
- 20 beef patties (small size, about 50 g each)
- 10 eggs, medium-sized
- 1/2 cup heavy cream
- 2 avocados, cubed
- 10 oz cheddar cheese, cubed
- Black pepper, to taste

Instructions
1. Preheat oven to 350°F.
2. Take a large muffin tin and put one sausage patty in each cup, shaping with a shot glass to line the entire inside.
3. Evenly divide the avocado and cheese in the cups.
4. Beat eggs and heavy cream together in a bowl, then pour into each cup until cheese and avocado are covered. Top with black pepper to taste.
5. Bake for 20 minutes at 350°; if desired, broil for an additional 1-2 minutes until top is browned. Enjoy!

Cheddar Biscuits
Nutrition: Cal 284;Fat 25g;Carb 2g;Protein 20 g
Serving 4; Cook time 20 min

Ingredients
- 1 cup cheddar cheese, shredded
- 1/4 cup butter melted and slightly cooled
- 4 eggs
- 1/3 cup coconut flour
- 1/4 teaspoon baking powder
- 1/4 teaspoon garlic powder
- 1 teaspoon dried parsley (optional)
- 1/4 teaspoon Old Bay Seasoning (optional)
- 1/4 teaspoon salt

Instructions
1. Set the oven to 400°F to preheat.
2. Crack the eggs in a bowl. Add the garlic powder, melted butter, dried parsley, and seasoning powder if you have some. Salt to taste.
3. Combine the cheese into the mixture together with the baking powder and coconut flour. Fold until you obtain a lump-free mixture.
4. Grease a cookie sheet before adding the batter into it. Place ice cream size scoops into the sheet.
5. Lightly brown the biscuits in the oven for 15 minutes.
6. Serve with any meal or eat them alone.
7. If you like to keep them for later, allow them to cool completely before storing in a jar to preserve the crispness.

Bacon and Mushroom Omelette

Nutrition: Cal 313;Fat 24g;Carb 1,5g;Protein 23g
Serving 2; Cook time 10min

Ingredients
- 3 medium mushrooms, raw
- 2 slices bacon
- 3 eggs
- 2 tbsp onion, chopped
- 2 slices cheddar cheese
- Lettuce or watercress, to taste (optional)
- Pinch salt
- Pinch pepper

Instructions
1. Brunoise cut the onion. Slice the mushrooms and bacon into small chunks as well.
2. Heat an 8-inch non-stick skillet coated with cooking spray over medium-high heat. Cook the onion and bacon in the pan. Once the bacon is toasted enough, toss in the mushrooms and remove from the heat.
3. Beat the eggs in a mixing bowl. Flavor with sea salt and black pepper then add the cooked bacon, mushroom, and onion.
4. Gently pour the egg mixture into the pan. Once the omelette starts to firm up, ease around the edges with a spatula. Lay the slices of cheddar cheese on one half of the omelette. Fold the other half onto the cheese.
5. Leave in the pan for another 2 minutes, then let the cooked omelette slide onto a plate.
6. Fill the inside of the omelette with lettuce leaves if preferred. Serve immediately while still crispy and warm.

Scrambled Eggs with Mushrooms and Cottage Cheese

Nutrition: Cal 210;Fat 19g;Carb 3g;Protein 9g
Serving 3; Cook time 20min

Ingredients
- 3 eggs
- 1 cup button mushrooms, rinsed and sliced
- 1/2 medium-sized onion, finely chopped
- 3 tbsp olive oil
- 1/4 tsp oregano
- 1/4 cup cottage cheese
- 1/2 tsp sea salt
- 1/4 tsp black pepper

Instructions
1. Place a large skillet over medium-high heat. Let the olive oil heat in the pan. Sauté the finely chopped onions in the oil until they become translucent. Drop in the sliced mushrooms and let it simmer until the liquid in the pan evaporates. Stir well with oregano, pepper, and salt. Put aside.
2. Beat the eggs in a bowl. Flavor with a dash of salt and pepper enough to taste. Fry in the skillet and fold with a wooden spoon for a minute until slightly underdone.

Vegetable Tart

Nutrition: Cal 250;Fat 22g;Carb 5.5g;Protein 10 g
Serving 8; Cook time 70 min

Ingredients

- 6 eggs
- ½ cup heavy cream
- 8 oz cream cheese
- ½ cup shredded cheese
- ½ cup almond milk (or coconut milk)
- 12 oz zucchini
- 4 oz cauliflower
- 2 oz broccoli
- 8 oz red pepper
- 3 oz jalapeno
- 3 oz onion
- 3 cloves garlic
- Seasoning of your choice

Instructions
1. Mince the cauliflower, broccoli, garlic, onion, red pepper, and jalapeño into small cubes. Dice the zucchini as well.
2. Sauté the diced vegetables in a heated oil on a large skillet. Remove from the heat when they become soft enough but not mushy.
3. Crack the eggs in another bowl. Combine the almond milk, softened cream cheese, and heavy cream in the bowl. Mix everything to combine well.
4. Mix the vegetables into the cream cheese bowl. Stir with the cheese and seasonings of choice. Fold together until uniform.
5. Lay a foil on the base of the springform you will use to avoid seeping the mixture through the bottom. Cover with parchment paper and brush some oil on the sides and on the base. Pour the batter into the form. Bake for one hour or up till the surface of the tart is golden brown in color. The oven must be preheated to 350°F.
6. Generously dust with cheese on top after baking. Slice into wedges and serve.

Zucchini Breakfast Muffins

Nutrition: Cal 185;Fat 16g;Carb 2g;Protein 9g
Serving 12; Cook time 35min

Ingredients
- 6 eggs
- 1 zucchini, medium-sized
- 5 slices bacon
- 2 tbsp sour cream
- 1 cup heavy cream
- 1 cup shredded cheddar cheese
- 1 tbsp mayonnaise
- 1 tbsp mustard
- 1/2 cup coconut milk
- 1 oz dill
- 1 jalapeno small size
- 4 oz red pepper
- Salt and pepper, to taste

Instructions
1. Shred your zucchini into thin pieces and dust with some salt. Put aside for a few minutes to release the moisture.
2. Chop the dill into fine pieces, then mince your jalapeno and red pepper.

3. Crispy fry the bacon slices for around 5 minutes or simply heat them in the microwave. Cut into bits.
4. Strain all the unnecessary liquids from the grated zucchini. Press it with your hands to squeeze out the extracts. Alternatively, use a cheesecloth to do this. Transfer all of the chopped vegetables in a bowl and toss to mix well. Add in the cheese and bacon bits.
5. Crack the eggs in a separate bowl. Blend together with the sour cream, mustard, heavy cream, and mayo. Include the coconut milk as well. Adjust the flavor with salt and pepper.
6. Transfer the vegetable mix into 12 muffin forms. Distribute evenly. Gently add in the egg mixture into the cups. Remember to fill only ⅔ of the cup. Combine the two mixture with a spoon. Stir well.
7. Bake in the oven preheated at 370°F for 20-25 minutes. Make sure the muffins are golden and firm before removing from the oven.
8. Unmold from the cups and serve on a plate

Keto Cereal
Nutrition: Cal 250;Fat 10 g;Carb 15 g;Protein 10 g
Serving 3; Cook time 45 min

Ingredients
- Cooking spray
- 1 c. almonds, chopped
- 1 c. walnuts, chopped
- 1 c. unsweetened coconut flakes
- 1/4 c. sesame seeds
- 2 tbsp. flax seeds
- 2 tbsp. chia seeds
- 1/2 tsp. ground clove
- 1 1/2 tsp. ground cinnamon
- 1 tsp. pure vanilla extract
- 1/2 tsp. kosher salt
- 1 large egg white
- 1/4 c. melted coconut oil

Instructions
1. Preheat oven to 350° and grease a baking sheet with cooking spray. In a large bowl, mix together almonds, walnuts, coconut flakes, sesame seeds, flax seeds, and chia seeds. Stir in cloves, cinnamon, vanilla, and salt.
2. Beat egg white until foamy then stir into granola. Add coconut oil and stir until everything is well coated. Pour onto prepared baking sheet and spread into an even layer. Bake for 20 to 25 minutes, or until golden, gently stirring halfway through. Let cool completely.

Keto Sausage Breakfast Sandwich
Nutrition: Cal 350;Fat 25 g;Carb 2 g;Protein 12 g
Serving 3; Cook time 20 min

Ingredients
- 6 large eggs
- 2 tbsp. heavy cream
- Pinch red pepper flakes
- Kosher salt
- Freshly ground black pepper
- 1 tbsp. butter
- 3 slices cheddar
- 6 frozen sausage patties, heated according to package instructions
- 1 Avocado, sliced

Instructions
1. In a small bowl beat eggs, heavy cream, and red pepper flakes together. Season generously with salt and pepper. In a nonstick skillet over medium heat, melt butter. Pour about ⅓ of the eggs into the skillet. Place a slice of cheese in the middle and let sit about 1 minute. Fold the sides of the egg into the middle, covering the cheese. Remove from pan and repeat with remaining eggs.
2. Serve eggs between two sausage patties with avocado.

Cabbage Hash Browns
Nutrition: Cal 250;Fat 22 g;Carb 5.5 g;Protein 10 g
Serving 2; Cook time 35 min

Ingredients
2 large eggs
1/2 tsp. garlic powder
1/2 tsp. kosher salt
Freshly ground black pepper
2 c. shredded cabbage
1/4 small yellow onion, thinly sliced
1 tbsp. vegetable oil

Instructions
1. In a large bowl, whisk together eggs, garlic powder, and salt. Season with black pepper. Add cabbage and onion to egg mixture and toss to combine.
2. In a large skillet over medium-high heat, heat oil. Divide mixture into 4 patties in the pan and press with spatula to flatten. Cook until golden and tender, about 3 minutes per side.

Omelet-Stuffed Peppers
Nutrition: Cal 280;Fat 12 g;Carb 8 g;Protein 25 g
Serving 4; Cook time 60 min

Ingredients
- 2 bell peppers, halved and seeds removed
- 8 eggs, lightly beaten
- 1/4 c. milk
- 4 slices bacon, cooked and crumbled
- 1 c. shredded cheddar
- 2 tbsp. finely chopped chives, plus more for garnish
- Kosher salt
- Freshly cracked black pepper

Instructions
1. Preheat oven to 400°. Place peppers cut side up in a large baking dish. Add a little water to the dish and bake peppers for 5 minutes.
2. Meanwhile, beat together eggs and milk. Stir in bacon, cheese, and chives and season with salt and pepper.
3. When peppers are done baking, pour egg mixture into peppers. Place back in the oven and bake 35 to 40 minutes more, until eggs are set. Garnish with more chives and serve.

Zucchini Egg Cups
Nutrition: Cal 280;Fat 12g;Carb 8g;Protein 25 g
Serving 12; Cook time 50 min

Ingredients
- Cooking spray, for pan
- 2 zucchini, peeled into strips
- 1/4 lb. ham, chopped
- 1/2 c. cherry tomatoes, quartered
- 8 eggs
- 1/2 c. heavy cream
- Kosher salt
- Freshly ground black pepper
- 1/2 tsp. dried oregano
- 1 c. Pinch red pepper flakes
- 1 c. shredded cheddar

Instructions
1. Preheat oven to 400° and grease a muffin tin with cooking spray. Line the inside and bottom of the muffin tin with zucchini strips, to form a crust. Sprinkle ham and cherry tomatoes inside each crust.
2. In a medium bowl whisk together eggs, heavy, cream, oregano, and red pepper flakes then season with salt and pepper. Pour egg mixture over ham and tomatoes then top with cheese.
3. Bake until eggs are set, 30 minutes.

Bacon Avocado Bombs
Nutrition: Cal 250;Fat 19 g;Carb 2,5 g;Protein 17 g
Serving 4; Cook time 30min

Ingredients
- 2 avocados
- 1/3 c. shredded Cheddar
- 8 slices bacon

Instructions
1. Heat broiler and line a small baking sheet with foil.
2. Slice each avocado in half and remove the pits. Peel the skin off of each avocado.
3. Fill two of the halves with cheese, then replace with the other avocado halves. Wrap each avocado with 4 slices of bacon.
4. Place bacon-wrapped avocados on the prepared baking sheet and broil until the bacon is crispy on top, about 5 minutes. Very carefully, flip the avocado using tongs and continue to cook until crispy all over, about 5 minutes per side.
5. Cut in half crosswise and serve immediately.

Ham & Cheese Egg Cups
Nutrition: Cal 340;Fat 30 g;Carb 10 g;Protein 12 g
Serving 12; Cook time 30min

Ingredients
- Cooking spray, for pan
- 12 slices ham
- 1 c. shredded cheddar
- 12 large eggs
- Kosher salt
- Freshly ground black pepper
- Chopped fresh parsley, for garnish

Instructions
1. Preheat oven to 400° and grease a 12-cup muffin tin with cooking spray. Line each cup with a slice of ham and sprinkle with cheddar. Crack an egg into each ham cup and season with salt and pepper.
2. Bake until eggs are cooked through, 12 to 15 minutes (depending on how runny you like your yolks).
3. Garnish with parsley and serve.

Keto Fat Bombs
Nutrition: Cal 290;Fat 28 g;Carb 5 g;Protein 5 g
Serving 16; Cook time 35 min

Ingredients
- 8 oz. cream cheese, softened to room temperature
- 1/2 c. keto-friendly peanut butter
- 1/4 c. coconut oil, plus 2 tbsp.
- 1/4 tsp. kosher salt
- 1/2 c. keto-friendly dark chocolate chips (such as Lily's)

Instructions
1. Line a small baking sheet with parchment paper. In a medium bowl, combine cream cheese, peanut butter, 1/4 cup coconut oil, and salt. Using a hand mixer, beat mixture until fully combined, about 2 minutes. Place bowl in freezer to firm up slightly, 10 to 15 minutes.
2. When peanut butter mixture has hardened, use a small cookie scoop or spoon to create tablespoon-sized balls. Place in refrigerator to harden, 5 minutes.
3. Meanwhile, make chocolate drizzle: combine chocolate chips and remaining coconut oil in a microwave safe bowl and microwave in 30 second intervals until fully melted. Drizzle over peanut butter balls and place back in refrigerator to harden, 5 minutes.
4. To store, keep covered in refrigerator.

Keto pizza egg wrap
Nutrition: Cal 350;Fat 10 g;Carb 2 g;Protein 25 g
Serving 1; Cook time 15 min

Ingredients
- 2 large eggs
- ½ tbsp butter
- ½ tbsp tomato sauce
- ½ oz. (2 tbsp) mozzarella cheese, shredded
- 1½ oz. salami, sliced

Instructions
1. Heat a large, non-stick frying pan to medium heat. Add the butter.
2. Crack the eggs into a bowl, and whisk until smooth in color.
3. Slowly pour the eggs into the pan, allowing the mixture to go right to the edges.
4. Cook until the edges begin to lift off the side of the frying pan. Using a spatula all around the edge, lift the egg from the pan.
5. Flip and cook on the other side for 30 seconds.
6. Remove from the pan. Layer tomato sauce, mozzarella cheese, andsalami in the middle. Roll it together into a wrap.

Green eggs
Nutrition: Cal 300;Fat 20 g;Carb 8 g;Protein 18 g
Serving 2; Cook time 20 min

Ingredients

- 1½ tbsp rapeseed oil , plus a splash extra
- 2 trimmed leeks , sliced
- 2 garlic cloves , sliced
- ½ tsp coriander seeds
- ½ tsp fennel seeds
- pinch of chilli flakes , plus extra to serve
- 200g spinach
- 2 large eggs
- 2 tbsp Greek yogurt
- squeeze of lemon

Instructions

1. Heat the oil in a large frying pan. Add the leeks and a pinch of salt, then cook until soft. Add the garlic, coriander, fennel and chilli flakes. Once the seeds begin to crackle, tip in the spinach and turn down the heat. Stir everything together until the spinach has wilted and reduced, then scrape it over to one side of the pan. Pour a little oil into the pan, then crack in the eggs and fry until cooked to your liking.
2. Stir the yogurt through the spinach mix and season. Pile onto two plates, top with the fried egg, squeeze over a little lemon and season with black pepper and chilli flakes to serve.

Masala frittata with avocado salsa
Nutrition: Cal 350;Fat 25 g;Carb 12 g;Protein 16 g
Serving 4; Cook time 40 min

Ingredients

- 2 tbsp rapeseed oil
- 3 onions, 2½ thinly sliced, ½ finely chopped
- 1 tbsp Madras curry paste
- 500g cherry tomatoes, halved
- 1 red chilli, deseeded and finely chopped
- small pack coriander, roughly chopped
- 8 large eggs, beaten
- 1 avocado, stoned, peeled and cubed
- juice 1 lemon

Instructions

1. Heat the oil in a medium non-stick, ovenproof frying pan. Tip in the sliced onions and cook over a medium heat for about 10 mins until soft and golden. Add the Madras paste and fry for 1 min more, then tip in half the tomatoes and half the chilli. Cook until the mixture is thick and the tomatoes have all burst.
2. Heat the grill to high. Add half the coriander to the eggs and season, then pour over the spicy onion mixture. Stir gently once or twice, then cook over a low heat for 8-10 mins until almost set. Transfer to the grill for 3-5 mins until set.
3. To make the salsa, mix the avocado, remaining chilli and tomatoes, chopped onion, remaining coriander and the lemon juice together, then season and serve with the frittata.

Tarragon, mushroom & sausage frittata
Nutrition: Cal 433;Fat 32g;Carb 8g;Protein 25 g
Serving 2; Cook time 20 min

Ingredients

- 1 tbsp olive oil
- 200g chestnut mushrooms , sliced
- 2 pork sausages
- 1 garlic clove , crushed
- 100g fine asparagus
- 3 large eggs
- 2 tbsp half-fat soured cream
- 1 tbsp wholegrain mustard
- 1 tbsp chopped tarragon
- mixed rocket salad , to serve (optional)

Instructions

1. Heat the grill to high. Heat the oil in a medium-sized, non-stick frying pan, add the mushrooms and fry over a high heat for 3 mins. Squeeze the sausage-meat out of their skins into nuggets, add to the pan and fry for a further 5 mins until golden brown. Add the garlic and asparagus and cook for another 1 min.
2. Whisk the eggs, soured cream, mustard and tarragon in a jug. Season well, then pour the egg mixture in to the pan. Cook for 3-4 mins, then grill for a further 1-2 mins or until the top has just set with a slight wobble in the middle. Serve with the salad leaves, if you like.

Keto Chia Pudding
Nutrition: Cal 336;Fat 27 g;Carb 16 g;Protein 8 g
Serving 2; Cook time 35 min

Ingredients

- 2 tbsp low carb sugar (Sukrin:1, Swerve, Lakanto, Truvia, or Besti)
- 1 tbsp Cocoa Powder (sift before measuring)
- 1 tsp Vanilla Extract
- 1 cup Coconut Milk (from a can) (or Almond Milk for less calories)
- 1/4 cup Chia Seeds

Instructions

1. Add the cocoa powder and sweetener to a mason jar. Close the lid and shake well to remove any lumps.
2. Add the coconut milk and vanilla extract to the mason jar. Close the lid and shake to combine.
3. Add the chia seeds to the jar and shake again. Once the mixture is well combined, transfer the jar to the fridge.
4. Chill for at least 30 minutes.
5. Serve the chocolate chia pudding in your favourite jars, with coconut yogurt and seasonal fruit. Enjoy!

Keto Breakfast Parfait
Nutrition: Cal 335;Fat 29 g;Carb 10 g;Protein 11 g
Serving 2; Cook time 10 min

Ingredients

- ½ cup Greek Yogurt full fat
- ¼ cup Heavy Cream
- 1 teaspoon Vanilla Essence
- ½ cup Keto Chocolate Almond Clusters
- 2 Strawberries diced
- 8 Blueberries

Instructions

1. In a mixing bowl, add together the yogurt, cream and vanilla. Whisk together until thick and smooth.

2. Spoon half the yogurt between two glasses, then sprinkle over half the granola.
3. Add the remaining yogurt, followed by the remaining granola.
4. Top with the berries and enjoy!

KETO SAUSAGE & EGG BOWLS
Nutrition: Cal 435;Fat 29 g;Carb 8 g;Protein 27 g
Serving 2; Cook time 10 min

Ingredients
- 1/4 cup sausage – cooked and crumbled
- 2 whole eggs
- sprinkle of cheddar cheese
- salt & pepper to taste
- 1 tbs butter

Instructions
1. Start by cracking two eggs into a bowl and scramble with a fork until all mixed together
2. Add butter to skillet over medium high heat
3. Once melted, add eggs to pan – stirring around often – careful not to over cook
4. Once the eggs are mostly set but still glossy, add the sausage and cheese.
5. Remove from heat and mix in well.
6. Add salt and pepper to taste.

Cheese and Egg Stuffed Peppers
Nutrition: Cal 285;Fat 7 g;Carb 7g;Protein 14 g
Serving 8; Cook time 50 min

Ingredients
- 4 large bell peppers, cut in half lengthwise and remove inner seeds and stems
- 1 tablespoon olive oil
- 1 cup white onion
- 1 pound gluten free pork sausage, casing removed
- 2 cups spinach
- 4 large eggs
- 1/4 teaspoon salt & pepper, each
- 3/4 cup shredded mozzarella

Instructions
1. Preheat oven to 350°F/180°C. Lightly grease a 9x13 baking dish.
2. Arrange the bell peppers side-by-side in the greased baking dish - cut side up. Set aside
3. Warm the olive oil to a large skillet over a medium heat. Add the onions and cook about 5 minutes to soften. Add the sausage and cook until no longer pink. Stir in the spinach and cook an addition 1-2 minutes until wilted. Remove from the heat.
4. In a medium sized mixing bowl whisk together the eggs, salt and pepper. Stir in 1/2 cup of the cheese.
5. Spoon the sausage mixture evenly into your prepared peppers. Pour the egg mixture over the top of the sausage. Top with the remaining 1/4 cup cheese.
6. Return to the oven and bake an additional 35-40 minutes until the cheese has goldened.

Keto Croque Madame
Nutrition: Cal 566;Fat 46.7g;Carb 3.1g;Protein 33 g
Serving 4; Cook time 30 min

Ingredients
Chaffles:
- 2 large egg
- 1 cup cheddar cheese, grated

Sandwich:
- 4 slice deli-sliced black forest ham
- 2/3 cup gruyere cheese, shredded
- 2 tablespoon butter
- 4 large egg

Bechemel Sauce:
- 1/2 cup heavy cream
- 1/4 cup parmesan cheese
- 1/3 cup gruyere cheese, shredded

Instructions
1. Measure out and prepare the ingredients. Preheat oven to 425F.
2. In a bowl, make the chaffles by whisking together the eggs and grated cheese.
3. Using a small waffle iron that is greased, make the chaffles.
4. On a parchment lined baking sheet, add the chaffles, topped with the deli sliced ham, and the shredded gruyere cheese. Bake in the oven for 10-15 minutes or until cheese is melted.
5. While the chaffles are in the oven, fry up the eggs in a frying pan with butter. Then top the baked chaffle with the fried eggs.
6. In a saucepan on medium heat, make the bechemel sauce by adding the heavy cream. Slowly add in the parmesan cheese and gruyere cheese a small handful at a time and wait until it is melted before adding in more.
7. Drizzle the bechemel sauce on top of the chaffles, serve with a small side salad and enjoy!

Keto Spinach Shakshuka
Nutrition: Cal 318;Fat 23 g;Carb 5 g;Protein 19 g
Serving 4; Cook time 25 min

Ingredients
- 3 tablespoon olive oil
- 1/2 medium onion, minced
- 2 teaspoon fresh garlic, minced
- 1 medium jalapeno pepper, seeded + minced
- 16 ounce frozen spinach, thawed
- 1 teaspoon cumin
- 3/4 teaspoon ground coriander
- 2 tablespoon harissa
- Salt and pepper to taste
- 1/2 cup vegetable broth
- 8 large eggs
- 1/4 cup fresh parsley, chopped, for garnish
- 1 teaspoon crushed red pepper flakes, for garnish

Instructions
1. Measure out and prepare all the ingredients. Preheat oven to 350F.

2. In a skillet, add the olive oil to the skillet over medium heat. Saute the minced onion in until fragrant.
3. Add the thawed spinach into the skillet and let it cook until it's wilted.
4. Add the cumin, coriander, harissa, and salt and pepper. Stir together well and let cook for another 1-2 minutes.
5. Transfer the seasoned spinach mixture to a food processor. Pulse until coarse. Then, add the vegetable broth and pulse until smooth. Wipe out your skillet.
6. Drizzle oil in the bottom of the skillet or spray some cooking spray. Pour the smooth spinach mixture into the skillet. Using a spoon, press the back of the spoon into parts of the spinach mixture.
7. Gently crack the eggs into these parts of the mixture. Cook in the oven until the egg whites are set and the yolk is a little runny. This should take about 20-25 minutes.

Keto Sausage Cream Cheese Rolls
Nutrition: Cal 203;Fat 16 g;Carb 3 g;Protein 12 g
Serving 10; Cook time 25 min

Ingredients
For the Rolls:
- 2 cups shredded mozzarealla cheese
- 2 ounces cream cheese
- 3/4 cup almond flour
- 2 tablespoons ground flax meal

For the Filling:
- 1/2 pound cooked breakfast sausage, drained
- 3 ounces of cream cheese

Instructions
Preheat oven to 400F.
For the Rolls:
1. In a microwave-safe mixing bowl, combine the shredded mozzarella cheese and cream cheese. Heat in 30 second increments, stirring in between until completely melted.
2. Add the almond flour and ground flax meal.
3. Mix the dough well until you have a soft ball
4. Between two silicone baking mats or parchment paper roll the dough into a rectangle roughly 12x9 inches.

For the filling:
1. Combine the sausage and cream cheese.
2. Spread the sausage cream cheese mixture evenly on the dough.
3. Starting at one end roll the dough as tightly as you can into a log.
4. Slice into rolls about the width of two fingers, be careful not to slice them too thick because it will be difficult for the dough in the center to cook through.
5. Place the rolls on a greased baking sheet.
6. Bake 12-15 minutes until golden brown.

Preheat oven to 400F.
Nutrition: Cal 353;Fat 23 g;Carb 4 g;Protein 18 g
Serving 12; Cook time 25 min

Ingredients
For the Keto Almond Flour Biscuits

- 3 ounces cream cheese,softened
- 1 cup shredded cheddar cheese
- 2 eggs
- 2 cups almond flour
- 1 teaspoon baking powder
- 1/4 teaspoon salt
- 1/4 cup heavy cream (scrape the measuring cup out since it is thick, make sure you get ALL of the liquid)
- 1 tablespoon melted butter

Sausage Patties
- 1 1/2 pounds breakfast sausage, formed into 12 patties

Instructions
1. Preheat the oven to 350 degrees.
2. In a mixing bowl combine the softened cream cheese, cheddar cheese and eggs. Stir until cream cheese is smooth with no clumps.
3. Add almond flour, baking powder, salt, heavy cream and melted butter.
4. Stir until combined. Do not overmix or biscuits will be tough.
5. Chill the dough 10-15 minutes.
6. Lightly sprinkle almond flour onto a cutting board and turn the dough onto the floured surface. Pat the biscuits to about 1/2 inch thick and use a biscuit cutter or the top of a mason jar to cut out your biscuits.
7. Place the biscuits onto a greased or silicone lined baking sheet.
8. Bake 15-18 minutes until golden.
9. Cook the sausage patties in a skillet over medium heat until cooked through.
10. To assemble slice the warm biscuits in half and add the sausage patty.

Keto Biscuits and Gravy
Nutrition: Cal 203;Fat 16g;Carb 3g;Protein 12 g
Serving 6; Cook time 40 min

Ingredients
Keto Biscuits
- ¼ cup unsalted butter melted
- 4 large eggs
- ⅓ cup coconut flour
- 1 cup cheddar cheese shredded
- 1 tbsp cream cheese
- ¼ tsp salt
- ¼ tsp baking powder

Keto Sausage Gravy
- 1 lb ground sausage
- ½ cup chicken broth
- 1 cup heavy cream
- salt & pepper to taste
- 4 tbsp cream cheese
- ½ tsp chili flakes optional
- ¼ tsp xanthan gum optional

Instructions
To make the keto biscuits
1. Preheat the oven to 350°F / 180°C and line a baking sheet with parchment paper.

2. In a large bowl add the eggs, one tablespoon cream cheese, and salt. Whisk for 30 seconds.
3. Pour the melted butter over the egg mixture and continue whisking.
4. Add the shredded cheddar cheese, coconut flour, and baking powder and combine well. Let the biscuits dough sit for about 5 minutes so the coconut flour can absorb the liquid and make the dough thick.
5. Divide the dough into 9 equal biscuits. Place them 2 inches apart on the baking sheet.
6. Bake in the preheated oven for about 15 minutes or until they get a beautiful golden color.

To make the sausage gravy

1. In a large skillet add the ground sausage. Brown and crumble the meat into smaller pieces over medium heat until fully cooked.
2. Add the chicken broth, cream cheese and whipping cream. Stir to combine well and let it simmer until it becomes thicker. Season with salt and pepper to taste (if necessary).
3. Serve one or two keto biscuits with 1/2 cup of gravy. Enjoy!

Keto Protein Breakfast Scramble
Nutrition: Cal 511;Fat 41g;Carb 6g;Protein 28 g
Serving 4; Cook time 20 min

Ingredients
- 6 links breakfast sausage sliced
- 6 slices bacon chopped
- 4 oz hard salami (such as Genoa) cubed
- 1 small onion sliced
- 1 medium bell pepper sliced
- 6 large eggs
- ¼ cup sour cream
- ½ cup cheddar cheese grated
- 2 stalks green onion (scallion) sliced
- salt and pepper

Instructions
1. Place a frying pan over medium-high heat. Once hot add raw sliced bacon and sausage. Fry until cooked through, and just starting to brown and crisp. (5 - 8 minutes)
2. 6 slices bacon
3. Add chopped salami and continue to fry until the salami, bacon, and sausage have reached a level of crispness you are satisfied with. If the pan contains a lot of rendered fat, drain off a portion now to avoid greasy eggs (2 - 3 minutes)
4. 6 links breakfast sausage,4 oz hard salami (such as Genoa)
5. Next add the sliced onions and pepper to fry until softened. (1 minute)
6. 1 small onion,1 medium bell pepper
7. Stir in egg mixture, and using a spatula begin to combine and scramble everything in the pan. Cook eggs to desired doneness. (3-5 minutes)
8. Stir in grated cheese, top with sliced green onion, and season to taste with salt and pepper.
9. 2 stalks green onion (scallion),salt and pepper

Egg Wraps with Ham and Greens
Nutrition: Cal 371;Fat 26 g;Carb 5 g;Protein 28 g
Serving 6; Cook time 20 min

Ingredients
- 8 large eggs
- 4 teaspoons water
- 2 teaspoons all-purpose flour or cornstarch
- 1/2 teaspoon fine salt
- 4 teaspoons vegetable or coconut oil
- 1 1/3 cups shredded Swiss cheese
- 4 ounces very thinly sliced ham
- 1 1/3 cups loosely packed watercress

Instructions
1. Place the eggs, water, flour or cornstarch, and salt in a medium bowl and whisk until broken up and the flour or cornstarch is completely dissolved.
2. Heat 1 teaspoon of the oil in a 12-inch nonstick frying pan over medium heat until shimmering. Swirl the pan to coat the bottom with the oil. Add 1/2 cup of the egg mixture and swirl to coat the bottom of the pan in a thin layer. Cook until the wrap is completely set on the edges and on the bottom (the top can be a little wet, but should be mostly set), 3 to 6 minutes.
3. Using a flat spatula, loosen the edges of the wrap and slide it underneath the wrap, making sure it can slide easily around the pan. Flip the wrap with the spatula. Immediately sprinkle 1/3 cup of the cheese over the wrap and cook until the second side is set, about 1 minute. Slide it onto a work surface or cutting board (the cheese might not be fully melted yet). While still warm, place a single layer of ham over the egg. Place 1/3 cup of the watercress across the center of the wrap. Roll it up tightly.
4. Repeat with cooking and filling the remaining wraps. Using a serrated knife, cut each wrap crosswise into 6 (1-inch) pieces.

Bacon Gruyère Egg Bites
Nutrition: Cal 208;Fat 17,5 g;Carb 1 g;Protein 11 g
Serving 9; Cook time 60 min

Ingredients
- Bacon fat or butter, for coating the pan
- 9 large eggs
- 3/4 cup grated Gruyère cheese (2 1/4 ounces)
- 1/3 cup cream cheese (about 2 1/2 ounces)
- 1/2 teaspoon kosher salt
- 6 slices thick-cut bacon, cooked and crumbled

Instructions
1. Arrange a rack in the middle of the oven and heat to 350°F. Coat an 8x8-inch (broiler-safe if you want a browned top) baking dish generously with bacon fat or butter.
2. Place the eggs, Gruyère, cream cheese, and salt in a blender and blend on medium-high speed until very smooth, about 1 minute. Pour into the baking dish. Sprinkle with the bacon. Cover tightly with aluminum foil.
3. Pull the oven rack halfway out of the oven. Place a roasting pan on the oven rack. Pour in 6 cups of very hot

tap water. Set the baking dish of eggs into the roasting pan. Bake until just set in the middle, 55 minutes to 1 hour.

4. Carefully remove the roasting pan from the oven. Remove the baking dish from the roasting pan and uncover. (For a browned top: Heat the oven to broil. Broil until the top is golde- brown, 4 to 5 minutes.) Cut into 9 squares and serve.

Radish and Turnip Hash with Fried Eggs
Nutrition: Cal 391;Fat 33,9 g;Carb 10 g;Protein 12 g
Serving 2; Cook time 20 min

Ingredients
- 2 to 3 small turnips, trimmed, peeled, and cut into 3/4-inch cubes (about 1 1/2 cups cubed)
- 4 to 5 small radishes, scrubbed and trimmed, and cut into 3/4-inch cubes (about 1 1/2 cups cubed)
- Coarse sea salt
- Freshly ground pepper
- 2 tablespoons grapeseed oil, or other neutral, heat-tolerant oil
- 1 stalk green garlic, trimmed and chopped (white and light green parts only)
- 2 tablespoons unsalted butter
- 4 eggs
- 1 tablespoon minced parsley

Instructions
1. Fill a large saucepan with water and bring to a boil. Add 2 teaspoons sea salt. Boil turnip cubes just until tender, 3 to 4 minutes; remove to a bowl with a slotted spoon, pour off any excess water, and set aside. Next, boil radishes briefly, 30 to 60 seconds; remove to a bowl with a slotted spoon, pour off any excess water, and set aside.
2. Set a large cast iron skillet over medium-high heat. Add grapeseed oil and when hot, add turnips and radishes, and a pinch each sea salt and pepper. Turning vegetables only once or twice, cook 8 minutes or until golden-brown. Turn heat to medium and fold in green garlic, cooking for about a minute. Push vegetables to the sides, melt butter in the center of pan, and add the eggs, salting each individually. For over-easy eggs, cook uncovered 4 to 6 minutes; for over-medium eggs, cover pan for 3 minutes, then uncover and continue cooking just until whites are set, 2 to 3 minutes longer. Finish with minced parsley and sea salt and pepper to taste. Serve immediately.

Keto Loaf Bread
Nutrition: Cal 239;Fat 22 g;Carb 4 g;Protein 8 g
Serving 1; Cook time 60 min

Ingredients
- 2 cups finely ground almond flour, such as Bob's Red Mill or King Arthur brands
- 1 teaspoon baking powder
- 1/2 teaspoon xanthan gum
- 1/2 teaspoon kosher salt
- 7 large eggs, at room temperature
- 8 tablespoons (1 stick) unsalted butter, melted and cooled
- 2 tablespoons refined coconut oil, melted and cooled

Instructions
1. Arrange a rack in the middle of the oven and heat to 350°F. Line the bottom and sides of a 9x5-inch metal loaf pan with parchment paper, letting the excess hang over the long sides to form a sling. Set aside.
2. Whisk together the almond flour, baking powder, xanthan gum, and salt in a medium bowl. Set aside.
3. Place the eggs in the bowl of a stand mixer fitted with the whisk attachment. Beat on medium-high speed until light and frothy. Reduce the speed to medium, slowly add the melted butter and coconut oil, and beat until until fully combined. Reduce the speed to low, slowly add the almond flour mixture, and beat until combined. Increase the speed to medium high and beat until mixture thickens, about 1 minute.
4. Pour into the prepared pan and smooth the top. Bake until a knife inserted in the center comes out clean, 45 to 55 minutes. Let cool in the pan for about 10 minutes. Grasping the parchment paper, remove the loaf from the pan and transfer to a wire rack. Cool completely before slicing.

Kale and Goat Cheese Frittata Cups
Nutrition: Cal 179;Fat 14,7 g;Carb 1 g;Protein 10 g
Serving 8; Cook time 40 min

Ingredients
- 2 cups chopped lacinato kale
- 1 garlic clove, thinly sliced
- 3 tablespoons olive oil
- 1/4 teaspoon red pepper flakes
- 8 large eggs
- 1/4 teaspoon salt
- Dash ground black pepper
- 1/2 teaspoon dried thyme
- 1/4 cup goat cheese, crumbled

Instructions
1. Preheat the oven to 350°F. To get 2 cups kale, remove the leaves from the kale ribs. Wash and dry the leaves and cut them into 1/2-inch-wide strips.
2. In a 10-inch nonstick skillet, cook the garlic in 1 tablespoon of oil over medium-high heat for 30 seconds. Add the kale and red pepper flakes and cook until wilted, 1 to 2 minutes.
3. In a medium bowl, beat the eggs with the salt and pepper. Add the kale and thyme to the egg mixture.
4. Using a 12-cup muffin tin, use the remaining 2 tablespoons of oil to grease 8 of the cups (you may also use butter or nonstick spray if you'd prefer). Sprinkle the tops with goat cheese. Bake until they are set in the center, about 25 to 30 minutes.
5. Frittata is best eaten warm from the oven or within the next day, but leftovers can be kept refrigerated and reheated for up to a week.

Roasted Radish and Herbed Ricotta Omelet

Nutrition: Cal 350;Fat 27 g;Carb 5,3 g;Protein 20 g
Serving 2; Cook time 15 min

Ingredients
For the roasted radishes:
- 1 cup thinly-sliced French Breakfast radishes, or other radish variety
- 2 teaspoons olive oil
- 1/4 teaspoon sea salt

For the ricotta:
- 1/4 cup plus 2 tablespoons fresh whole milk ricotta
- 2 teaspoons minced fresh chives
- 1 teaspoon minced fresh thyme
- 1 teaspoon minced fresh flat leaf parsley, plus extra for topping

For the eggs:
- 4 large or extra-large eggs
- 2 tablespoons whole milk
- 1/2 teaspoon sea salt
- 1/4 teaspoon black pepper
- 1 tablespoon butter

Instructions
1. To make the radishes, preheat the oven to 400°F. Toss the radishes with the olive oil and salt. Spread in a thin layer in a roasting dish and bake until soft and tender, 10 to 12 minutes (any longer and you may end up with radish chips).
2. In a small bowl, combine the ricotta with the minced herbs.
3. To make the omelet, whisk together the eggs, milk, salt, and pepper. Heat 1/2 tablespoon of butter in an 8-inch non-stick skillet over medium-low heat. Pour in half the egg mixture and cook for 1 to 2 minutes, allowing the bottom to set slightly. Run a spatula under the edges, lifting up and tilting the pan to allow uncooked eggs to run under the cooked part. Continue to do this until the majority of the egg is set. Carefully flip the omelet and remove from heat.
4. Spread half the ricotta mixture over half of the omelet and sprinkle with half of the radishes. Fold the omelet over over the filling and sprinkle with a few more roasted radish slices and minced parsley.
5. Repeat to make the second omelet. Serve both omelets immediately.

Mixed Mushroom Egg Bakes

Nutrition: Cal 287;Fat 21 g;Carb 8,3 g;Protein 16 g
Serving 4; Cook time 35 min

Ingredients
- Butter or cooking spray
- 2 tablespoons extra-virgin olive oil
- 1/3 cup minced shallot (from about 2 small shallots)
- 8 ounces sliced mixed fresh mushrooms (cremini, oyster or shiitake, stems removed before slicing)
- 2 tablespoons chopped fresh thyme
- 6 large eggs
- 3/4 cup whole milk
- 1/2 teaspoon kosher salt
- 1/2 teaspoon ground black pepper
- 1/2 cup shredded mozzarella cheese

Instructions
1. Arrange a rack in the middle of the oven and heat to 400°F. Coat 4 (8-ounce) ramekins with a little butter, or use cooking spray instead. Place the ramekins on a rimmed baking sheet so they'll be easier to move to and from the oven; set aside.
2. Heat the olive oil in a medium saucepan over medium-high heat until shimmering. Add the shallot and sauté until soft and translucent, about 3 minutes. Add the mushrooms and a pinch of salt and cook until softened and fragrant, about 5 minutes. Stir in the thyme and remove from the heat.
3. Whisk the eggs, milk, salt, and pepper together in a medium bowl. Divide the mushroom mixture evenly between the ramekins. Divide the cheese over the mushrooms. Pour the egg mixture over the top, stopping just below the top of the ramekin.
4. Place the baking sheet in the oven and bake until the tops are golden and have puffed slightly and the eggs are completely set, 20 to 25 minutes.

3-Ingredient Pesto Zoodle Bowl

Nutrition: Cal 400;Fat 38 g;Carb 8,3 g;Protein 10 g
Serving 1; Cook time 10 min

Ingredients
- 2 tablespoons olive oil, divided
- 1 medium zucchini (about 6 ounces), ends trimmed and spiralized, or 1 heaping cup of store-bought zucchini noodles
- 1 tablespoon basil pesto
- 1 large egg
- Kosher salt
- Freshly ground black pepper
- Red pepper flakes or hot sauce, for serving (optional)

Instructions
1. Heat 1 tablespoon of the oil in a medium nonstick skillet over medium heat until shimmering. Add the zucchini noodles and sauté until just tender, about 2 minutes. Add the pesto and toss until the noodles are well-coated. Transfer the noodles to a plate or shallow bowl.
2. Heat the remaining 1 tablespoon oil in the skillet until shimmering. Add the egg, season with salt and pepper, and cook undisturbed until the outer white edges are opaque, about 1 minute. Cover and cook until the yolk is set but still runny, 2 to 3 minutes.
3. Gently slide a spatula under the egg and place it on top of the zoodles. Sprinkle with a pinch of red pepper flakes or finish with a little hot sauce, if using.

Chocolate Protein Pancakes

Nutrition: Cal 380;Fat 31 g;Carb 5.4 g;Protein 19 g
Serving 2; Cook time 20 min

Ingredients
Dry ingredients
- 1scoop vanilla protein powder
- 1 tablespoon cocoa powder

- 2 teaspoon baking powder
- 1 tablespoon coconut flour
- 1 tablespoon granulated sweetener
- 1 pinch salt

Wet ingredients
- 2 eggs
- 4 tablespoon unsalted butter (softened)
- 1 tablespoon cream cheese
- 1/4 teaspoon vanilla extract

Instructions
1. Whisk together all of the dry ingredients in a mixing bowl until no lumps remain.
2. Make a well in the middle of the dry ingredients and add the eggs, butter, cream cheese, and vanilla extract into the middle.
3. Fold the batter together gently and set aside for 5 minutes.
4. Heat a non-stick frying pan over medium to high heat.
5. Add 1/4 cup of the batter to the pan at a time. Cook until bubbles form on the top surface, then flip over to cook on the other side, cooking for about 3 – 4 minutes per side.

Keto Breakfast Sandwich
Nutrition: Cal 603;Fat 54 g;Carb 4 g;Protein 22 g
Serving 2; Cook time 35 min

Ingredients
- 4 sausage patties
- 2 egg
- 2 tbsp cream cheese
- 4 tbsp sharp cheddar
- 1/2 medium avocado, sliced
- 1/2–1 tsp sriracha (to taste)
- Salt, pepper to taste

Instructions
1. In skillet over medium heat, cook sausages per package instructions and set aside
2. In small bowl place cream cheese and sharp cheddar. Microwave for 20-30 seconds until melted
3. Mix cheese with sriracha, set aside
4. Mix egg with seasoning and make small omelette
5. Fill omelette with cheese sriracha mixture and assemble sandwich

Poached Eggs Mytilene
Nutrition: Cal 275;Fat 23.6 g;Carb 6 g;Protein 13 g
Serving 1; Cook time 20 min

Ingredients
- 4 sausage patties
- 2 egg
- 2 tbsp cream cheese
- 4 tbsp sharp cheddar
- 1/2 medium avocado, sliced
- 1/2–1 tsp sriracha (to taste)
- Salt, pepper to taste

Instructions
1. In skillet over medium heat, cook sausages per package instructions and set aside

2. Combine lemon juice and oil in a small serving bowl; whisk to combine.
3. Add water and vinegar to a medium saute pan or small saucepan and bring to a slow boil. Reduce the heat to medium-low. Crack 1 egg into a small bowl, being careful not to break the yolk. Gently slip egg into the simmering water, holding the bowl just above the surface of water. Repeat with the remaining egg. Cook eggs until the whites are firm and the yolks are lightly cooked outside, but liquid inside, 2 to 3 minutes. Remove the eggs from the water with a slotted spoon, and place into a serving bowl.
4. Break the yolks with a fork and drizzle with lemon juice mixture. Stir yolks twice; season with salt and pepper.

Healthy Breakfast Cheesecake
Nutrition: Cal 152;Fat 12.6 g;Carb 3 g;Protein 6 g
Serving 1; Cook time 1 hour 5 min

Ingredients
- Crust Ingredients:
- 2 cups whole almonds
- 2 tablespoon Joy Filled Eats Sweetener (or see alternatives in recipe notes)
- 4 tablespoon salted butter

Filling Ingredients:
- 16 oz 4% fat cottage cheese
- 8 oz cream cheese
- 6 eggs
- ¾ cup Joy Filled Eats Sweetener (or see alternatives in recipe notes)
- ½ teaspoon almond extract
- ½ teaspoon vanilla extract

Topping when serving:
- ¼ cup frozen mixed berries per cheesecake thawed

Instructions
1. Preheat the oven to 350. In a large food processor pulse the almonds, 2 tablespoon sweetener, and 4 tablespoon butter until a coarse dough forms. Grease two twelve hole standard silicone muffin pans or line metal tins with paper or foil cupcake liners. I used a silicone muffin pan for this and the cheesecakes popped out really easily. Divide the dough between the 24 holes and press into the bottom to form a crust. Bake for 8 minutes.
2. Meanwhile, combine the Friendship Dairies 4% cottage cheese and the cream cheese in the food processor (you don't need to wash the bowl). Pulse the cheeses until smooth. Add the sweetener and extracts. Mix until combined.
3. Add the eggs. Blend until smooth. You will need to scrape down the sides. Divide the batter between the muffin cups.
4. Bake for 30-40 minutes until the centers no longer jiggly when the pan is lightly shaken. Cool completely. Refrigerate for at least 2 hours before trying to remove them if you didn't use paper or foil liners. Serve with thawed frozen berries.

Blueberry Pancakes

Nutrition: Cal 202;Fat 16 g;Carb 9 g;Protein 10 g
Serving 3; Cook time 10 min

Ingredients

- 2 eggs
- 2/3 cup almond flour
- 1 tsp baking powder
- 1/2 tsp vanilla
- 1 tsp Swerve sweetener
- 3 tbsp milk or almond milk
- 1/4 cup blueberries
- Keto pancake syrup for serving, optional

Instructions

1. Whisk the eggs in a bowl, then add vanilla, Swerve and milk and mix until combined. Add almond flour and baking powder and mix until combined. Stir in the blueberries.
2. Spray a non-stick frying pan or pancake griddle with a non-stick cooking spray and heat over medium-high heat. Laddle the pancake batter on a frying pan, making 6 small pancakes.
3. Cook for 3-4 minutes (or until the bottom is golden-brown and bubbles begin to form on top of the pancakes), then flip the pancakes over with a spatula and cook for another 2 minutes, or until the other side is golden-brown.

Low Carb Pumpkin Cheesecake Pancakes

Nutrition: Cal 202;Fat 16 g;Carb 9 g;Protein 10 g
Serving 16; Cook time 10 min

Ingredients

- 4 ounces Cream Cheese
- 4 large Eggs
- 2 Tablespoons Pure Pumpkin Puree
- 1 teaspoon Pure Vanilla Extract
- 1 teaspoon Pyure Sugar Substitute (or your choice)
- 1/2 teaspoon Baking Powder
- 1/4 teaspoon Pumpkin Pie Spice
- 1/8 teaspoon Ground Cinnamon
- 2 teaspoons Butter

Instructions

1. Add all ingredients except butter to blender and process until smooth. Let sit while the skillet is heating.
2. Heat a cast iron skillet or griddle with a medium flame until hot and then add 1 teaspoon of butter.
3. Slowly pour pancake mix into skillet to make 3 inch pancakes. When bubbles begin to form, flip pancakes. Continue until all batter has been used. Use the second teaspoon of butter, half way through, to grease pan.
4. Serve with butter and maple syrup.

Mediterranean Keto Quiche

Nutrition: Cal 133;Fat 8 g;Carb 9 g;Protein 7 g
Serving 8; Cook time 50 min

Ingredients

- 1 tsp olive oil or butter
- 1/2 cup red onion, chopped
- 2 tsp (1 large clove) garlic, minced
- 2/3 to 3/4 cup unsweetened almond or coconut milk
- 4 eggs
- 2 tbsp grated Parmesan cheese + extra for topping
- 3 tbsp coconut flour, sifted
- 3 tbsp tapioca starch or non-GMO cornstarch
- 1 tsp baking powder
- 1/4 tsp kosher salt or fine sea salt
- 1 tsp smoked paprika
- 1 cup chopped/sliced zucchini, divided
- 1/2 to 2/3 cup crumbled feta cheese, divided
- 1 red bell pepper, roasted and diced (fresh and roasted in oven or roasted red bell peppers from a jar both work)
- Fresh basil for garnish.
- Optional black pepper, to season.

Instructions

1. Grease or line a 9-inch pie or cake pan with parchment paper.
2. Coat small skillet with 1 tsp butter or oil. Add onion and garlic to the pan and cook over medium to medium high for 5 minutes (or until fragrant). Set aside.
3. To a large mixing bowl or bowl of stand mixer, add milk, eggs, and Parmesan cheese. Whisk/blend until smooth.
4. In a separate bowl, sift the coconut flour, then add tapioca flour, spices, salt, baking powder. Mix together.
5. Mix the dry ingredients with the blended egg/milk batter. Whisk together until smooth.
6. Layer your onion and garlic at the bottom of the pie pan.
7. Layer 2/3 cup zucchini on top, roasted pepper slices, and 1/3 cup feta crumbles.
8. Evenly pour the egg/flour mixture into your prepared pie or cake pan. Add remaining zucchini slices and cheese on top (Parmesan and/or feta)
9. Bake at 400F for 35 -45 minutes. Check at 25 minutes for doneness. The edges will be crispy brown and a knife or toothpick inserted into the center of the quiche will come out clean. Check the middle to make sure it's no longer soft.
10. When the crustless quiche is finished cooking, remove it from the oven and garnish with fresh basil before serving.

Keto Sausage Balls

Nutrition: Cal 363;Fat 8 g;Carb 9 g;Protein 7 g
Serving 6; Cook time 30 min

Ingredients

FATHEAD DOUGH

- cups mozzarella cheese
- 1 oz cream cheese
- 3/4 cup almond flour
- 1 large egg
- 12 oz ground breakfast sausage

Instructions

1. Preheat your oven to 400 degrees F and line a baking sheet with parchment paper.
2. Preheat a medium skillet to medium high heat.

3. Divide the sausage into 6 and roll into balls. Add to the hot skillet and cook through. Set aside on a plate to cool.

FATHEAD DOUGH

1. Add the mozzarella cheese and cream cheese to a microwave safe mixing bowl and microwave on high for 30 seconds. Combine using a fork until evenly mixed.
2. Add the almond flour and egg and combine as thoroughly as possible. If it does not combine well microwave for another 20 seconds.
3. Switch to a spatula if necessary and combine. Pour the dough onto a piece of parchment paper. If it is not evenly combined use your hands to incorporate everything.
4. Portion the dough out into 6 even balls.
5. Flatten out each ball using your hands or roll it out with another piece of parchment on top (so there is no sticking) and place the cooked sausage in the center. Pull up the side and place the sausage ball, seam side down, on a lined baking sheet.
6. Repeat until all 6 sausage balls are complete and on the baking sheet.
7. Bake for 10-15 minutes, until browned on top.
8. Best stored in a air tight sealed container in the fridge up to 5 days.

Turkish-Style Breakfast Recipe
Nutrition: Cal 359;Fat 27 g;Carb 7 g;Protein 17 g
Serving 4; Cook time 25 min

Ingredients
• 4 eggs
• 250g halloumi, sliced thickly into 8 pieces
• 250g yogurt
• 400g tomatoes, roughly chopped
• 400g cucumber, sliced
For The Zhoug:
• 1 bunch parsley
• ½ bunch coriander
• 2 green chillies
• 2 cloves garlic
• 200ml olive oil
• Pinch of sugar
• ½ tsp ground cumin
• ¼ tsp cardamom
Instructions
1. To make the zhoug blitz all the ingredients in a food processor until finely chopped, adding water to get the consistency of a loose pesto. Season to taste.
2. Bring a pan of water to a rolling boil. Add the eggs and cook for 6 mins for soft boiled. Immediately plunge in cool water and peel.
3. Bring a griddle pan to a high heat. Add the halloumi and fry on each side for 2 mins, until golden and slightly charred.
4. Swirl the zhoug into the yogurt and spoon onto plates. Top with the tomatoes, cucumber and halloumi.

Poached Egg and Bacon Salad
Nutrition: Cal 311;Fat 22 g;Carb 12 g;Protein 15 g
Serving 2; Cook time 20 min

Ingredients
• 100g (3½oz) unsmoked bacon lardons
• 1 slice bread, cut into small cubes
• 2 medium or large eggs
• 2 good handfuls of mixed salad leaves (we used rocket and chard)
• 10 baby plum tomatoes, halved
• 1 stick celery, chopped
• For The Dressing:
• 1tbsp olive oil
• 1tsp white wine vinegar
• ½tsp Dijon mustard
• Salt and ground black pepper
Instructions
1. Heat a frying pan, add the bacon and fry until golden and crispy. Take out of the pan with a draining spoon and set aside. Add the bread cubes to the pan, and fry in the bacon fat until browned and crispy.
2. Meanwhile poach the eggs, pour boiling water, 10cm (4in) in depth, into a small pan, over a high heat. Add a dash of white wine vinegar. When water boils again, break egg into pan.
3. As water comes back to the boil, gather egg white round yolk, using a draining spoon. Turn down heat. Simmer for a minute for a soft egg, longer for a firmer one.
4. Lift the egg out of the pan with the draining spoonand put into a bowl of warm water if cooking more than one or two eggs. Add another egg to the pan.How to poach an egg video
5. Mix together the dressing ingredients. Put a good handful of salad leaves on to 2 plates. Divide the bacon, croutons, tomatoes and celery between them. Spoon drained eggs on top, drizzle the salad with dressing and sprinkle with salt and pepper.

Chicken liver salad
Nutrition: Cal 450;Fat 33 g;Carb 9 g;Protein 28 g
Serving 4; Cook time 25 min

Ingredients
• 400g (14oz) fresh chicken livers
• Salt and ground black pepper
• 2 thick slices white bread
• 3 tbsp clarified butter
• 4-6 rashers streaky bacon, chopped
• 4 good handfuls of salad leaves
For The Dressing
• 1 tbsp cider vinegar
• 1 tsp Dijon mustard
• Pinch of sugar
• 2 tbsp light olive oil
• 1 tbsp walnut oil
Instructions
1. Remove sinews from the livers and, if large, cut livers into bite-sized pieces. Season well.

2. Cut the crusts off the bread and cut the bread into 1cm (½in) cubes.
3. Heat 2 tablespoons of butter in a frying pan over a medium heat. Add the bread, stir well to coat in butter and fry for a few mins until crisp and golden. Drain them on kitchen paper and keep them warm in the oven.
4. Add the chopped bacon to the hot pan and fry until crispy. Put on the baking tray with the fried bread. Heat the rest of the butter in the pan with any fat from the bacon, add the chicken livers in one layer and fry for a couple of mins each side. Take the frying pan off the heat.
5. Mix the dressing ingredients in a small bowl or jug and season. Put a handful of leaves on each plate, then divide the chicken livers, bacon and croutons between the plates. Drizzle with the dressing and serve warm.

Spinach pancakes
Nutrition: Cal 186;Fat 15 g;Carb 5 g;Protein 7 g
Serving 4; Cook time 15 min

Ingredients
For The Batter:
- 30g or ⅓ cup gram (chickpea) flour
- 85ml/⅓ cup water
- A pinch of sea salt
- 1 garlic clove
- 2 handfuls of spinach
- 2 tbsp olive oil
- 1 tbsp no-taste coconut oil or unrefined rapeseed oil

For The Filling:
- 50g Parmesan cheese, grated
- ½ avocado, sliced lengthways
- 1 tbsp chopped chives
- Chopped chillies (if liked)

Instructions
1. Add all of the batter ingredients to a blender and mix until smooth. Heat the coconut oil or rapeseed oil in a frying pan.
2. Pour a thin layer of the mixture into the pan. Top with most of the avocado slices, chives and most of the grated cheese – leaving some to decorate with later.
3. Cook a few minutes, loosen edges with a spatula then flip over.
4. Top with the remaining cheese, chives and avocados – plus a few slices of red chilli, if preferred

Halloumi salad with roasted plums
Nutrition: Cal 382;Fat 32 g;Carb 11 g;Protein 28 g
Serving 4; Cook time 30 min

Ingredients
- 4 whole plums, quartered and de-stoned
- 1tbsp olive oil
- 2tsp butter
- 1 pack halloumi cheese, sliced into 8 pieces

For The Dressing
- 4tbsp olive oil
- Zest and juice of 1 lime, plus 1 lime cut into wedges to serve
- 1tsp sugar
- 1tsp Dijon mustard
- Small bunch of each mint and coriander, finely chopped

Instructions
1. Preheat the oven to 220C. Place the plums on a baking tray, drizzle with olive oil and season well with salt and pepper. Roast in the oven for 15-18 mins until they are slightly charred and just beginning to soften.
2. Mix the dressing ingredients together in a small bowl and season well. Heat the butter in a frying pan and pan-fry the halloumi slices for a few mins on each side until golden brown and starting to melt slightly.
3. Plate up the halloumi slices with the roasted plums, and drizzle over the dressing. Serve with lime wedges on the side.

Griddled halloumi and watermelon salad
Nutrition: Cal 386;Fat 30 g;Carb 16 g;Protein 16 g
Serving 4; Cook time 20 min

Ingredients
- ½ x 1.5kg watermelon
- 4tbsp extra virgin olive oil
- 1tbsp balsamic vinegar
- 250g halloumi
- 150g Mixed baby leaf salad leaves
- 1tbsp fresh basil, finely sliced
- Edible flowers, optional

Instructions
1. Remove the rind and pips from the watermelon, and cut into 2.5cm cubes. Mix 3tbsp of olive oil and the balsamic vinegar together and season with salt and pepper.
2. Cut the halloumi lengthways into eight slices and toss in the remaining 1tbsp olive oil. Place a griddle pan over a medium heat and cook each slice for 30-60 seconds on each side, or until there are golden brown griddle marks on each side.
3. To serve divide the salad leave between four plates, scatter with watermelon cubes and top each salad with 2 slices of halloumi. Drizzle over the dressing, add a few slices of basil leaves and some edible flowers.

<u>POULTRY</u>

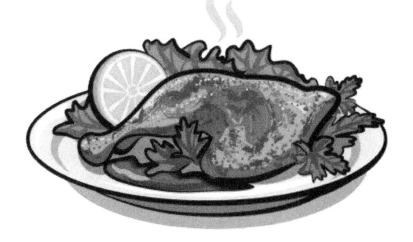

CHICKEN EGG SALAD WRAPS

Nutrition: Cal 545;Fat 38g;Carb 23g;Protein33 g
Serving 3; Cook time 10 min

Ingredients
- 2 romaine lettuce heads, chopped
- 2 cups chopped Baked Boneless Chicken Thighs
- 1 cup grape tomatoes
- 2 cucumbers, diced
- ½ cup chopped red onion
- 4 slices Perfectly Cooked Bacon , chopped
- ½ cup crumbled blue cheese
- 4 Hard-boiled Eggs , sliced
- ½ cup Dairy-Free Ranch Dressing

Instructions
1. Evenly divide the lettuce between 4 storage containers.
2. Evenly distribute and arrange the chicken, tomatoes, cucumbers, onion, bacon, blue cheese, and eggs over the lettuce.
3. Divide the dressing into 2-tablespoon servings and store on the side.

COBB SALAD

Nutrition: Cal 545;Fat 38g;Carb 23g;Protein33 g
Serving 4; Cook time 20 min

Ingredients
- 1½ cups chopped Baked Boneless Chicken Thighs
- 6 Hard-boiled Eggs , chopped
- 3 celery stalks, minced
- 2 tablespoons minced red onion
- 1 tablespoon Dijon mustard
- 2 cups Mayonnaise
- Salt
- Freshly ground black pepper
- 8 leaves butter or romaine lettuce

Instructions
1. In a large bowl, combine the chicken, eggs, celery, onion, and mustard. Add the Mayonnaise and stir until mixed. Season with salt and pepper.
2. Divide the egg salad and lettuce between 3 storage containers. To serve, make egg salad wraps by filling the lettuce leaves with the salad and wrapping the lettuce around it.

Baked Chicken Nuggets

Nutrition: Cal 400;Fat 26g;Carb 2g;Protein 43g
Serving 4; Cook time 30 min

Ingredients:
- ¼ cup almond flour
- 1 teaspoon chili powder
- ½ teaspoon paprika
- 2 pounds boneless chicken thighs, cut into 2-inch chunks
- Salt and pepper
- 2 large eggs, whisked well

Instructions:
1. Preheat the oven to 400°F and line a baking sheet with parchment.
2. Stir together the almond flour, chili powder, and paprika in a shallow dish.
3. Season the chicken with salt and pepper, then dip in the beaten eggs.
4. Dredge the chicken pieces in the almond flour mixture, then arrange on the baking sheet.
5. Bake for 20 minutes until browned and crisp. Serve hot.

Coconut Chicken Tenders

Nutrition: Cal 325;Fat 9.5.5g;Carb 2g;Protein 45g
Serving 4; Cook time 40 min

Ingredients:
- ¼ cup almond flour
- 2 tablespoons shredded unsweetened coconut
- ½ teaspoon garlic powder
- 2 pounds boneless chicken tenders
- Salt and pepper
- 2 large eggs, whisked well

Instructions:
1. Preheat the oven to 400°F and line a baking sheet with parchment.
2. Stir together the almond flour, coconut, and garlic powder in a shallow dish.
3. Season the chicken with salt and pepper, then dip into the beaten eggs.
4. Dredge the chicken tenders in the almond flour mixture, then arrange on the baking sheet.
5. Bake for 25 to 30 minutes until browned and cooked through. Serve hot.

Cheesy Buffalo Chicken Sandwich

Nutrition: Cal 555;Fat 33.5.5g;Carb 3.5g;Protein 55g
Serving 1; Cook time 30 min

Ingredients:
- 1 large egg, separated into white and yolk
- Pinch cream of tartar
- Pinch salt
- 1 ounce cream cheese, softened
- 1 cup cooked chicken breast, shredded
- 2 tablespoons hot sauce
- 1 slice Swiss cheese

Instructions:
1. For the bread, preheat the oven to 300°F and line a baking sheet with
2. parchment.
3. Beat the egg whites with the cream of tartar and salt until soft peaks form.
4. Whisk the cream cheese and egg yolk until smooth and pale yellow.
5. Fold in the egg whites a little at a time until smooth and well combined.
6. Spoon the batter onto the baking sheet into two even circles.
7. Bake for 25 minutes until firm and lightly browned.
8. Shred the chicken into a bowl and toss with the hot sauce.
9. Spoon the chicken onto one of the bread circles and top with cheese.
10. Top with the other bread circle and enjoy.

Sesame Chicken Avocado Salad

Nutrition: Cal 540;Fat 47.5g;Carb 10.5g;Protein 23g
Serving 2; Cook time 10 min

Ingredients:
- 1 tablespoon sesame oil
- 8 ounces boneless chicken thighs, chopped
- Salt and pepper
- 4 cups fresh spring greens
- 1 cup sliced avocado
- 2 tablespoons olive oil
- 2 tablespoons rice wine vinegar
- 1 tablespoon sesame seeds

Instructions:
1. Heat the sesame oil in a skillet over medium-high heat.
2. Season the chicken with salt and pepper, then add to the skillet.
3. Cook the chicken until browned and cooked through, stirring often.
4. Remove the chicken from the heat and cool slightly.
5. Divide the spring greens onto two salad plates and top with avocado.
6. Drizzle the salads with olive oil and rice wine vinegar.
7. Top with cooked chicken and sprinkle with sesame seeds to serve.

Curried Chicken Soup

Nutrition: Cal 390;Fat 22g;Carb 14g;Protein 34g
Serving 4; Cook time 30 min

Ingredients:
- 2 tablespoons olive oil, divided
- 4 boneless chicken thighs (about 12 ounces)
- 1 small yellow onion, chopped
- 2 teaspoons curry powder
- 2 teaspoons ground cumin
- Pinch cayenne
- 4 cups chopped cauliflower
- 4 cups chicken broth
- 1 cup water
- 2 cloves minced garlic
- ½ cup canned coconut milk
- 2 cups chopped kale
- Fresh chopped cilantro

Instructions:
1. Chop the chicken into bite-sized pieces then set aside.
2. Heat 1 tablespoon oil in a saucepan over medium heat.
3. Add the onions and cook for 4 minutes then stir in half of the spices.
4. Stir in the cauliflower and sauté for another 4 minutes.
5. Pour in the broth then add the water and garlic and bring to a boil.
6. Reduce heat and simmer for 10 minutes until the cauliflower is softened.
7. Remove from heat and stir in the coconut milk and kale.
8. Heat the remaining oil in a skillet and add the chicken – cook until
9. browned.
10. Stir in the rest of the spices then cook until the chicken is done.
11. Stir the chicken into the soup and serve hot, garnished with fresh cilantro.

Kale Caesar Salad with Chicken

Nutrition: Cal 390;Fat 30g;Carb 13g;Protein 15g
Serving 2; Cook time 20 min

Ingredients:
- 1 tablespoon olive oil
- 6 ounces boneless chicken thigh, chopped
- Salt and pepper
- 3 tablespoons mayonnaise
- 1 tablespoon lemon juice
- 1 anchovy, chopped
- 1 teaspoon Dijon mustard
- 1 clove garlic, minced
- 4 cups fresh chopped kale

Instructions:
1. Heat the oil in a skillet over medium-high heat.
2. Season the chicken with salt and pepper, then add to the skillet.
3. Cook until the chicken is no longer pink, then remove from heat.
4. Combine the mayonnaise, lemon juice, anchovies, mustard, and garlic in a blender.
5. Blend smooth, then season with salt and pepper.
6. Toss the kale with the dressing, then divide in half and top with chicken to serve.

Chicken Enchilada Soup

Nutrition: Cal 390;Fat 27g;Carb 12g;Protein 24g
Serving 4; Cook time 60 min

Ingredients:
- 2 tablespoons coconut oil
- 2 medium stalks celery, sliced
- 1 small yellow onion, chopped
- 1 small red pepper, chopped
- 2 cloves garlic, minced
- 1 cup diced tomatoes
- 2 teaspoons ground cumin
- 1 teaspoon chili powder
- ½ teaspoon dried oregano
- 4 cups chicken broth
- 1 cup canned coconut milk
- 8 ounces cooked chicken thighs, chopped
- 2 tablespoons fresh lime juice
- ¼ cup fresh chopped cilantro

Instructions:
1. Heat the oil in a saucepan over medium-high heat then add the celery,
2. onion, peppers, and garlic – sauté for 4 to 5 minutes.
3. Stir in the garlic and cook for a minute until fragrant.
4. Add the tomatoes and spices then cook for 3 minutes, stirring often.
5. Add the broth and bring the soup to a boil, then reduce heat and simmer for about 20 minutes.
6. Stir in the coconut milk and simmer for another 20 minutes, then add the chicken.
7. Cook until the chicken is heated through, then stir in the lime juice and cilantro.

Bacon-Wrapped Chicken Rolls

Nutrition: Cal 350;Fat 16g;Carb 0,5g;Protein 46g
Serving 2; Cook time 40 min

Ingredients:
• 6 boneless, skinless, chicken breast halves
• 6 slices uncooked bacon

Instructions:
1. Preheat the oven to 350°F.
2. Pound the chicken breast halves with a meat mallet to flatten.
3. Roll the chicken breast halves up then wrap each one with bacon.
4. Place the rolls on a foil-lined baking sheet.
5. Bake for 30 to 35 minutes until the chicken is done and the bacon crisp.

Slow-Cooker Chicken Fajita Soup
Nutrition: Cal 325;Fat 17g; Carb 17g;Protein 28g
Serving 4; Cook time 60 hours

Ingredients:
• 12 ounces chicken thighs
• 1 cup diced tomatoes
• 2 cups chicken stock
• ½ cup enchilada sauce
• 2 ounces chopped green chiles
• 1 tablespoon minced garlic
• 1 medium yellow onion, chopped
• 1 small red pepper, chopped
• 1 jalapeno, seeded and minced
• 2 teaspoons chili powder
• ¾ teaspoon paprika
• ½ teaspoon ground cumin
• Salt and pepper
• 1 small avocado, sliced thinly
• ¼ cup chopped cilantro
• 1 lime, cut into wedges

Instructions:
1. Combine the chicken, tomatoes, chicken stock, enchilada sauce, chiles, and garlic in the slow cooker and stir well.
2. Add the onion, bell peppers, and jalapeno.
3. Stir in the seasonings then cover and cook on low for 5 to 6 hours.
4. Remove the chicken and chop or shred then stir it back into the soup.
5. Spoon into bowls and serve with sliced avocado, cilantro, and lime wedges.

Chicken Enchilada Bowl
Nutrition: Cal 356;Fat 35g; Carb 6g;Protein 28g
Serving 4; Cook time 30 min

Ingredients
• 2 tablespoons coconut oil (for searing chicken)
• 1 pound of boneless skinless chicken thighs
• 3/4 cup red enchilada sauce
• 1/4 cup water
• 1/4 cup chopped onion
• 1 4 ounce can diced green chiles
• **Toppings (feel free to customize)**
• 1 whole avocado, diced
• 1 cup shredded cheese (I used mild cheddar)
• 1/4 cup chopped pickled jalapenos
• 1/2 cup sour cream

• 1 roma tomato, chopped

Instructions
1. In a pot or dutch oven over medium heat melt the coconut oil. Once hot, sear chicken thighs until lightly brown.
2. Pour in enchilada sauce and water, then add onion and green chiles. Reduce heat to a simmer and cover. Cook chicken for 17-25 minutes or until chicken is tender and fully cooked through to at least 165° internal temperature.
3. Carefully remove the chicken and place onto a work surface. Chop or shred chicken (your preference), then add it back into the pot. Let the chicken simmer uncovered for an additional 10 minutes to absorb flavor and allow the sauce to reduce a little.
4. To serve, top with avocado, cheese, jalapeno, sour cream, tomato, and any other desired toppings. Feel free to customize these to your preference. Serve alone or over cauliflower rice if desired, just be sure to update your personal nutrition info as needed.

Chicken Philly Cheesesteak
Nutrition: Cal 263;Fat 12g; Carb 5g;Protein 27g
Serving 3; Cook time 15 min

Ingredients
• 10 ounces boneless chicken breasts (about 2)
• 2 tablespoons worcestershire sauce
• 1/2 teaspoon onion powder
• 1/2 teaspoon garlic powder
• 1 dash of ground pepper
• 2 teaspoons olive oil, divided
• 1/2 cup diced onion, fresh or frozen
• 1/2 cup diced bell pepper, fresh or frozen
• 1/2 teaspoon minced garlic
• 3 slices provolone cheese or queso melting cheese

Instructions
1. Slice chicken breasts into very thin pieces (freeze slightly, if desired, to make this easier) and place in a medium bowl. Add next 4 ingredients (worcestershire through ground pepper) and stir to coat chicken.
2. Heat 1 teaspoon olive oil in a large (9") ovenproof skillet. Add chicken pieces and cook until browned - about 5 minutes. Turn pieces over and cook about 2-3 minutes more or until brown. Remove from skillet.
3. Add remaining 1 teaspoon olive oil to warm skillet. Then add onions, bell pepper, and garlic. Cook and stir to heated and tender, 2-3 minutes.
4. Turn heat off and add chicken back to skillet and stir with veggies to combine. Place sliced cheese over all and cover 2-3 minutes to melt.

Easy Cashew Chicken
Nutrition: Cal 330;Fat 24g; Carb 8g;Protein 22g
Serving 3; Cook time 15 min

Ingredients
• 3 raw chicken thighs, boneless and skinless
• 2 tablespoons coconut oil (for cooking)
• 1/4 cup raw cashews
• 1/2 medium green bell pepper
• 1/2 teaspoon ground ginger

- 1 tablespoon rice wine vinegar
- 1 1/2 tablespoons liquid aminos
- 1/2 tablespoon chili garlic sauce
- 1 tablespoon minced garlic
- 1 tablespoon sesame oil
- 1 tablespoon sesame seeds
- 1 tablespoon green onions
- 1/4 medium white onion
- Salt and pepper, to taste

Instructions

1. Heat a pan over low heat and toast the cashews for 8 minutes, or until they start to lightly brown and become fragrant. Remove and set aside.
2. Dice chicken thighs into 1 inch chunks. Cut onion and pepper into equally large chunks.
3. Increase heat to high and add coconut oil to pan.
4. Once oil is up to temperature, add in the chicken thighs and allow them to cook through (about 5 minutes).
5. Once the chicken is fully cooked add in the pepper, onions, garlic, chili garlic sauce, and seasonings (ginger, salt, pepper). Allow to cook on high for 2-3 minutes.
6. Add liquid aminos, rice wine vinegar, and cashews. Cook on high and allow the liquid to reduce down until it is a sticky consistency. There should not be excess liquid in the pan upon completing cooking.

Thai Chicken Lettuce Wraps

Nutrition: Cal 270;Fat 14g; Carb 12g;Protein 21g
Serving 4; Cook time 10 min

Ingredients

- 1 lb ground chicken
- 1 tablespoon olive oil
- 2 tablespoons red curry paste
- 1 tablespoon ginger, minced
- 4 cloves garlic, minced
- 1 red bell pepper, sliced thinly
- 4 green onions, chopped
- 1 cup cabbage, shredded or coleslaw mix
- 1/4 cup hoisin sauce
- 1/4 teaspoon salt, or to taste
- 1/4 teaspoon pepper, or to taste
- 5 leaves basil, chopped
- 1/2 head iceberg lettuce, cut into half

Instructions

1. Add olive oil to a large skillet and heat until oil is very hot. Add ground chicken and cook until no longer pink and starts to brown, break it up with a wooden spoon as necessary. Should take about 3 minutes.
2. Add red curry paste, ginger, garlic, peppers, coleslaw mix, and stir-fry for another 3 minutes. Add hoisin sauce and green onions, and toss. Remove from heat then add basil and toss. Transfer cooked chicken to a bowl.
3. Serve by placing spoonfuls of chicken into pieces of lettuce, fold lettuce over like small tacos, and eat.

Crispy Chipotle Chicken Thighs

Nutrition: Cal 400;Fat 20g; Carb 8g;Protein 25g
Serving 2; Cook time 22 min

Ingredients

- ½ teaspoon chipotle chili powder
- ¼ teaspoon garlic powder
- ¼ teaspoon onion powder
- ¼ teaspoon ground coriander
- ¼ teaspoon smoked paprika
- 12 ounces boneless chicken thighs
- Salt and pepper
- 1 tablespoon olive oil
- 3 cups fresh baby spinach

Instructions

1. Combine the chipotle chili powder, garlic powder, onion powder, coriander, and smoked paprika in a small bowl.
2. Pound the chicken thighs out flat, then season with salt and pepper on both sides.
3. Cut the chicken thighs in half and heat the oil in a heavy skillet over medium-high heat.
4. Add the chicken thighs skin-side-down to the skillet and sprinkle with the spice mixture.
5. Cook the chicken thighs for 8 minutes then flip and cook on the other side for 3 to 5 minutes.
6. During the last 3 minutes, add the spinach to the skillet and cook until wilted. Serve the crispy chicken thighs on a bed of wilted spinach.

Easy Cashew Chicken

Nutrition: Cal 330;Fat 24g; Carb 8g;Protein 22g
Serving 3; Cook time 15 min

Ingredients

- 3 raw chicken thighs, boneless and skinless
- 2 tablespoons coconut oil (for cooking)
- 1/4 cup raw cashews
- 1/2 medium green bell pepper
- 1/2 teaspoon ground ginger
- 1 tablespoon rice wine vinegar
- 1 1/2 tablespoons liquid aminos
- 1/2 tablespoon chili garlic sauce
- 1 tablespoon minced garlic
- 1 tablespoon sesame oil
- 1 tablespoon sesame seeds
- 1 tablespoon green onions
- 1/4 medium white onion
- Salt and pepper, to taste

Instructions

1. Heat a pan over low heat and toast the cashews for 8 minutes, or until they start to lightly brown and become fragrant. Remove and set aside.
2. Dice chicken thighs into 1 inch chunks. Cut onion and pepper into equally large chunks.
3. Increase heat to high and add coconut oil to pan.
4. Once oil is up to temperature, add in the chicken thighs and allow them to cook through (about 5 minutes).
5. Once the chicken is fully cooked add in the pepper, onions, garlic, chili garlic sauce, and seasonings (ginger, salt, pepper). Allow to cook on high for 2-3 minutes.

6. Add liquid aminos, rice wine vinegar, and cashews. Cook on high and allow the liquid to reduce down until it is a sticky consistency. There should not be excess liquid in the pan upon completing cooking.
7. Serve in a bowl, top with sesame seeds, and drizzle with sesame oil.

Roasted Turkey Breast with Mushrooms & Brussels Sprouts
Nutrition: Cal 210;Fat 9g; Carb 6g;Protein 27g
Serving 4; Cook time 50 min

Ingredients
- •2 tbsp olive oil
- •1 tsp salt
- •1 tsp black pepper
- •1 tsp garlic powder
- •1 pound turkey breast raw, cut into 1 inch cubes
- •1/2 pound brussels sprouts cleaned, cut in half
- •1 cups mushrooms cleaned

Instructions
1. Preheat oven to 350 degrees Fahrenheit.
2. In a small mixing bowl, combine olive oil, salt, black pepper, and garlic powder.
3. In a 9 x 6-inch casserole dish, combine turkey, brussels sprouts, and mushrooms. Pour the olive oil mixture over the top.
4. Cover with foil and bake for 45 minutes or until the turkey is cooked through and no longer pink. An internal temperature of 165 degrees Fahrenheit is a safe bet.

Turkey and Bacon Lettuce Wraps
Nutrition: Cal 305;Fat 20g; Carb 22g;Protein 11g
Serving 4; Cook time 15 min

Ingredients
Wraps
- •1 head iceberg lettuce
- •4 slices deli turkey
- •4 slices bacon cooked
- •1 avocado thinly sliced
- •1 roma tomato thinly sliced
- •1 cucumber thinly sliced
- •1 carrot thinly sliced

Basil Mayo
- •1/2 cup mayo
- •6 basil leaves chopped
- •1 tsp lemon juice
- •1 garlic clove minced
- •salt and pepper to taste

Instructions
Basil Mayo
1. Combine all of the ingredients in a food processor, blend until smooth

Wraps
1. Lay out two large lettuce leaves then layer on 1 slice of turkey and slather with Basil-Mayo.
2. Layer on a second slice of turkey followed by the bacon, and a few slices of avocado, tomato, cucumber and carrot.

3. Season lightly with salt and pepper then fold the bottom up, the sides in, and roll like a burrito.
4. Slice in half and serve cold.

Chiken Stir-Fry
Nutrition: Cal 312;Fat 14g; Carb 11g;Protein 31g
Serving 4; Cook time 40 min

Ingredients
- •3 boneless, skinless chicken breasts, trimmed and cut into pieces at least 1 inch square
- •2 red bell peppers
- •2 cups sugar snap peas
- •1 1/2 T peanut oil
- •1-2 T sesame seeds, preferably black

Marinade ingredients:
- •1/3 cup soy sauce (gluten-free if needed)
- •2 T unseasoned (unsweetened) rice vinegar
- •2 T low-carb sweetener of your choice (see notes)
- •1 T sesame oil
- •1/2 tsp. garlic powder

Instructions
1. Trim the chicken breasts and cut into pieces at least 1 inch square.
2. Combine soy sauce, rice vinegar, Stevia, agave or maple syrup, sesame oil and garlic powder.
3. Put the chicken into a Ziploc bag and pour in HALF the marinade. Let chicken marinate in the fridge for at least 4 hours (or all day while you're at work would be even better.)
4. When you're ready to cook, cover a large baking sheet with foil, then put it in the oven and let the pan get hot while the oven heats to 425F/220C.
5. Drain the marinated chicken well in a colander placed in the sink.
6. Remove the hot baking sheet from the oven and spread the chicken out over the surface (so pieces are not touching). Put baking sheet into the oven and cook chicken 8 minutes.
7. While the chicken cooks, trim ends of the sugar snap peas. Cut out the core and seeds of the red bell peppers and discard; then cut peppers into strips about the same thickness as the sugar snap peas.
8. Put veggies into a bowl and toss with the peanut oil.
9. After 8 minutes, remove pan from the oven and arrange the veggies around the chicken, trying to have each vegetable piece touching the pan as much as you can.
10. Put back into the oven and cook about 11 minutes more, or until the chicken is cooked through and lightly browned.
11. Brush cooked chicken and vegetables with the remaining marinade and sprinkle with black sesame seeds. Serve hot.

Garlic, Lemon & Thyme Roasted Chicken Breasts
Nutrition: Cal 230;Fat 27g; Carb 4g;Protein 26g
Serving 4; Cook time 2 hours 45 min

Ingredients
- •4 boneless skinless chicken breasts
- •zest of 1 lemon

- juice of 1 lemon
- 1/2 cup extra virgin olive oil
- 4 cloves garlic minced
- 1 tablespoon fresh thyme
- 1 teaspoon salt
- 1/2 teaspoon ground black pepper
- 1 tablespoon olive oil for sauteing

Instructions

1. Create the marinade by mixing the lemon juice, zest, 1/2 cup of olive oil, garlic, thyme, salt, and pepper. Place the chicken breasts in a non-reactive glass dish, or plastic ziptop bag, and pour the marinade over the chicken. Make sure to evenly coat the chicken, then cover and refrigerate for 2 hours.
2. Preheat your oven to 400 degrees F. Remove the chicken from the marinade and wipe off the excess. Heat 1 tablespoon of olive oil, and sear the chicken breasts for 2 minutes on each side, until they're golden brown.
3. Place the chicken breasts on a baking sheet lined with a baking rack, and roast at 400 degrees F for 20-30 minutes depending on the thickness of the chicken breast, or until the internal temperature reads 165 degrees F.

Grilled Chicken Kabobs

Nutrition: Cal 278;Fat 12g; Carb 26g;Protein 27g
Serving 2; Cook time 30 min

Ingredients

- 0.5 pound boneless skinless chicken breasts cut into 1 inch pieces
- 0.13 cup olive oil
- 0.17 cup soy sauce
- 0.13 cup honey
- 0.5 teaspoon minced garlic
- salt and pepper to taste
- 0.5 red bell pepper cut into 1 inch pieces
- 0.5 yellow bell pepper cut into 1 inch pieces
- 1 small zucchini cut into 1 inch slices
- 0.5 red onion cut into 1 inch pieces
- 0.5 tablespoon chopped parsley

Instructions

1. Place the olive oil, soy sauce, honey, garlic and salt and pepper in a large bowl.
2. Whisk to combine.
3. Add the chicken, bell peppers, zucchini and red onion to the bowl. Toss to coat in the marinade.
4. Cover and refrigerate for at least 1 hour, or up to 8 hours.
5. Soak wooden skewers in cold water for at least 30 minutes. Preheat grill or grill pan to medium high heat.
6. Thread the chicken and vegetables onto the skewers.
7. Cook for 5-7 minutes on each side or until chicken is cooked through.
8. Sprinkle with parsley and serve.

Keto Barbeque Chicken Soup

Nutrition: Cal270;Fat 24 g; Carb 18 g;Protein 22 g
Serving 2; Cook time 60 min

Ingredients
The Base:

- 3 medium Chicken Thighs
- 2 teaspoon Chili Seasoning
- Salt and Pepper to Taste
- 2 tablespoon Chicken Fat or Olive Oil
- 1 1/2 cup Chicken Broth
- 1 1/2 cup Beef Broth
- Salt and Pepper to Taste

BBQ Sauce:

- 1/4 Cup Reduced Sugar Ketchup
- 1/4 cup Tomato Paste
- 2 tablespoon Dijon Mustard
- 1 tablespoon Soy Sauce
- 1 tablespoon hot sauce
- 2 1/2 teaspoon Liquid Smoke
- 1 teaspoon Worcestershire Sauce
- 1 1/2 teaspoon Garlic Powder
- 1 teaspoon Onion Powder
- 1 teaspoon Chili Powder
- 1 teaspoon Red Chili Flakes
- 1 teaspoon Cumin
- 1/4 cup Butter

Instructions

1. Preheat oven to 400F.
2. De-bone chicken thighs, set bones aside, and season well with your favorite chili seasoning.
3. Line a cookie sheet with foil and bake for 50 minutes.
4. While that is cooking, add 2 tablespoons of Chicken Fat or Olive Oil in a pot.
5. Heat this to a medium high heat and once hot, add chicken bones.
6. Let these cook for at least 5 minutes and then add broths.
7. Season with salt and pepper to taste.
8. Once the chicken is done, remove the skins and set aside.
9. Add all of the fat from the chicken thighs into the broth and stir.
10. Make the BBQ sauce by combining all ingredients above.
11. Add barbeque sauce to the pot and stir together.
12. Let this simmer in a pot for 20-30 minutes.
13. Use an immersion blender to emulsify all of the fats and liquids together.
14. Then, shred chicken thighs and add to the soup. You can optionally add spring onion or bell pepper here.
15. Simmer for another 10-20 minutes.

Serve with yellow bell pepper, spring onion, or cheddar cheese and the crispy chicken skins

Avocado Chicken Salad

Nutrition: Cal 267;Fat 20 g; Carb 4 g;Protein 19 g
Serving 3; Cook time 30 min

Ingredients

- 2 cups poached chicken finely diced (10 oz)

- 1 medium Hass Avocado, mashed
- 1/3 cup celery, finely diced (1 large rib)
- 2 tbsp red onion or scallion, minced
- 2 tbsp cilantro, finely chopped
- 2 tbsp avocado oil (or your favorite)
- 1 tbsp fresh lemon juice (or lime juice)
- salt and pepper to taste

Instructions

1. Prepare the celery, onion, and cilantro, placing in a medium bowl. Dice the chicken and add it to the bowl with the vegetables.
2. Cut into the avocado with a chef's knife until the blade hits the pit. Slide the knife around the pit, cutting the avocado in half. Twist the halves to separate. Remove the pit by tapping the knife into the pit until it sticks, make sure the avocado half is held steadily on a cutting board before attempting. Scoop out the avocado flesh with a spoon and place into a small bowl. Mash with a fork until smooth and creamy. Stir in the lemon juice and oil.
3. Add the mashed avocado to the to the chicken and vegetables and stir to mix. Serve over lettuce or enjoy on a low carb bagel.

Makes 3, 3/4-1 cup servings.

Keto Chicken Soup
Nutrition: Cal 267;Fat 20 g; Carb 9 g;Protein 22 g
Serving 4; Cook time 60 min

Ingredients
- 2 tbsp. vegetable oil
- 1 medium onion, chopped
- 5 cloves garlic, smashed
- 2" piece fresh ginger, sliced
- 1 small cauliflower, cut into florets
- 3/4 tsp. crushed red pepper flakes
- 1 medium carrot, peeled and thinly sliced on a bias
- 6 c. low-sodium chicken broth
- 1 stalk celery, thinly sliced
- 2 boneless skinless chicken breasts
- Freshly chopped parsley, for garnish

Instructions

1. In a large pot over medium heat, heat oil. Add onion, garlic and ginger. Cook until beginning to brown.
2. Meanwhile, pulse cauliflower in a food processor until broken down into rice-sized granules. Add cauliflower to pot with onion mixture and cook over medium high heat until beginning to brown, about 8 minutes.
3. Add pepper flakes, carrots, celery and chicken broth and bring to a simmer. Add chicken breasts and let cook gently until they reach an internal temperature of 165°, about 15 minutes. Remove from pan, let cool until cool enough to handle, and shred. Meanwhile, continue simmering until vegetables are tender, 3 to 5 minutes more.

Remove ginger from pot, and add shredded chicken back to soup. Season to taste with salt and pepper, then garnish with parsley before serving.

Keto White Chicken Chili
Nutrition: Cal 480;Fat 30 g; Carb 5 g;Protein 38 g
Serving 4; Cook time 45 min

Ingredients
- 1 lb chicken breast
- cups chicken broth
- 2 garlic cloves, finely minced
- 1 4.5oz can chopped green chiles
- 1 diced jalapeno
- 1 diced green pepper
- 1/4 cup diced onion
- 4 tbsp butter
- 1/4 cup heavy whipping cream
- 4 oz cream cheese
- 2 tsp cumin
- 1 tsp oregano
- 1/4 tsp cayenne (optional)
- Salt and Pepper to taste

Instructions

1. In large pot, season chicken with cumin, oregano, cayenne, salt and pepper
2. Sear both sides over medium heat until golden
3. Add broth to pot, cover and cook chicken for 15-20 minutes or until fully cooked
4. While chicken is cooking, melt butter in medium skillet
5. Add chiles, diced jalapeno, green pepper and onion to skillet and saute until veggies soften
6. Add minced garlic and saute additional 30 seconds and turn off heat, set aside
7. Once chicken is fully cooked, shred with fork and add back into broth
8. Add sauteed veggies to pot with chicken and broth and simmer for 10 minutes
9. In medium bowl, soften cream cheese in microwave until you can stir it (~20 sec)
10. Mix cream cheese with heavy whipping cream
11. Stirring quickly, add mixture into pot with chicken and veggies
12. Simmer additional 15 minutes
13. Serve with favorite toppings such as: pepper jack cheese, avocado slices, cilantro, sour cream

CHICKEN WITH SPINACH AND FETA
Nutrition: Cal 300;Fat 12 g; Carb 2 g;Protein 40 g
Serving 4; Cook time 30 min

Ingredients
- Chicken breasts (no bones and skin, 4 pieces)
- Spinach (half cup)
- Coconut oil (2 tbsp)
- Feta cheese (1/3 cup)
- Garlic powder (¼ teaspoon)
- Salt (¼ teaspoon)
- Dry oregano (¼ teaspoon)
- Parsley (¼ teaspoon, dry or fresh)
- Water (1 cup)

Instructions

1. Pound the chicken breasts but don't make these to thin; cut "pockets" inside meat.
2. In a bowl mix the feta along with the spinach and add the salt. Put this mix inside the "pockets" and after that close it with toothpicks.
3. Add the remainder in the seasoning all on the meat.
4. Set the pressure cooker to "Sauté" and squeeze coconut oil inside; fry the chicken breasts till they have a golden color. When the meat is cooked, press "Cancel."
5. Put the chicken breasts over a plate and pour water inside the pressure cooker; place the steaming rack inside and put the meat onto it. Steam the meat for fifteen minutes.
6. Release the stress naturally for fifteen minutes. Serve while still warm.

SALSA CHICKEN
Nutrition: Cal 244;Fat 10 g; Carb 4.2 g;Protein 30 g
Serving 6; Cook time 35 min

Ingredients
• Chicken thighs without bones (2 lbs)
• Chicken broth (1/4 cup)
• Cream cheese (4 oz.)
• Salsa (1 cup)
• Taco seasoning (3 tbsp)
• Salt, Pepper

Instructions
1. Put the chicken thighs inside pressure cooker and add the taco seasoning, salt, and pepper.
2. Add the salsa, chicken broth and cream cheese, close and seal the lead. Press "Manual" and set it to prepare for 20 mins on questionable.
3. When it's over, release pressure naturally for quarter-hour.
4. Put the chicken thighs inside a plate; blend the sauce until it's smooth.
5. With a fork shred the meat and place it back inside the creamy sauce. Stir so the meat coats well inside the sauce.
6. Serve with lettuce and avocados and other

CHICKEN WINGETTES WITH CILANTRO DIP
Nutrition: Cal 296;Fat 22 g; Carb 11 g;Protein 10 g
Serving 6; Cook time 60 min

Ingredients
• 10 fresh cayenne peppers, trimmed and chopped
• 3 garlic cloves, minced
• 1 ½ cups white wine vinegar
• ½ teaspoon black pepper
• 1 teaspoon sea salt
• 1 teaspoon onion powder
• 12 chicken wingettes
• 2 tablespoons olive oil
• **DIPPING SAUCE:**
• ½ cup mayonnaise
• ½ cup sour cream
• ½ cup cilantro, chopped

• 2 cloves garlic, minced
• 1 teaspoon smoked paprika
Instructions
1. Place cayenne peppers, 3 garlic cloves, white vinegar, black pepper, salt, and onion powder in the container. Add chicken wingettes, and allow them marinate, covered, for one hour inside the refrigerator.
2. Add the chicken wingettes, along while using marinade and extra virgin olive oil on the Instant Pot.
3. Secure the lid. Choose the "Manual" setting and cook for 6 minutes. Once cooking is complete, use a quick pressure release; carefully take away the lid.
4. In a mixing bowl, thoroughly combine mayonnaise, sour cream, cilantro, garlic, and smoked paprika.
5. Serve warm chicken with all the dipping sauce privately.

TURKEY TACO BOWLS
Nutrition: Cal 366;Fat 10 g; Carb 42 g;Protein 23 g
Serving 4; Cook time 70 min

Ingredients
• cheese cheddar or mozzarella
Rice
• 3/4 cup uncooked brown rice
• 1/8 tsp salt
• Zest of 1 lime
• Turkey
• 3/4 lb lean ground turkey
• 2 tablespoons taco seasoning of choice
Salsa
• 1 pint cherry tomatoes quartered
• 1 jalapeno minced
• 1 1/4 cup red onion minced
• Juice from 1/2 a lime
• 1/8 tsp salt
Other:
• One 12 oz/341 mL can corn kernels drained & rinsed
• 1/4 cup shredded chee
Instructions
1. Cook brown rice according to package directions, adding the lime zest and salt to the cooking water.
2. Cook turkey over medium heat, tossing in the taco seasoning and breaking it up as you cook. Cook for 10 or so minutes, until cooked through.
3. Combine all salsa ingredients and toss together.
4. To assemble lunch bowls:
5. 1/4 portion of cooked rice (roughly ½ cup)
6. 1/2 cup corn kernels
7. 1/2 cup cooked taco meat
8. 1/4 portion of salsa (just over ½ cup)

TURKEY BREAST
Nutrition: Cal 268 ;Fat 10 g; Carb 8 g;Protein 30 g
Serving 2; Cook time 15 min

Ingredients
• 2 turkey breast fillets
• 1 cup water
• 1 tbsp. rosemary

- 1 tbsp. garlic powder
- 1 tbsp. sage
- ¼ tsp. pepper
- ½ tsp. salt
- ½ tsp. thyme

Instructions

1. Arrange the rack within the Instant Pot or just add the breast to the river for poaching.
2. Use the spices and herbs to rub the turkey and place them in to the pot. Secure the lid using the "Poultry" function (7-10 min).
3. Quick release pressure if the time is completed and eliminate the meat.
4. You can use the juices with all the meat or save it for the broth later.

TURKEY WITH BROCCOLI
Nutrition: Cal 268 ;Fat 10 g; Carb 8 g;Protein 30 g
Serving 2; Cook time 15 min

Ingredients
- ½ pound ground turkey
- 1 spring onion, finely chopped
- 1 cup broccoli, chopped
- 1 cup shredded mozzarella
- 3 tbsps. sour cream
- ¼ cup Parmesan cheese, grated
- 2 tbsps. essential olive oil
- ¼ cup chicken stock
- ¼ tsp. dried oregano
- ¼ tsp. white pepper, freshly ground
- ½ tsp. dried thyme
- ½ tsp. salt

Instructions

1. Plug inside the Instant Pot and press the "Sauté" button. Add organic olive oil and warm up.
2. Now add spring onions and cook for 1 minute, stirring constantly.
3. Add turkey and broccoli. Pour inside the stock and cook for 12 - quarter-hour, stirring occasionally. Season with salt, pepper, thyme, and oregano and stir in the cheese.
4. Press the "Cancel" button and remove from your pot. Transfer a combination to a small baking dish as well as set aside.
5. Preheat the oven to 3500 F and bake for 15 - 20 mins, or until lightly charred.
6. Remove through the oven and chill for a while. Top with sour cream and serve.

JALAPENO CHICKEN
Nutrition: Cal 358 ;Fat 12 g; Carb 3 g;Protein 55 g
Serving 4; Cook time 30 min

Ingredients
5 chicken thighs, skin on
1 large onion, chopped
3 jalapeno peppers, chopped
¾ cup cauliflower, chopped into florets

1 chili pepper, chopped
3 tbsps. fish sauce
1 tbsps. Swerve
5 cups chicken stock
2 tbsps. extra virgin olive oil
3 bay leaves
1 tsp peppercorn
1 tsp dried thyme
1½ tsp salt

Instructions

1. Combine all ingredients inside instant pot and stir well. Seal the lid and hang the steam release handle for the "Sealing" position.
2. Press the "Poultry" button and hang up the timer for twenty minutes on high heat.
3. When done, release the stress naturally and open the lid. Remove the meat in the bones and stir well again. Serve by incorporating grated Parmesan cheese.

TURKEY STEW RECIPE
Nutrition: Cal 386 ;Fat 20 g; Carb 12 g;Protein 36 g
Serving 5; Cook time 30 min

Ingredients
- 2 lbs turkey breast, chopped into smaller pieces
- 2 cups cherry tomatoes, chopped
- 1 onion, finely chopped
- 4 cups chicken broth
- ¾ cup heavy cream
- 2 celery stalks, chopped
- 4 tbsps. butter
- 1 tsp. dried thyme
- 1 tsp. peppercorn
- 2 tsps. Salt

Instructions

1. Combine the constituents in the instant pot and seal the lid
2. Set the steam release handle towards the "Sealing" position and press the "Stew" button. Set the timer for twenty minutes on high heat.

When done; release pressure to succeed naturally and open the lid. Chill for a while and stir in most sour cream. To enjoy, serve it immediately.

TURKEY LASAGNA WITH RICOTTA
Nutrition: Cal 740 ;Fat 56 g; Carb 7.8 g;Protein 47 g
Serving 8; Cook time 60 min

Ingredients
- 2 lbs ground turkey
- 5 cups baby spinach leaves
- 1 cup ricotta
- 1 cup mozzarella cheese, grated
- 1 can crushed tomatoes
- 3 tsp dried oregano
- 2 tsp thyme
- 3 tbsp fresh parsley, finely chopped
- 1 tsp salt
- 1 tsp freshly ground black pepper

- 1 tsp onion powder
- 1 tsp garlic powder
- 8 lasagna sheets
- 3 cups water

Instructions

1. In a bowl mix together the ricotta and mozzarella and place aside.
2. In another bowl, mix the crushed tomatoes using the oregano, thyme, parsley, salt, pepper, onion and garlic powder.
3. Start layering the lasagna in a very heatproof dish that fits inside Instant Pot.
4. Spread one tablespoon of the tomatoes sauce and layer some with the lasagna sheets. Spread more of the tomatoes sauce around the sheets and top using a layer of each one in the following: cheese, minced meat and spinach. Top with more sauce and set the remainder in the lasagna. Repeat the layering process before you uses up lasagna sheets. Sprinkle with leftover cheese and cover tightly with aluminum foil.
5. Place the Instant Pot over medium heat, pour in water and punctiliously position the lasagna dish inside pot on the trivet.
6. Cover the pot and manually set the timer for a half-hour. When time is conducted, carefully release pressure.
7. Uncover the pot and eliminate the foil. To allow the lasagna to brown.

Carefully remove the lasagna dish out of the pot and serve hot.

Keto Tandoori Chicken Wings
Nutrition: Cal 420 ;Fat 16 g; Carb 8 g;Protein 25 g
Serving 2 Cook time 2 hours 10 min

Ingredients
- 2-1/2 lbs. chicken wings, trimmed and separated
- 1 cup Homemade Yogurt*
- 2 tbsp. ginger
- 6 cloves garlic, minced
- 1-1/2 tsp. curry powder
- ¼ tsp. turmeric
- ½ tsp. cumin
- ½ tsp. dry mustard
- 2 tsp. red pepper flakes
- 1 lemon, juiced
- 3 tbsp. vegetable oil
- Salt, pepper

Instructions
1. Add all ingredients in a a bowl and mix well
2. Marinade for at least two hours at room temperature. (saving marinade)
3. Place wings on broiling rack and broil until browned, about 20 minutes
4. Baste wings with marinade about every 10 minutes.
5. Transfer to platter and serve.

Keto Riced Cauliflower & Curry Chicken
Nutrition: Cal 420 ;Fat 16 g; Carb 8 g;Protein 25 g
Serving 4 Cook time 30 min

Ingredients
1. 2 Lbs. of Chicken (4 breasts)
2. 1 packet of Curry Paste
3. 1 Cup Water
4. 3 Tablespoons Ghee (can substitute butter)
5. ½ Cup Heavy Cream
6. 1 Head Cauliflower (around 1 kg)

Instructions
1. In a large pot, melt the Ghee
2. Add the curry paste and mix to combine
3. Once combined, add the water and simmer for an additional 5 minutes
4. Add the chicken, cover, and simmer for 20 minutes.
5. Meanwhile, chop up a head of cauliflower into florets and pulse in the food processor to make riced cauliflower, (cauliflower doesn't need to be cooked)
6. Once the chicken is cooked, uncover, add the cream, and cook for an additional 5 minutes.

Sun-Dried Tomato and Goat Cheese Chicken
Nutrition: Cal 460 ;Fat 17 g; Carb 14 g;Protein 22 g
Serving 4 Cook time 20 min

Ingredients
- 1/3 cup sun-dried tomatoes, packed without oil, finely chopped
- 2 tsp. olive oil, divided
- 1/2 cup chopped shallots, divided
- 1 tsp. Splenda
- 3 garlic cloves, minced
- 2 1/2 Tablespoon balsamic vinegar, divided
- 1/2 cup (2 oz.) crumbled goat cheese - to cut down on the fat, find the lowest-fat variety
- 2 Tablespoon chopped fresh basil
- 3/4 tsp. salt, divided
- 4 (6-oz) skinless, boneless chicken breast halves
- 1/8 tsp. freshly ground black pepper
- 3/4 cup fat-free, less-sodium chicken broth
- 1/4 tsp. dried thyme

Instructions
1. Heat 1 tsp. oil in a large non-stick skillet over medium heat.
2. Add 1/3 cup shallots, Splenda, and garlic.
3. Cook 4 minutes or until golden brown, stirring often.
4. Spoon into a mixing bowl and stir in 1 1/2 tsp. vinegar.
5. Incorporate chopped tomatoes, shallot mixture, cheese, basil, and 1/4 tsp. salt together and mix well.
6. Cut a horizontal slit through each chicken breast half.
7. Stuff 2 Tbsps. cheese mixture into each newly formed pocket.
8. Season with 1/2 tsp. salt and black pepper.
9. Heat 1 tsp. oil in pan over medium-high heat and add stuffed chicken.
10. Cook approximately 6 minutes on each side or until juices run clear.
11. Remove chicken from pan and add broth, remaining shallots, 2 Tbsps. vinegar, and thyme.
12. Bring to a boil and stir until thickened.

13. Serve over chicken.

Zoodles and Turkey balls
Nutrition: Cal 360 ;Fat 14 g; Carb 12 g;Protein 25 g
Serving 2 Cook time 30 min

Ingredients
1 zucchini cut into spirals
1 can vodka pasta sauce
1 package of frozen Armour Turkey meatballs
Instructions
1. Cook meatballs and sauce on medium heat for 22-25 minutes and stir occasionally.
2. Clean zucchini and put through a vegetable spiral maker.
3. Boil water and blanch raw zoodles 45 seconds.
4. Remove and drain.
Combine zoodles and prepared saucy meatballs

Creamy Italian Chicken Scampi
Nutrition: Cal 360 ;Fat 14 g; Carb 12 g;Protein 25 g
Serving 2 Cook time 30 min

Ingredients
• 1 1/2 lbs. Chicken Breast – Cut into tenders sized pieces
• 6 Large Cloves garlic – Minced
• 6 Tbsp. Butter – Divided
• 1 Cup Chicken Stock
• 1 Cup Heavy Cream
• 1/4 Cup Parmesan Cheese – Grated
• 6 oz. Mixed Bell Peppers – Sliced
• A Few Slices Red Onion
• 1 tsp. Italian Seasoning
• 1/2 tsp. Red Pepper Flakes
• Salt and Pepper – To Taste
Instructions
1. In a large sauté pan, over medium-high heat, pan-sear seasoned chicken in 4 Tbsp. butter.
2. Sear on both sides until golden brown approximately 3-4 minutes each side.
3. Remove chicken from pan and set aside.
4. Using the same pan, reduce heat to medium and brown remaining 2 Tbs. butter, and minced garlic about 1-2 minutes.
5. Add sliced red onion and sauté until transparent.
6. De-glaze the pan with chicken stock. And add Italian seasoning and red pepper flakes.
7. Bring to a boil over medium heat and reduce to low.
8. Let simmer 2-3 minutes.
9. Add heavy cream and continue to simmer and thicken 5-10 minutes.
10. Mix in Parmesan cheese and salt and pepper to taste.
11. Stir in peppers and add chicken.
Simmer on low until chicken is fully cooked.

CHICKEN MEATBALLS
Nutrition: Cal 357 ;Fat 28 g; Carb 3 g;Protein 23 g
Serving 6 Cook time 30 min

Ingredients

• Chicken (1.5 lb., grounded)
• Ghee (2 tbsp)
• Garlic (2 cloves, minced)
• Onion (2, thin sliced)
• Almond meal (¾ cup)
• Hot sauce (6 tbsp)
• Butter (4 tbsp)
Instructions
1. Mix the almond meal, chicken, salt, garlic, and onions in the bowl; put ghee on the hands and form the meatballs.
2. Set the stress cooker to "Sauté" and place two tablespoons of ghee inside; squeeze meatballs inside and fry until they turn brown (roll them every minute, so either side is well fried).
3. Mix 4 tablespoons of butter and hot sauce and heat this mixture within the microwave (this will likely serve like a buffalo sauce for the meatballs). Pour this sauce within the meatballs; secure the lid over pressure cooker and hang up it to "Poultry."
4. Once the cooking is conducted (within 20 minutes), the sound will inform you, and it is possible to press "Cancel." Release the stress valve (protect your hand having a towel or possibly a kitchen glove).
5. Serve with any food you want or take in the meatballs on their own.

COCONUT MILK CHICKEN CURRY
Nutrition: Cal 357 ;Fat 28 g; Carb 3 g;Protein 23 g
Serving 6 Cook time 4 hours 20 min

Ingredients
• Chicken breasts (1 lb.)
• Curry powder (3 tbsp)
• Ground coriander (half teaspoon)
• Turmeric powder (1 teaspoon)
• Butter (2 tbsp)
• Garlic (2 cloves)
• Sweet potatoes (4 pieces, chopped in cubes)
• Rice
• Onion (1, chopped)
• Sugar (1 teaspoon)
• Salt (1 teaspoon)
• Coconut milk (2 cans of 15 oz.)
• Water (1 cup)
Instructions
1. Put the spices (turmeric, coriander, sugar, salt and curry powder) in a bowl and mix them well.
2. Put the chicken breasts inside the pressure cooker and fry them, but ensure they don't burn. Add coconut milk (and a few water when the coconut milk is thick).
3. Add the butter and garlic and also the seasoning mix and stir well, and so the chicken breasts soak in everything.
4. Add the onion and sweet potatoes and stir.
5. Close the lid and set it to high pressure for 4-6 hours.

6. In the final half hour of cooking, receive the chicken out with the pressure cooker, cut it which has a fork and send it back prior to the cooking is complete.

7. Turn pressure cooker off and allow the meal to put for 25 minutes before eating. Serve it with rice.

CHICKEN WINGETTES WITH CILANTRO DIP
Nutrition: Cal 300 ;Fat 22 g; Carb 11 g;Protein 10 g
Serving 4 Cook time 65 min

Ingredients
- 10 fresh cayenne peppers, trimmed and chopped
- 3 garlic cloves, minced
- 1 ½ cups white wine vinegar
- ½ teaspoon black pepper
- 1 teaspoon sea salt
- 1 teaspoon onion powder
- 12 chicken wingettes
- 2 tablespoons olive oil

DIPPING SAUCE:
- ½ cup mayonnaise
- ½ cup sour cream
- ½ cup cilantro, chopped
- 2 cloves garlic, minced
- 1 teaspoon smoked paprika

Instructions
1. Place cayenne peppers, 3 garlic cloves, white vinegar, black pepper, salt, and onion powder in the container. Add chicken wingettes, and allow them marinate, covered, for one hour inside the refrigerator.
2. Add the chicken wingettes, along while using marinade and extra virgin olive oil on the Instant Pot.
3. Secure the lid. Choose the "Manual" setting and cook for 6 minutes. Once cooking is complete, use a quick pressure release; carefully take away the lid.
4. In a mixing bowl, thoroughly combine mayonnaise, sour cream, cilantro, garlic, and smoked paprika.
5. Serve warm chicken with all the dipping sauce privately.

CHICKEN LEGS WITH PIQUANT MAYO SAUCE
Nutrition: Cal 485 ;Fat 42 g; Carb 2.5 g;Protein 22 g
Serving 4 Cook time 25 min

Ingredients
- 4 chicken legs, bone-in, skinless
- 2 garlic cloves, peeled and halved
- ½ teaspoon coarse sea salt
- ¼ teaspoon ground black pepper, or maybe more to taste
- ½ teaspoon red pepper flakes, crushed
- 1 tablespoon essential olive oil
- ¼ cup chicken broth

DIPPING SAUCE:
- ¾ cup mayonnaise
- 2 tablespoons stone ground mustard
- 1 teaspoon fresh freshly squeezed lemon juice
- ½ teaspoon Sriracha

TOPPING:

- ¼ cup fresh cilantro, roughly chopped

Instructions
1. Rub the chicken legs with garlic halves; then, season with salt, black pepper, and red pepper flakes. Press the "Sauté" button.
2. Once hot, heat the oil and sauté chicken legs for four or five minutes, turning once during cooking time. Add a a little chicken broth to deglaze the bottom of the pan.
3. Secure the lid. Choose "Manual" mode and questionable; cook for 14 minutes. Once cooking is complete, work with a natural pressure release; carefully eliminate the lid.
4. Meanwhile, mix all
5. Ingredients for that dipping sauce; place inside the refrigerator until ready to offer.
6. Garnish chicken legs with cilantro. Serve with the piquant mayo sauce quietly.

CHICKEN SHAWARMA
Nutrition: Cal 267 ;Fat 15 g; Carb 5 g;Protein 28 g
Serving 4 Cook time 25 min

Ingredients
- 1-pound boneless, skinless chicken thighs or breasts, cut into large bite-size chunks
- 3 teaspoons extra-virgin essential olive oil, divided
- 3 tablespoons Shawarma Spice Mix
- 1 cup thinly sliced onions
- ¼ cup water
- 4 large lettuce leaves
- 1 cup Tzatziki Sauce

Instructions
1. Place the chicken inside a zip-top bag and add 1 teaspoon of extra virgin olive oil and the shawarma spice mix. Mash it all together, so the chicken is evenly coated within the oil and spices.
2. At this aspect, it is possible to freeze the chicken to get a meal later inside week, or you'll get forced out inside the refrigerator to marinate for about twenty four hours. (I like to create half the chicken now and freeze one other half for an additional meal. Clearly this "now and later" is one area beside me.)
3. Select "Sauté" to preheat the Instant Pot and conform to high heat. When the hot, add the remainder 2 teaspoons of oil and let it shimmer. Add the chicken in a very single layer. Let it sear, then flip the pieces to the other side, about 4 minutes in whole.
4. Add the onion.
5. Pour inside water and scrape up any browned bits from your bottom in the pot.
6. Latch the lid. Select "Pressure Cook" or "Manual" as well as set pressure to high and cook for ten minutes. After some time finishes, allow ten minutes to naturally release the pressure. For any remaining pressure, just quick-release it. Open the lid. To serve, wrap the chicken inside lettuce leaves and serve with all the tzatziki sauce.

THAI GREEN CURRY

Nutrition: Cal 290 ;Fat 20 g; Carb 12 g;Protein 17 g
Serving 6 Cook time 10 min

Ingredients
- 1 tablespoon coconut oil
- 2 tablespoons Thai green curry paste (adjust in your preferred spice level)
- 1 tablespoon minced fresh ginger
- 1 tablespoon minced garlic
- ½ cup sliced onion
- 1-pound boneless, skinless chicken thighs
- 2 cups peeled, chopped eggplant
- 1 cup chopped green, yellow, or orange bell pepper
- ½ cup fresh basil leaves, preferably Thai basil
- 1½ cups unsweetened coconut milk
- 1 tablespoon fish sauce
- 2 tablespoons soy sauce
- 2 teaspoons Truvia or Swerve
- salt, to taste

Instructions
1. Select "Sauté" to preheat the Instant Pot and adapt to high heat. When the hot, add coconut oil and let it shimmer. Add the curry paste and cook for one to two minutes, stirring occasionally.
2. Add the ginger and garlic and stir-fry for a few seconds. Add the onion and stir all of it together.
3. Add the chicken, eggplant, bell pepper, basil, coconut milk, fish sauce, soy sauce, and Truvia or Swerve. Stir to blend.
4. Press "Cancel" to make off "Sauté" mode, and switch to "Slow Cook" mode. Adjust to cook for 8 hours on medium (not low).
5. When the curry has finished cooking, add salt to taste.

SWEET AND SPICY CHICKEN TINGA

Nutrition: Cal 260 ;Fat 16 g; Carb 9 g;Protein 24 g
Serving 6 Cook time 40 min

Ingredients
- 4 teaspoons vegetable oil
- 2 tomatillos, cut into thin slices
- ½ onion, cut into thin slices
- 3 garlic cloves
- 1 (0.9 lb.) can fire-roasted tomatoes
- ⅓ cup chicken broth
- 1 chipotle chile with adobo sauce coming from a can, chopped
- ½ teaspoon ground cumin
- ¼ teaspoon ground cinnamon
- ½ teaspoon dried oregano
- 1 teaspoon Truvia or Swerve
- 1 tablespoon fish sauce or soy sauce
- 1 tablespoon cider vinegar
- 1½ pounds boneless, skinless chicken thighs
- ½ cup sour cream
- 2 teaspoons fresh lemon juice
- 1 avocado, sliced

Instructions
1. Select "Sauté" to preheat the Instant Pot and accommodate high heat. When the hot, add oil and allow it shimmer.
2. Add the tomatillo slices inside a single layer and atart exercising . the onions as being a flat layer between your tomatillo slices. Nestle inside garlic cloves. You're gonna let them char, so not stir them.
3. Once the thinner slices start to look somewhat burned, flip the vegetables. The bottom of the pot may have large black spots where the vegetables have charred, but this is a great sign.
4. Once the vegetables are very well charred, add the tomatoes and broth and deglaze the pan, scraping up all of the lovely brown bits from the bottom. Do this very well and make certain there isn't any burned bits remaining around the bottom. Otherwise, your Instant Pot will not arrive at pressure.
5. Add the chipotle, cumin, cinnamon, oregano, sweetener, fish sauce, and vinegar. Cook for one to two minutes allowing the spices to bloom. Add the chicken.
6. Latch the lid. Select "Pressure Cook" or "Manual" as well as set pressure to high and cook for fifteen minutes. After the time finishes, allow 10 mins to naturally release pressure to succeed. For any remaining pressure, just quick-release it. Open the lid.
7. Remove the chicken and shred it.
8. Tilting the pot, readily immersion blender to purée the sauce until the mixture is smooth.
9. Turn the pot to "Sauté" and adapt to high heat; then cook to thicken the sauce for approximately ten minutes. Once it's thickened a little, add inside chicken and also heat.
10. While the chicken heats, make a crema inside a small bowl by mixing together the sour cream and lemon juice.
11. Top the chicken while using crema and avocado slices. Serve over cauliflower rice or wrapped in lettuce leaves to get a low-carb option. You can also use low-carb corn tortillas.

CHICKEN FAJITAS

Nutrition: Cal 322 ;Fat 6 g; Carb 12 g;Protein 4 5g
Serving 4 Cook time 30 min

Ingredients
- 1 lb. chicken white meat, chopped into bite-sized pieces
- 1 onion, finely chopped
- 1 tbsp lime juice
- 6 large leaves Iceberg lettuce
- 2 tbsps. homemade taco seasoning
- 1 cup cherry tomatoes, chopped
- 3 garlic cloves, minced
- 1 bell pepper, cut into strips

TACO SEASONING:
- 1 tbsp. smoked paprika
- ½ tsp. coriander powder
- ½ tsp. black pepper, freshly ground
- 3 tbsps. chili powder

- 1 tsp onion powder
- 2 tbsps. pink Himalayan salt
- 2 tsps. garlic powder
- 2 tsps. Oregano

Instructions

1. Ingredients for taco seasoning in a jar and shake well. Set aside.
2. Rinse the meat well and place in a deep bowl. Generously sprinkle with taco seasoning. Place in the pot and add tomatoes, garlic, sliced peppers, onions, and lime juice
3. Seal the lid and press the "Poultry" button. Set the timer for 8 minutes on underhand.
4. When done, perform a quick release and open the lid. Remove a combination in the pot and set in a bowl. Cool completely.
5. Spread about 2 - 3 tablespoons with the mixture at the center of every lettuce leaf and wrap tightly. Secure each wrap with a toothpick and serve immediately.
6. Cut the chicken into bite-size pieces. Add it back to the sauce.
7. Preheat the Instant Pot by selecting "Sauté" and adjust to less for low heat. Let the chicken heat through. Break it up into smaller pieces if you like, but don't shred it.
8. Serve over cauliflower rice or raw cucumber noodles.

SHORTCUT DAN DAN–STYLE CHICKEN

Nutrition: Cal 300 ;Fat 17 g; Carb 10 g;Protein 26 g
Serving 4 Cook time 15 min

Ingredients

- 2 tablespoons extra virgin olive oil
- 1 tablespoon doubanjiang
- 2 teaspoons soy sauce
- 2 teaspoons rice wine vinegar
- ½ to 2 teaspoons red pepper flakes
- 1 teaspoon ground Sichuan peppercorns
- ¼ cup warm water
- 1-pound boneless, skinless chicken, cut into bite-size pieces
- ¼ cup room-temperature water
- 1 (½ pound) package shirataki noodles, rinsed
- 1 tablespoon sesame oil
- ¼ cup chopped fresh cilantro (optional) 2 tablespoons extra virgin olive oil
- 1 tablespoon doubanjiang
- 2 teaspoons soy sauce
- 2 teaspoons rice wine vinegar
- ½ to 2 teaspoons red pepper flakes
- 1 teaspoon ground Sichuan peppercorns
- ¼ cup warm water
- 1-pound boneless, skinless chicken, cut into bite-size pieces
- ¼ cup room-temperature water
- 1 (½ pound) package shirataki noodles, rinsed
- 1 tablespoon sesame oil
- ¼ cup chopped fresh cilantro (optional)

Instructions

1. In a medium bowl, mix together the olive oil, doubanjiang, soy sauce, vinegar, red pepper flakes, peppercorns, and hot water.
2. Put the chicken in the bowl and mix, so the chicken is well coated. For the best results, permit the chicken marinate for 30 minutes.
3. Put the chicken and marinade inside the inner cooking pot. Pour inside room-temperature water.
4. Latch the lid. Select "Pressure Cook" or "Manual" and set pressure to high and cook for 7 minutes. After the time finishes, allow 10 minutes to naturally release pressure. For any remaining pressure, just quick-release it. Open the lid. While the chicken is cooking, prepare the shirataki noodles as outlined by the package instructions.
5. Mix the chicken while using noodles. Just before serving, stir within the sesame oil. Serve garnished using the peanuts and cilantro (if using).

CHICKEN BRATWURST MEATBALLS WITH CABBAGE

Nutrition: Cal 338 ;Fat 23 g; Carb 10 g;Protein 23 g
Serving 4 Cook time 20 min

Ingredients

- 1-pound ground chicken
- ¼ cup heavy (whipping) cream
- 2 teaspoons salt, divided
- ½ teaspoon ground caraway seeds
- 1½ teaspoons freshly ground black pepper, divided
- ¼ teaspoon ground allspice
- 4 to 6 cups thickly chopped green cabbage
- 2 tablespoons unsalted butter

Instructions

1. To make meatballs, place the chicken in the bowl. Add the cream, 1 teaspoon of salt, the caraway, ½ teaspoon of pepper, as well as the allspice. Mix thoroughly. Refrigerate a combination for a half-hour. Once the amalgamation has cooled, it is simpler to make up the meatballs.
2. Using a tiny scoop, make up the chicken mixture into small-to medium-size meatballs. Place half the meatballs inside inner cooking pot of the Instant Pot and cover them half the cabbage. Place the remaining meatballs at the top from the cabbage, then cover them while using rest of the cabbage.
3. Place pats from the butter randomly and sprinkle with all the remaining 1 teaspoon of salt and 1 teaspoon of pepper.
4. Latch the lid. Select "Pressure Cook" or "Manual" as well as set pressure to high and cook for 4 minutes. After time finishes, allow 10 mins to naturally release the stress. For any remaining pressure, just quick-release it. Open the lid. Serve the meatballs ahead in the cabbage.

CHICKEN LIVER PTÉ

Nutrition: Cal 109 ;Fat 7 g; Carb 5 g;Protein 10 g
Serving 8 Cook time 15 min

Ingredients
- 1 lb. chicken liver
- ½ cup leeks, chopped
- 2 garlic cloves, crushed
- 2 tablespoons essential olive oil
- 1 tablespoon poultry seasonings
- 1 teaspoon dried rosemary
- ½ teaspoon dried marjoram
- ¼ teaspoon dried dill weed
- ½ teaspoon paprika
- ½ teaspoon red pepper flakes
- salt, to taste
- ½ teaspoon ground black pepper
- 1 cup water
- 1 tablespoon stone ground mustard

Instructions
1. Press the "Sauté" button to warm up the Instant Pot. Now, heat the oil. Once hot, sauté the chicken livers until no longer pink.
2. Add the rest of the
3. Ingredients, apart from the mustard, for a Instant Pot.
4. Secure the lid. Choose the "Manual" setting and cook for 10 minutes at High pressure. Once cooking is complete, work with a quick pressure elease; carefully remove the lid.
5. Transfer the cooked mixture to some blender; add stone ground mustard. Process until smooth and uniform.

Roasted Turkey Breast with Mushrooms & Brussels Sprouts

Nutrition: Cal 210;Fat 9 g; Carb 6 g;Protein 27 g
Serving 4; Cook time 50 min

Ingredients
- 2 tbsp olive oil
- 1 tsp salt
- 1 tsp black pepper
- 1 tsp garlic powder
- 1 pound turkey breast raw, cut into 1 inch cubes
- 1/2 pound brussels sprouts cleaned, cut in half
- 1 cups mushrooms cleaned

Instructions
1. Preheat oven to 350 degrees Fahrenheit.
2. In a small mixing bowl, combine olive oil, salt, black pepper, and garlic powder.
3. In a 9 x 6-inch casserole dish, combine turkey, brussels sprouts, and mushrooms. Pour the olive oil mixture over the top.
4. Cover with foil and bake for 45 minutes or until the turkey is cooked through and no longer pink. An internal temperature of 165 degrees Fahrenheit is a safe bet.

Turkey and Bacon Lettuce Wraps

Nutrition: Cal 305;Fat 20 g; Carb 22 g;Protein 11 g
Serving 4; Cook time 15 min

Ingredients
Wraps
- 1 head iceberg lettuce
- 4 slices deli turkey
- 4 slices bacon cooked
- 1 avocado thinly sliced
- 1 roma tomato thinly sliced
- 1 cucumber thinly sliced
- 1 carrot thinly sliced

Basil Mayo
- 1/2 cup mayo
- 6 basil leaves chopped
- 1 tsp lemon juice
- 1 garlic clove minced
- salt and pepper to taste

Instructions
Basil Mayo
1. Combine all of the ingredients in a food processor, blend until smooth

Wraps
2. Lay out two large lettuce leaves then layer on 1 slice of turkey and slather with Basil-Mayo.
3. Layer on a second slice of turkey followed by the bacon, and a few slices of avocado, tomato, cucumber and carrot.
4. Season lightly with salt and pepper then fold the bottom up, the sides in, and roll like a burrito.
5. Slice in half and serve cold.

Chiken Stir-Fry

Nutrition: Cal 312;Fat 14 g; Carb 11 g;Protein 31 g
Serving 4; Cook time 40 min

Ingredients
- 3 boneless, skinless chicken breasts, trimmed and cut into pieces at least 1 inch square
- 2 red bell peppers
- 2 cups sugar snap peas
- 1 1/2 T peanut oil
- 1-2 T sesame seeds, preferably black

Marinade ingredients:
- 1/3 cup soy sauce (gluten-free if needed)
- 2 T unseasoned (unsweetened) rice vinegar
- 2 T low-carb sweetener of your choice (see notes)
- 1 T sesame oil
- 1/2 tsp. garlic powder

Instructions
1. Trim the chicken breasts and cut into pieces at least 1 inch square.
2. Combine soy sauce, rice vinegar, Stevia, agave or maple syrup, sesame oil and garlic powder.
3. Put the chicken into a Ziploc bag and pour in HALF the marinade. Let chicken marinate in the fridge for at least 4 hours (or all day while you're at work would be even better.)
4. When you're ready to cook, cover a large baking sheet with foil, then put it in the oven and let the pan get hot while the oven heats to 425F/220C.
5. Drain the marinated chicken well in a colander placed in the sink.

6. Remove the hot baking sheet from the oven and spread the chicken out over the surface (so pieces are not touching). Put baking sheet into the oven and cook chicken 8 minutes.
7. While the chicken cooks, trim ends of the sugar snap peas. Cut out the core and seeds of the red bell peppers and discard; then cut peppers into strips about the same thickness as the sugar snap peas.
8. Put veggies into a bowl and toss with the peanut oil.
9. After 8 minutes, remove pan from the oven and arrange the veggies around the chicken, trying to have each vegetable piece touching the pan as much as you can.
10. Put back into the oven and cook about **11** minutes more, or until the chicken is cooked through and lightly browned.
11. Brush cooked chicken and vegetables with the remaining marinade and sprinkle with black sesame seeds. Serve hot.

Garlic, Lemon & Thyme Roasted Chicken Breasts
Nutrition: Cal 230;Fat 27 g; Carb 4 g;Protein 26 g
Serving 4; Cook time 2 hours 45 min

Ingredients
- 4 boneless skinless chicken breasts
- zest of 1 lemon
- juice of 1 lemon
- 1/2 cup extra virgin olive oil
- 4 cloves garlic minced
- 1 tablespoon fresh thyme
- 1 teaspoon salt
- 1/2 teaspoon ground black pepper
- 1 tablespoon olive oil for sauteing

Instructions
1. Create the marinade by mixing the lemon juice, zest, 1/2 cup of olive oil, garlic, thyme, salt, and pepper. Place the chicken breasts in a non-reactive glass dish, or plastic ziptop bag, and pour the marinade over the chicken. Make sure to evenly coat the chicken, then cover and refrigerate for 2 hours.
2. Preheat your oven to 400 degrees F. Remove the chicken from the marinade and wipe off the excess. Heat 1 tablespoon of olive oil, and sear the chicken breasts for 2 minutes on each side, until they're golden brown.
3. Place the chicken breasts on a baking sheet lined with a baking rack, and roast at 400 degrees F for 20-30 minutes depending on the thickness of the chicken breast, or until the internal temperature reads 165 degrees F.

Grilled Chicken Kabobs
Nutrition: Cal 278;Fat 12 g; Carb 26 g;Protein 27 g
Serving 2; Cook time 30 min

Ingredients
- 0.5 pound boneless skinless chicken breasts cut into 1 inch pieces
- 0.13 cup olive oil
- 0.17 cup soy sauce
- 0.13 cup honey

- 0.5 teaspoon minced garlic
- salt and pepper to taste
- 0.5 red bell pepper cut into 1 inch pieces
- 0.5 yellow bell pepper cut into 1 inch pieces
- 1 small zucchini cut into 1 inch slices
- 0.5 red onion cut into 1 inch pieces
- 0.5 tablespoon chopped parsley

Instructions
1. Place the olive oil, soy sauce, honey, garlic and salt and pepper in a large bowl.
2. Whisk to combine.
3. Add the chicken, bell peppers, zucchini and red onion to the bowl. Toss to coat in the marinade.
4. Cover and refrigerate for at least 1 hour, or up to 8 hours.
5. Soak wooden skewers in cold water for at least 30 minutes. Preheat grill or grill pan to medium high heat.
6. Thread the chicken and vegetables onto the skewers.
7. Cook for 5-7 minutes on each side or until chicken is cooked through.
8. Sprinkle with parsley and serve.

Chicken Cordon Bleu with Cauliflower
Nutrition: Cal 420;Fat 24 g; Carb 7 g;Protein 45 g
Serving 4; Cook time 55 min

Ingredients
- 4 boneless chicken breast halves (about 12 ounces)
- 4 slices deli ham
- 4 slices Swiss cheese
- 1 large egg, whisked well
- 2 ounces pork rinds
- ¼ cup almond flour
- ¼ cup grated parmesan cheese
- ½ teaspoon garlic powder
- Salt and pepper
- 2 cups cauliflower florets

Instructions
1. Preheat the oven to 350°F and line a baking sheet with foil.
2. Sandwich the chicken breast halves between pieces of parchment and
pound flat.
3. Lay the pieces out and top with sliced ham and cheese.
4. Roll the chicken up around the fillings then dip in the beaten egg.
5. Combine the pork rinds, almond flour, parmesan, garlic powder, salt and pepper in a food processor and pulse into fine crumbs.
6. Roll the chicken rolls in the pork rind mixture then place on the baking sheet.
7. Toss the cauliflower with melted butter then add to the baking sheet.
Bake for 45 minutes until the chicken is cooked through.

Chicken Tikka with Cauliflower Rice
Nutrition: Cal 350;Fat 21 g; Carb 8 g;Protein 35 g
Serving 4; Cook time 15 min

Ingredients
- 2 pounds boneless chicken thighs, chopped
- 1 cup canned coconut milk
- 1 cup heavy cream
- 3 tablespoons tomato paste
- 2 tablespoons garam masala
- 1 tablespoon fresh grated ginger
- 1 tablespoon minced garlic
- 1 tablespoon smoked paprika
- 2 teaspoons onion powder
- 1 teaspoon guar gum
- 1 tablespoon butter
- 1 ½ cup riced cauliflower

Instructions
1. Spread the chicken in a slow cooker, then stir in the remaining ingredients except for the cauliflower and butter.
2. Cover and cook on low heat for 6 hours until the chicken is done and the sauce thickened.
3. Melt the butter in a saucepan over medium-high heat.
4. Add the riced cauliflower and cook for 6 to 8 minutes until tender.
5. Serve the chicken tikka with the cauliflower rice.

Sesame Wings with Cauliflower
Nutrition: Cal 400;Fat 28,5 g; Carb 4 g;Protein 31 g
Serving 4; Cook time 35 min

Ingredients
- 2 ½ tablespoons soy sauce
- 2 tablespoons sesame oil
- 1 ½ teaspoons balsamic vinegar
- 1 teaspoon minced garlic
- 1 teaspoon grated ginger
- Salt
- 1 pound chicken wing, the wings itself
- 2 cups cauliflower florets

Instructions
1. Combine the soy sauce, sesame oil, balsamic vinegar, garlic, ginger, and salt in a freezer bag, then add the chicken wings.
2. Toss to coat, then chill for 2 to 3 hours.
3. Preheat the oven to 400°F and line a baking sheet with foil.
4. Spread the wings on the baking sheet along with the cauliflower.
5. Bake for 35 minutes, then sprinkle with sesame seeds to serve.

Spicy Chicken Enchilada Casserole
Nutrition: Cal 550;Fat 31 g; Carb 12 g;Protein 54 g
Serving 6; Cook time 1 hour 15 min

Ingredients
- 2 pounds boneless chicken thighs, chopped
- Salt and pepper
- 3 cups tomato salsa
- 1 ½ cups shredded cheddar cheese
- ¾ cup sour cream
- 1 cup diced avocado

Instructions
1. Preheat the oven to 375°F and grease a casserole dish.
2. Season the chicken with salt and pepper then spread into the dish.
3. Spread the salsa over the chicken and sprinkle with cheese.
4. Cover with foil, then bake for 60 minutes until the chicken is done.
5. Serve with sour cream and chopped avocado.

White Cheddar Broccoli Chicken Casserole
Nutrition: Cal 435;Fat 32 g; Carb 6 g;Protein 29 g
Serving 6; Cook time 45 min

Ingredients
- 2 tablespoons olive oil
- 1 pound boneless chicken thighs, chopped
- 1 medium yellow onion, chopped
- 1 clove garlic, minced
- 1 ½ cups chicken broth
- 8 ounces cream cheese, softened
- ¼ cup sour cream
- 2 ½ cups broccoli florets
- ¾ cup shredded white cheddar cheese

Instructions
1. Preheat the oven to 350°F and grease a casserole dish.
2. Heat the oil in a large skillet over medium-high heat.
3. Add the chicken and cook for 2 to 3 minutes on each side to brown.
4. Stir in the onion and garlic, and season with salt and pepper.
5. Sauté for 4 to 5 minutes until the chicken is cooked through.
6. Pour in the chicken broth, then add the cream cheese and sour cream.
7. Simmer until the cream cheese is melted, then stir in the broccoli.
8. Spread the mixture in the casserole dish and sprinkle with cheese.
9. Bake for 25 to 30 minutes until hot and bubbling

Lemon Chicken Kebabs with Veggies
Nutrition: Cal 360;Fat 21,5 g; Carb 8 g;Protein 34 g
Serving 4; Cook time 25 min

Ingredients
- 1 pound boneless chicken thighs, cut into cubes
- ¼ cup olive oil
- 2 tablespoons lemon juice
- 1 teaspoon minced garlic
- Salt and pepper
- 1 large yellow onion, cut into 2-inch chunks
- 1 large red pepper, cut into 2-inch chunks
- 1 large green pepper, cut into 2-inch chunks

Instructions
1. Toss the chicken with the olive oil, lemon juice, garlic, salt, and pepper.
2. Slide the chicken onto skewers with the onion and peppers.
3. Preheat a grill to medium-high heat and oil the grates.

4. Grill the skewers for 2 to 3 minutes on each side until the chicken is done.

Lemon ButTer Chicken

Nutrition: Cal 300;Fat 26 g; Carb 4 g;Protein 12 g
Serving 4; Cook time 50 min

Ingredients

- 4 bone-in, skin-on chicken thighs
- Sea salt
- Freshly ground black pepper
- 2 tablespoons butter, divided
- 2 teaspoons minced garlic
- ½ cup chicken stock
- ½ cup heavy (whipping) cream
- Juice of ½ lemon

Instructions

1. Preheat the oven to 400°F.
2. Lightly season the chicken thighs with salt and pepper.
3. Place a large ovenproof skillet over medium-high heat and add 1 tablespoon of buter.
4. Brown the chicken thighs until golden on both sides, about 6 minutes in total. Remove the thighs to a plate and set aside.
5. Add the remaining 1 tablespoon of buter and sauté the garlic until translucent, about 2 minutes.
6. Whisk in the chicken stock, heavy cream, and lemon juice.
7. Bring the sauce to a boil and then return the chicken to the skillet.
8. Place the skillet in the oven, covered, and braise until the chicken is cooked through, about 30 minutes

Chicken Bacon Burgers

Nutrition: Cal 375;Fat 33 g; Carb 3 g;Protein 18 g
Serving 6; Cook time 25 min

Ingredients

- 1 pound ground chicken
- 8 bacon slices, chopped
- ¼ cup ground almonds
- 1 teaspoon chopped fresh basil
- ¼ teaspoon sea salt
- Pinch freshly ground black pepper
- 2 tablespoons coconut oil
- 4 large lettuce leaves
- 1 avocado, peeled, pitted, and sliced

Instructions

1. Preheat the oven to 350°F. Line a baking sheet with parchment paper and set aside.
2. In a medium bowl, combine the chicken, bacon, ground almonds, basil, salt, and pepper until well mixed.
3. Form the mixture into 6 equal paties.
4. Place a large skillet over medium-high heat and add the coconut oil.
5. Pan sear the chicken paties until brown on both sides, about 6 minutes in total.
6. Place the browned paties on the baking sheet and bake until completely cooked through, about 15 minutes.

7. Serve on the letuce leaves, topped with the avocado slices.

Paprika Chicken

Nutrition: Cal 390;Fat 30 g; Carb 4 g;Protein 25 g
Serving 4; Cook time 35 min

Ingredients

- 4 (4-ounce) chicken breasts, skin-on
- Sea salt
- Freshly ground black pepper
- 1 tablespoon olive oil
- ½ cup chopped sweet onion
- ½ cup heavy (whipping) cream
- 2 teaspoons smoked paprika
- ½ cup sour cream
- 2 tablespoons chopped fresh Parsley

Instructions

1. Lightly season the chicken with salt and pepper.
2. Place a large skillet over medium-high heat and add the olive oil.
3. Sear the chicken on both sides until almost cooked through, about 15 minutes in total. Remove the chicken to a plate.
4. Add the onion to the skillet and sauté until tender, about 4 minutes.
5. Stir in the cream and paprika and bring the liquid to a simmer.
6. Return the chicken and any accumulated juices to the skillet and simmer the chicken for 5 minutes until completely cooked.
7. Stir in the sour cream and remove the skillet from the heat.
8. Serve topped with the parsley

StufFed Chicken Breasts

Nutrition: Cal 390;Fat 30 g; Carb 3 g;Protein 25 g
Serving 4; Cook time 30 min

Ingredients

- 1 tablespoon butter
- ¼ cup chopped sweet onion
- ½ cup goat cheese, at room temperature
- ¼ cup Kalamata olives, chopped
- ¼ cup chopped roasted red pepper
- 2 tablespoons chopped fresh basil
- 4 (5-ounce) chicken breasts, skin-on
- 2 tablespoons extra-virgin olive oil

Instructions

1. Preheat the oven to 400°F.
2. In a small skillet over medium heat, melt the buter and add the onion. Sauté until tender, about 3 minutes.
3. Transfer the onion to a medium bowl and add the cheese, olives, red pepper, and basil. Stir until well blended, then refrigerate for about 30 minutes.
4. Cut horizontal pockets into each chicken breast, and stuf them evenly with the filling. Secure the two sides of each breast with toothpicks.
5. Place a large ovenproof skillet over medium-high heat and add the olive oil.

6.Brown the chicken on both sides, about 10 minutes in total.

7.Place the skillet in the oven and roast until the chicken is just cooked through, about 15 minutes. Remove the toothpicks and serve.

7.Transfer the paties to the baking sheet and bake them until cooked through, flipping them once, about 15 minutes in total.

Turkey Meatloaf

Nutrition: Cal 216;Fat 20 g; Carb 1 g;Protein 15 g
Serving 6; Cook time 35 min

Ingredients

•1 tablespoon olive oil

•½ sweet onion, chopped

•1&½ pounds ground turkey

•⅓ cup heavy (whipping) cream

•¼ cup freshly grated Parmesan cheese

•1 tablespoon chopped fresh parsley

•Pinch sea salt

•Pinch freshly ground black pepper

Instructions

1.Heat the oven to 450°F.

2.Place a small skillet over medium heat and add the olive oil.

3.Sauté the onion until it is tender, about 4 minutes.

4.Transfer the onion to a large bowl and add the turkey, heavy cream,

5.Parmesan cheese, parsley, salt, and pepper.

6.Stir until the ingredients are combined and hold together. Press the mixture into a loaf pan.

7.Bake until cooked through, about 30 minutes.

8.Let the meatloaf rest for 10 minutes and serve.

Turkey RisSoles

Nutrition: Cal 440;Fat 34 g; Carb 7 g;Protein 27 g
Serving 4; Cook time 35 min

Ingredients

•1 pound ground turkey

•1 scallion, white and green parts,

•finely chopped

•1 teaspoon minced garlic

•Pinch sea salt

•Pinch freshly ground black pepper

•1 cup ground almonds

•2 tablespoons olive oil

Instructions

1.Preheat the oven to 350°F. Line a baking sheet with aluminum foil and set aside.

2.In a medium bowl, mix together the turkey, scallion, garlic, salt, and pepper until well combined.

3.Shape the turkey mixture into 8 paties and flaten them out.

4.Place the ground almonds in a shallow bowl and dredge the turkey paties in the ground almonds to coat.

5.Place a large skillet over medium heat and add the olive oil.

6.Brown the turkey paties on both sides, about 10 minutes in total.

Beef and Lamb

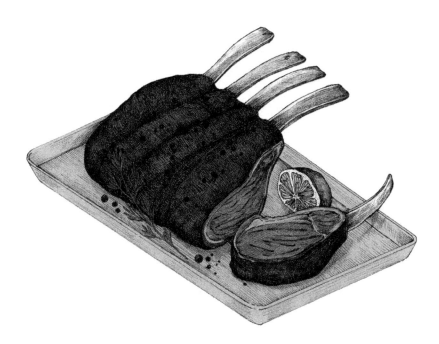

BLUE CHEESE BACON BURGERS

Nutrition: Cal 772;Fat 54g;Carb 6g;Protein61 g
Serving 4; Cook time 20 min

Ingredients

- 1½ pounds ground beef
- 4 slices Perfectly Cooked Bacon , crumbled
- ½ cup crumbled blue cheese
- 1 tablespoon Worcestershire sauce
- 2 large eggs
- Salt
- Freshly ground black pepper
- 1 romaine lettuce head, chopped
- 1 avocado, chopped
- 1 cup grape tomatoes

Instructions

1. In a large mixing bowl, combine the beef, bacon, blue cheese, Worcestershire sauce, and eggs. Season with salt and pepper. Use your hands to shape 4 patties. Cover with plastic and refrigerate for 30 minutes to 2 hours.
2. Heat the grill or broiler on high and cook for 4 to 5 minutes on each side, or until the burgers are cooked to your liking. Remove from the grill and let cool.
3. Into each of 4 storage containers, divide the lettuce, avocado, and tomatoes, and top with a burger patty.

FAJITA SALAD

Nutrition: Cal 893;Fat 60g;Carb 17g;Protein70 g
Serving 4; Cook time 30 min

Ingredients

FOR THE STEAK

- 1 (2-pound) flank steak
- ¼ cup extra-virgin olive oil
- 1 teaspoon garlic powder
- 1 teaspoon onion powder
- 1 teaspoon ground cumin
- Juice of 1 lime
- 1 bunch cilantro, leaves chopped
- Salt
- Freshly ground black pepper

FOR THE SALAD

- 2 tablespoons extra-virgin olive oil or coconut oil
- 1 yellow onion, sliced
- 1 green bell pepper, sliced
- 1 red bell pepper, sliced
- 6 cups chopped romaine lettuce
- ½ cup sour cream
- ½ cup shredded Cheddar cheese
- 2 limes, quartered
- 1 avocado

Instructions

1. In a large resealable bag, add the flank steak, oil, garlic powder, onion powder, cumin, lime juice, cilantro, salt, and pepper. Marinate for 30 minutes to 24 hours.

2. When ready to cook, turn the broiler on high and remove the flank steak from the marinade, discarding the remaining marinade. Place the steak on a baking sheet and bake for 3 to 5 minutes on each side. Let rest for 10 minutes before thinly slicing against the grain.

TO MAKE THE SALAD

1. Heat a large skillet over medium heat and combine the oil, onion, and peppers. Stir often and cook until the onion becomes translucent, 8 to 10 minutes.
2. Into each of 4 divided storage containers, place the steak, peppers, and onions in one side, and the lettuce, sour cream, cheese, and lime wedges in the other side. Before enjoying an individual serving, halve, pit, and chop an avocado. Top the steak with ¼ of the chopped avocado, along with the lettuce, sour cream, and cheese. Squeeze the lime juice over everything and mix.
3. the lettuce around it.

GROUND BEEF AND CABBAGE STIR-FRY

Nutrition: Cal 550;Fat 33g;Carb 13g;Protein49 g
Serving 4; Cook time 35 min

Ingredients

- 1 tablespoon coconut oil
- 1½ pounds ground beef
- 2 garlic cloves, minced
- 1 green cabbage head, cored and chopped
- 2 tablespoons coconut aminos
- 2 tablespoons apple cider vinegar
- Salt
- Freshly ground black pepper
- 4 scallions, both white and green parts, chopped
- Sesame seeds (optional)
- Sriracha (optional)
- Toasted sesame oil (optional)

Instructions

1. In a large skillet, heat the oil over medium heat. Cook the beef and garlic until the beef is browned, 5 to 7 minutes.
2. Add the cabbage to the skillet and continue to cook until the cabbage becomes slightly wilted, 8 to 10 minutes.
3. Add the coconut aminos and vinegar and season with salt and pepper.

Bacon Cheeseburger Soup

Nutrition: Cal 315;Fat 20g;Carb 6g;Protein 27g
Serving 4; Cook time 25 min

Ingredients:

- 4 slices uncooked bacon
- 8 ounces ground beef (80% lean)
- 1 medium yellow onion, chopped
- 1 clove garlic, minced
- 3 cups beef broth
- 2 tablespoons tomato paste
- 2 teaspoons Dijon mustard
- Salt and pepper
- 1 cup shredded lettuce
- ½ cup shredded cheddar cheese

Instructions:

4. Cook the bacon in a saucepan until crisp then drain on paper towels and chop.
5. Reheat the bacon fat in the saucepan and add the beef.
6. Cook until the beef is browned, then drain away half the fat.
7. Reheat the saucepan and add the onion and garlic – cook for 6 minutes.
8. Stir in the broth, tomato paste, and mustard then season with salt and
9. pepper.
10. Add the beef and simmer on medium-low for 15 minutes, covered.
11. Spoon into bowls and top with shredded lettuce, cheddar cheese and bacon.

Taco Salad with Creamy Dressing
Nutrition: Cal 470;Fat 36g;Carb 7g;Protein 28g
Serving 2; Cook time 20 min

Ingredients:
• 6 ounces ground beef (80% lean)
• Salt and pepper
• 1 tablespoon ground cumin
• 1 tablespoon chili powder
• 4 cups fresh chopped lettuce
• ½ cup diced tomatoes
• ¼ cup diced red onion
• ¼ cup shredded cheddar cheese
• 3 tablespoons mayonnaise
• 1 teaspoon apple cider vinegar
• Pinch paprika

Instructions:
1. Cook the ground beef in a skillet over medium-high heat until browned.
2. Drain half the fat, then season with salt and pepper and stir in the taco seasoning.
3. Simmer for 5 minutes, then remove from heat.
4. Divide the lettuce between two salad bowls, then top with ground beef.
5. Add the diced tomatoes, red onion, and cheddar cheese.
6. Whisk together the remaining ingredients, then drizzle over the salads to serve.

Beef and Pepper Kebabs
Nutrition: Cal 365;Fat 21g;Carb 6.5g;Protein 35.5g
Serving 2; Cook time40 min

Ingredients:
• 2 tablespoons olive oil
• 1 ½ tablespoons balsamic vinegar
• 2 teaspoons Dijon mustard
• Salt and pepper
• 8 ounces beef sirloin, cut into 2-inch pieces
• 1 small red pepper, cut into chunks
• 1 small green pepper, cut into chunks

Instructions:
1. Whisk together the olive oil, balsamic vinegar, and mustard in a shallow dish.
2. Season the steak with salt and pepper, then toss in the marinade.

3. Let marinate for 30 minutes, then slide onto skewers with the peppers.
4. Preheat a grill pan to high heat and grease with cooking spray.
5. Cook the kebabs for 2 to 3 minutes on each side until the beef is done.

Bacon-Wrapped Hot Dogs
Nutrition: Cal 500;Fat 4g;Carb 3g;Protein 24g
Serving 2; Cook time40 min

Ingredients:
• 4 all-beef hot dogs
• 2 slices cheddar cheese
• 4 slices uncooked bacon

Instructions:
1. Slice the hotdogs lengthwise, cutting halfway through the thickness.
2. Cut the cheese slices in half and stuff one half into each hot dog.
3. Wrap the hotdogs in bacon then place them on a foil-lined roasting pan.
4. Bake for 30 minutes or until the bacon is crisp.

Slow-Cooker Beef Chili
Nutrition: Cal 395; Fat 20g; Carb 12g; Protein 42g
Serving 4; Cook time 6 hours

Ingredients:
• 1 tablespoon coconut oil
• 1 medium yellow onion, chopped
• 3 cloves garlic, minced
• 1 pound ground beef (80% lean)
• 1 small red pepper, chopped
• 1 small green pepper, chopped
• 1 cup diced tomatoes
• 1 cup low-carb tomato sauce
• 1 tablespoon chili powder
• 2 teaspoons dried oregano
• 1 ½ teaspoons dried basil
• Salt and pepper
• ¾ cup shredded cheddar cheese
• ½ cup diced red onion

Instructions:
1. Heat the oil in a skillet over medium-high heat.
2. Add the onions and sauté for 4 minutes, then stir in the garlic and cook 1 minute.
3. Stir in the beef and cook until it is browned, then drain some of the fat.
4. Spoon the mixture into a slow cooker and add the spices.
5. Cover and cook on low heat for 5 to 6 hours, then spoon into bowls.
6. Serve with shredded cheddar and diced red onion.

Mexican Meatza
Nutrition. Cal 414;Fat 30g; Carb 2g;Protein 35g
Serving 4; Cook time 25 min

Ingredients
• 1 lb ground beef, lean
• 1/2 onion
• 1 egg

- 1 cup cauliflower, riced
- 2 teaspoons chili powder
- 1 teaspoon cumin
- 1 teaspoon salt
- 1/2 teaspoon pepper
- 1 teaspoon garlic powder
- 1/4 red onion, sliced thin
- 1 cup cheddar cheese, shredded
- 1/4 cup sweet pepper slices

Cilantro Crema (optional)
- 1/3 cup cilantro leaves, loosely packed
- 1/2 cup sour cream
- 1 tablespoon lime juice
- 1 clove garlic

Instructions

1. Preheat oven to 350°F.
2. Add onion to a food processor and pulse until finely chopped.
3. Place in a large bowl and then add cauliflower to food processor and pulse until it looks like grains of rice.
4. Add that to the large bowl along with meat, a beaten egg, chili powder, cumin, salt, pepper, and garlic powder.
5. Mix well and split meat into 4.
6. Take each piece and make into a very thin, round pizza-looking shell. Place on a sprayed cookie sheet. Continue with the rest of the meat mixture. May take 2 cookie sheets.
7. Bake for 20 minutes or until meat is cooked. (thickness of meat will affect cooking times. Try not to overcook.)
8. Take out of the oven, sprinkle cheese, and add onions and peppers on top.
9. Broil for 3 minutes or until cheese is melted.
10. Add avocado pieces onto each meatza, slice, and enjoy.
11. Note: You can use any topping you like such as tomatoes, lettuce, black olives, green onions, sour cream, hot sauce, etc.
12. Make crema.

Thai Beef Salad

Nutrition: Cal 350;Fat 18g; Carb 8g;Protein 27g
Serving 2; Cook time 15 min

Ingredients
Dressing
- 1 clove garlic
- 1 jalapeno, halved
- 1 lime, juiced
- 1 1/2 tablespoons fish sauce
- 2 tablespoons minced lemongrass (remove the tough outer leaves and slice the tender white core)
- 1 1/4 teaspoons brown sugar
- 1/4 teaspoon red chile flakes
Steak
- 1/2 tablespoon vegetable oil
- 1 1-inch thick New York strip steak, 9 to 10 ounces
- 2 medium shallots, thinly sliced
- 1/4 cup fresh mint leaves loosely packed, roughly chopped
- 3 tablespoons roughly chopped cilantro leaves and stems
Rice Powder

- 2 tablespoons uncooked rice

For Serving
- Lettuce of your choosing

Cherry tomatoes, halved

Instructions
Dressing

1. Mince the garlic and one of the chile halves and place in a small bowl. Slice the remaining chile half into thin rings and add it to the bowl, along with the lime juice, fish sauce, lemongrass, brown sugar, and red chile flakes. Taste and adjust seasonings with additional lime juice, fish sauce, sugar, if needed. Stir well and set aside.

Rice Powder

2. Put rice in a small frying pan over medium heat. Cook, stirring frequently, until the grains are toasted and golden, about 10 minutes. Let cool for a few minutes and then grind into a coarse powder in a spice grinder or with a mortar and pestle.

Steak

3. Heat the oil in a skillet over medium high heat. Sear the steak until it is well browned on one side, 5 to 6 min. Flip and cook until the second side is dark brown and the meat is medium rare, another 5 to 6 min. Transfer to a cutting board and let rest for 5 min. Slice the steak thinly and then cut into bite-size pieces.
4. In a medium bowl, combine the beef (and any accumulated juices), shallots, mint, and cilantro. Stir the dressing and pour it on top. Toss gently. Add the ground toasted rice, and toss.

Keto Asian Steak Salad

Nutrition: Cal 350;Fat 22g; Carb 6g;Protein 27g
Serving 2; Cook time 15 min

Ingredients
- 2 Ribeye Steaks
- 1/2 cup Soy sauce or coconut aminos divided
- For the asian sesame dressing
- 1/2 cup Olive oil
- 2 tbsp Soy sauce or coconut aminos
- 2 tbsp Apple Cider Vinegar
- 1 tsp Sesame Oil
- 1/8 tsp liquid stevia
- For assembling
- 4 cups Raw spinach
- 4 radishes sliced thin
- Sesame seeds for garnish

Instructions

1. Place each steak in a zip top bag with 1/4 cup of soy sauce. Zip up the bags and allow to marinate on the counter for 1 hour.
2. Remove the steaks from the bag and discard the marinade. In a cast iron skillet on high heat, cook the steaks to your desired doneness. I did 4 minutes on each side for medium.
3. Let the steaks rest for 10 minutes on a cutting board.
4. While the steaks are resting, make your dressing. Add all of the dressing ingredients to a jar with a lid and shake to combine.

5. Assemble the salads. Add 2 cups of spinach and half of the sliced radish to each of the 2 bowls. Slice the steaks into 1/2 in thick pieces and add those to the salads. Drizzle the dressing on top and garnish with sesame seeds.

Keto Mongolian Beef
Nutrition: Cal 350;Fat 14g; Carb 17g;Protein 30g
Serving 4; Cook time 25 min

Ingredients
- 1 Tablespoon avocado oil
- 2 teaspoons Minced ginger
- 1 Tablespoon Minced garlic
- 1/2 Cup Soy sauce or Coconut aminos
- 1/2 cup Water
- 3/4 cup Granulated sweetener
- 1 1/2 pounds Flank steak or Flatiron steak
- 1/4 teaspoon Red pepper flakes
- 5 Stems Green onions-cut diagonal into 2 inch pieces
- 1/4 teaspoon xanthan gum

Instructions
Making the sauce:
1. Heat 1 tablespoon Avocado Oil in a medium saucepan over medium heat.
2. Add ginger, garlic, red pepper flakes and stir for 30 seconds.
3. Add soy sauce, water and sweetener. Bring to a boil and simmer until thickened. Should take about 5 minutes.
4. Remove from skillet to a bowl and set aside.
5. For the Steak:
6. Slice flank steak against the grain into 1/4 inch slices with the knife held at a 45 degree angle. Some of the really long pieces I cut in half to make them more bite-sized.
7. Heat avocado oil in skillet over medium-high heat.
8. Add beef (may need to cook in 2 batches) and cook 2-3 minutes, until brown, flipping pieces over to cook both sides.
9. Add the sauce to the pan along with the xantham gum and cook over medium heat for a few minute, Stirring to coat meat.
10. Add green onions and remove from heat.

GROUND BEEF AND CABBAGE STIR-FRY
Nutrition: Cal 550;Fat 33 g;Carb 13 g;Protein 49 g
Serving 4; Cook time 35 min

Ingredients
- 1 tablespoon coconut oil
- 1½ pounds ground beef
- 2 garlic cloves, minced
- 1 green cabbage head, cored and chopped
- 2 tablespoons coconut aminos
- 2 tablespoons apple cider vinegar
- Salt
- Freshly ground black pepper
- 4 scallions, both white and green parts, chopped
- Sesame seeds (optional)
- Sriracha (optional)
- Toasted sesame oil (optional)

Instructions

1. In a large skillet, heat the oil over medium heat. Cook the beef and garlic until the beef is browned, 5 to 7 minutes.
2. Add the cabbage to the skillet and continue to cook until the cabbage becomes slightly wilted, 8 to 10 minutes.
3. Add the coconut aminos and vinegar and season with salt and pepper.

Keto Burrito Bowl
Nutrition: Cal 374;Fat 25 g; Carb 15 g;Protein 27 g
Serving 4; Cook time 20 min

Ingredients
- 1 cup Mexican Cauliflower Rice
- 1/2 cup Mexican Shredded Beef
- 1/4 cup Keto Guacamole
- 1/4 cup Pico de Gallo
- 1/4 cup shredded cheddar cheese
- 1 tablespoon chopped cilantro

Instructions
1. Arrange all of the ingredients in a shallow bowl and taste for seasoning.
2. Add salt and pepper or hot sauce, if desired.
3. Serve immediately.

EGG ROLL IN A BOWL
Nutrition: Cal 331;Fat 23.5 g; Carb 5 g;Protein 25 g
Serving 4; Cook time 15 min

Ingredients
- 1 lb (16 ounces) ground pork or beef
- 1 teaspoon minced garlic
- 14 ounces shredded cabbage or coleslaw mix
- 1/4 cup low-sodium soy sauce (or liquid aminos)
- 1 teaspoon ground ginger
- 1 whole egg
- 2 teaspoons sriracha
- 1 tablespoon sesame oil
- 2 tablespoons sliced green onions

Instructions
1. In a large skillet, brown the pork or beef until no longer pink. Drain the meat if it's really wet. Add the garlic and sautee for 30 seconds. Add the cabbage/coleslaw, soy sauce, ginger, and sautee until desired tenderness. You can add a little water if you need more liquid to sautee the coleslaw down.
2. Make a well in the center of the skillet and add the egg. Scramble until done over low heat.
3. Stir in sriracha. Drizzle with sesame oil and sprinkle with green onions. Add additional soy sauce and sriracha if desired.

Keto Bacon Cheeseburger Wraps
Nutrition: Cal 267;Fat 20 g; Carb 4 g;Protein 19 g
Serving 4; Cook time 30 min

Ingredients
- 7 oz. bacon
- 4 oz. mushrooms, sliced

95

- 1½ lbs ground beef or ground turkey
- ½ tsp salt
- ¼ tsp pepper
- 1 cup (4 oz.) shredded cheddar cheese
- 1 butterhead lettuce, leaves separated and washed
- 8 (5 oz.) cherry tomatoes, sliced

Instructions

1. Add the bacon to a large skillet and cook over medium heat for about 15 minutes, or until crispy. Remove the bacon from the pan and set aside.
2. Over medium-high heat, sauté the mushrooms in the bacon fat, for about 5 to 7 minutes, or until browned and tender. Set aside.
3. Add the ground beef, salt, and pepper. Sauté the beef (breaking up any chunks with the back of a wooden spoon) for about 10 minutes, or until evenly browned. For serving, spoon the ground beef onto the lettuce leaves and layer the cheddar cheese, bacon, mushrooms, and tomatoes on top.

MEATBALLS IN TOMATO SAUCE
Nutrition: Cal 388;Fat 27 g; Carb 11 g;Protein 23 g
Serving 8; Cook time 25 min

Ingredients
For meatballs
- Ground beef (2 lbs)
- Eggs (2)
- Garlic (3 cloves)
- Oregano (dry, 2 teaspoons)
- Salt (1 along with a half teaspoon)
- Pepper (1 teaspoon)
- Onion powder (2 teaspoons)

For the tomato sauce
- Coconut oil (2 teaspoons)
- Garlic (2 cloves)
- Tomatoes (grated or blended, around 30 oz.)
- Onion (1, chopped)
- Water (¼ cup)
- Tomato paste (2 tbsp)
- Salt (2 teaspoons)

Instructions
1. Mix the meatball
2. Ingredients and roll the meat in small balls.
3. Set the pressure cooker to "Sauté" and pour inside the coconut oil (it's ok to make use of avocado oil at the same time).
4. The garlic and onion come next and must be cooked for 5 minutes with occasional stirring (before the onion is tender).
5. Press Cancel and adding the lake, grated tomatoes, tomato paste, and salt. Put within the meatballs, stir everything together (the meatballs ought to be well covered with tomato sauce).
6. Close pressure cooker and seal the pressure valve; place it to "Manual" and cook the meatballs for 7 minutes.
7. When the cooking is complete, release pressure naturally for 10 minutes.
8. Serve the meatballs with pasta, vegetables, or alone.

BEEF STEW
Nutrition: Cal 310;Fat 14 g; Carb 26 g;Protein 3.8 g
Serving 6; Cook time 45 min

Ingredients
- Beef (16 oz)
- Beef broth (2 cups)
- Worchester Sauce (4 teaspoons)
- Butter (2 tbsp, unsalted)
- Brown sugar (2 teaspoons)
- Garlic (2 cloves)
- Soy sauce (1 tbsp)
- Onion (chopped, 1 cup)
- Carrots (chopped, 1 cup)
- Rosemary (1 teaspoon)
- Potatoes (2, chopped)

Instructions
1. Season the beef with salt and pepper.
2. Put the butter within the pressure cooker and set it to "Sauté" and permit the butter fully melt. Put the meat in the pot and cook on each side until it gets brown color.
3. Pour the beef broth and stir well; add the Worchester sauce, brown sugar, soy sauce, garlic, and rosemary.
4. Add the chopped potatoes and carrots in cubes. Add them along while using onion inside Pressure cooker and stir all the ingredients
5. Close the lid along with the steam valve. Set to "Meat/Stew" and let it cook for 35 minutes. Once the cooking is complete, release pressure to succeed naturally and allow it to cool.
6. Open the pot, stir the components, add salt and pepper by taste and serve hot.

POMEGRANATE MOLASSES ROASTED CHUCK
Nutrition: Cal 466 ;Fat 32 g; Carb 3 g;Protein 37 g
Serving 10; Cook time 55 min

Ingredients
- 3 lbs chuck steak, boneless
- 2 tsp salt
- 1 ½ tsp freshly grounded black pepper
- 1 ¼ tsp garlic powder
- 1 tbsp pomegranate molasses
- 2 tbsp balsamic vinegar
- 1 onion, finely chopped
- 2 cups regular water
- ½ tsp xanthan gum (it is possible to use 1 tsp of Agar Agar if unavailable)
- 1/3 cup fresh parsley, finely chopped

Instructions
1. On a cutting board, slice the meat in two and season each half, on each party with salt, pepper and garlic powder.
2. Place the Instant Pot over heat and hang up on "Sauté" mode.
3. Place the seasoned meat into the pot and cook until browned on both sides.

4. Once the meat has browned, start adding the remaining with the
5. Add the pomegranate molasses, balsamic vinegar, onion and half the water.
6. Cover the pot and hang up the timer on 35 minutes.
7. When enough time is finished, manually release pressure to succeed by pressing "venting".
8. Remove the lid once all the pressure may be released. Transfer the meat to some cutting board and remove any fat or refuse. Cut the meat into large slices.
9. Simmer the sauce that was left within the pot by setting the pot on "sauté". Allow it to simmer for ten mins before the liquid has reduced.
10. Stir within the xanthan gum and return the meat into the pot and stir.
11. Turn over heat and transfer the meat onto serving plate. Drizzle the sauce on the meat and garnish with parsley. Serve hot.

SPICY MINCED LAMB WITH PEAS AND TOMATO SAUCE
Nutrition: Cal 242 ;Fat 12 g; Carb 10 g;Protein 24 g
Serving 6; Cook time 55 min

Ingredients
- 2 lbs ground lamb
- 3 tbsp ghee
- 1 onion, finely chopped
- 5 cloves garlic, crushed
- 1 tsp ground ginger
- 1 Serrano pepper, chopped
- 2 tsp ground coriander
- 1 tsp red pepper flakes
- 1 tsp Kosher salt
- ½ tsp turmeric powder
- ¾ tsp freshly ground black pepper
- ½ tsp chat masala
- ¾ tsp ground cumin
- ¼ tsp cayenne powder
- 2 cardamom pods, shell removed
- 1 can diced tomatoes
- 1 can peas
- Fresh cilantro, finely chopped

Instructions
1. Place the Instant Pot over medium heat and set on "Sauté". Add the ghee and onion. Stir before onion is tender.
2. Stir inside ginger, garlic along with the spices. Stir for 3 minutes and then add the minced meat.
3. Stir the meat until browned and covered well using the spices.
4. Add in the tomatoes and peas and cover the pot. Set on "Keep Warm" then choose "Bean/Chili" option.
5. When time is completed, release the pressure from your pot. Set back on 'Sauté' and allow the liquid to simmer for ten mins until reduced.
6. Transfer the meat into serving bowl and sprinkle fresh cilantro and serve hot.

ROASTED LAMB SHANKS WITH VEGETABLES
Nutrition: Cal 422 ;Fat 20 g; Carb 35 g;Protein 48 g
Serving 4; Cook time 65 min

Ingredients
- 4 lbs lamb shanks
- 2 tsp salt
- 1 tsp freshly ground black pepper
- 3 tbsp ghee
- 3 carrots, diced
- 3 celery stalks, sliced
- 1 large onion, diced
- 2 tbsp tomato paste
- 4 cloves garlic, minced
- 1 can diced tomatoes
- 1 1/3 cup bone broth
- 2 tsp fish sauce (optional)
- 1 ½ tbsp balsamic vinegar
- ½ cup fresh parsley, finely chopped

Instructions
1. Season the lamb with salt and pepper from either side.
2. Place the Instant Pot over medium heat and hang on "Sauté" , stir within the ghee until melted and add the meat. Stir until browned for a few minutes.
3. Transfer the meat to your plate and add the vegetables to the pot and sauté for some minutes. Season with many salt and pepper.
4. Add the tomato paste and garlic and stir for any minute. Return the meat to the pot and add the diced tomatoes.
5. Pour within the broth, fish sauce and vinegar.
6. Cover the pot and press "Cancel/Keep Warm". Manually set the timer for 45 minutes. Lower the temperature after the first 5 minutes.
7. When some time ends, release pressure.
8. Transfer the meat onto serving platter and pour the rest of the sauce within the meat. Garnish with fresh parsley and serve hot.

CLASSIC MEATLOAF STUFFED WITH MOZZARELLA
Nutrition: Cal 537 ;Fat 17 g; Carb 30 g;Protein 63 g
Serving 8; Cook time 45 min

Ingredients
- 3 lbs minced beef
- 2 cups bread crumbs
- 4 eggs
- 1 tsp salt
- 1 tsp freshly ground black pepper
- 1 tsp garlic powder
- 4 oz mozzarella cheese, sliced
- ¼ cup fresh basil, finely chopped
- 1 cup beef broth
- ¼ cup light brown sugar
- ½ cup ketchup
- 2 tbsp Dijon mustard
- 1 tbsp Worcestershire sauce

Instructions

1. In a large bowl combine the meat with the breadcrumbs. Add the eggs and season with salt, pepper and garlic powder. It is best to use both your hands to mix the components to insure that they're fully incorporated.
2. In a another bowl, whisk together the brown sugar, ketchup, mustard and Worcestershire sauce.
3. Place Instant Pot over medium heat, position the rack provided with the pot inside and pour inside broth.
4. Cut a big part of aluminum foil and put half with the meatloaf mixture. Flatten it out just a little bit. Line the mozzarella slices over meatloaf, sprinkle the basil. Place the opposite half with the meatloaf and press the sides to seal.
5. Carefully place the wrapped meatloaf inside the pot, for the rack.
6. Using a spoon, spread half from the brown sugar mixture around the meatloaf.
7. Cover the pot and manually set the timer on 30 minutes. Once enough time is completed, manually release the pressure and remove the lid.
8. Take the meatloaf out with the pot and allow it to cool a little to start with serving.

BARACOA-STYLE SHREDDED BEEF
Nutrition: Cal 435 ;Fat 31 g; Carb 4.5 g;Protein 31 g
Serving 12; Cook time 75 min

Ingredients
- 3 lbs minced beef
- 2 cups bread crumbs
- 4 eggs
- 1 tsp salt
- 1 tsp freshly ground black pepper
- 1 tsp garlic powder
- 4 oz mozzarella cheese, sliced
- ¼ cup fresh basil, finely chopped
- 1 cup beef broth
- ¼ cup light brown sugar
- ½ cup ketchup
- 2 tbsp Dijon mustard
- 1 tbsp Worcestershire sauce

Instructions
1. Trim any body fat off the meat then cut into 4 large pieces. Season with salt and pepper on either side.
2. Place the Instant Pot over medium heat, then one tablespoon of olive oil. Cook the meat until browned for a couple minutes. You will add the meat in to the pot in two batches.
3. Meanwhile, inside a food processor, blend together the onion, vinegar, lime juice, garlic, peppers, broth, cumin, cloves and tomato paste until smooth no lumps are normally found.
4. Pour inside the blended mixture on the meet and add the bay leaves.
5. Cover the pot as well as set on "Beef/Stew" for an hour.
6. Once time is finished, manually release the pressure and uncover the pot.
7. Transfer the meat onto a cutting board, using two forks start shredding the meat.

8. Discard the bay leaves and return the shredded meat in to the pot. Cover the pot and enable the meat to take a seat for 10 mins.
9. Serve the shredded meat like a filling for tortilla wraps, tacos or sandwiches with your favorite sauce.

BEEF SHAWARMA WITH TAHINI SAUCE
Nutrition: Cal 787 ;Fat 23 g; Carb 90 g;Protein 63 g
Serving 8; Cook time 45 min

Ingredients
- 2 lbs ground turkey
- 5 cups baby spinach leaves
- 1 cup ricotta
- 1 cup mozzarella cheese, grated
- 1 can crushed tomatoes
- 3 tsp dried oregano
- 2 tsp thyme
- 3 tbsp fresh parsley, finely chopped
- 1 tsp salt
- 1 tsp freshly ground black pepper
- 1 tsp onion powder
- 1 tsp garlic powder
- 8 lasagna sheets
- 3 cups water

Instructions
1. Trim the extra fat off of the chuck roast and sear the meat lengthwise. Make about 4 cuts. Place the crushed garlic cloves into each cut.
2. In a bowl mix together every one of the spices together. Add the balsamic vinegar and one tablespoon in the extra virgin olive oil.
3. Rub the spices mixture on the meat, make certain you cover the whole surface area.
4. Place the meat in a shallow dish and cover with cling film. position the meat inside fridge for about 8 hours or overnight.
5. Once the meat has rested inside the fridge, squeeze Instant Pot over medium heat as well as set on "Sauté". Add the rest of the olive oil and grill the meat for 8 minutes until browned on either side. Pour inside broth and cover the pot.
6. Set on "Beef/Stew" and invite it in order to cook with an hour.
7. Once the time is fully gone, release pressure to succeed and get rid of the lid. Stir inside the onion rings. Allow the meat to sit down inside pot, while using lid off for 5 minutes.
8. Transfer the meat in to a cutting board or possibly a plate and initiate slicing or shredding it into small pieces.
To serve, spread some tahini sauce into each pita bread, fill with shawarma and wrap. Enjoy these Arabian wraps with many French fries or pickles.

AVOCADO BEEF CHILI WITH COCONUT YO-GURT

Nutrition: Cal 366 ;Fat 8.5 g; Carb 90 g;Protein 55 g
Serving 8; Cook time 25 min

Ingredients
- 2 tbsp avocado oil
- 1 onion, finely chopped
- 1 red bell pepper, diced
- 1 tsp salt
- 3 tbsp tomato paste
- 5 garlic cloves, crushed
- 3 lbs ground beef
- 4 tsp chili powder
- 2 tsp dried oregano
- 2 tsp ground cumin
- ½ tsp red pepper flakes
- 1 can roasted diced tomatoes
- 1/3 cup bone broth
- 1 tbsp fish sauce
- 2 tsp apple cider vinegar
- 1 ripe avocado, cubed
- 2 scallion, sliced
- 1/3 cup fresh parsley
- ½ cup coconut yogurt
- 1 lime, cut into wedges

Instructions
1. Place the Instant Pot over medium heat and set on "Sauté". Heat the avocado oil and stir in the onions and pepper. Season with salt and stir for a couple of minutes until tender.
2. Add the tomato paste and crushed garlic.
3. Stir inside the ground beef, season with increased salt and mix using a wooden spoon for 6 minutes.
4. Season the meat with chili powder, oregano, cumin and red pepper flakes.
5. Drain the tomatoes and stir into the meat. Pour inside broth, fish sauce and vinegar.
6. Cover the pot as well as set "Pressure Cook" and manually set the time for quarter-hour.
7. When the time is fully gone, manually release the stress and get rid of the lid.
8. To serve, transfer the chili for a serving bowls, top with avocado, scallion and a dollop of coconut yogurt. Garnish with fresh parsley, serve with lime wedges.

SPARE RIBS WITH CURRY SAUCE

Nutrition: Cal 522 ;Fat 23 g; Carb 15 g;Protein 71 g
Serving 4; Cook time 45 min

Ingredients
- 3 lbs lamb spare ribs
- 2 tbsp salt, divided
- 2 tbsp freshly ground black pepper
- 2 tbsp curry powder, divided
- 3 tsp coconut oil
- 1 onion, pureed
- 4 ripe tomatoes, pureed
- 5 cloves garlic, crushed
- Juice of 1 lemon
- 1 bunch fresh cilantro, finely chopped
- 5 scallion, finely chopped

Instructions
1. Start by seasoning the ribs with one tablespoon of salt, pepper and curry powder.
2. Place the ribs in a very shallow dish and cover. Refrigerate overnight.
3. To cook the ribs, put the Instant Pot over medium heat. Melt the oil inside the pot and add in half the ribs. You would want to prepare them by 50 % batches so that you can be certain they're cooked evenly.
4. When the ribs have browned on each side, transfer these phones a plate and repeat with all the remaining half.
5. When the subsequent batch of ribs are browned, transfer these to home plate and stir within the crushed garlic and stir for half a moment. Add the pureed tomato and onion. Add the remainder salt and pepper, lemon juice and half the cilantro.
6. Bring the sauce to your boil and add the ribs back into the pot. Cover the pot and turn heat. Set the timer on 20 minutes. Once the time is finished, allow pressure to be released naturally.
7. To serve, transfer the ribs onto serving platter and garnish with scallion and cilantro, serve hot.

RED PEPPER FLAKES BEEF RIBS WITH RICE

Nutrition: Cal 537 ;Fat 24 g; Carb 7g;Protein 67g
Serving 6; Cook time 45 min

Ingredients
- 3 lbs beef short ribs, boneless
- 2 tbsp red pepper flakes
- 2 tsp salt
- 2 tbsp butter
- 1 onion, finely chopped
- 2 tbsp tomato paste
- 5 garlic cloves, minced
- 2/3 cup roasted tomato salsa (accessible in supermarkets)
- 2/3 cup beef broth
- 1 tsp fish sauce
- ½ tsp freshly ground black pepper
- 1 small bunch fresh cilantro, finely chopped

Instructions
1. On a cutting board, cut the meat into cubes or slices. Place the meat right into a bowl and add inside the red pepper flakes and salt.
2. Place the Instant Pot over medium heat, set on "Sauté" and melt the butter. Stir inside onion, keep stirring until it will become translucent.
3. Add the tomato paste, garlic and salsa. Stir for any minute.
4. Drop the meat in the pot, and pour within the broth and fish sauce and stir.
5. Cover the pot and hang up on "Keep Warm" and "Meat/Stew". You only need in order to smoke it for a half-hour.

6. Once some time ends, allow the stress to be removed naturally.
7. Meanwhile cook the rice according to the instructions for the package.
8. To serve, put the rice into serving bowl and top with meat, drizzle using the meat sauce and garnish with fresh cilantro.

SIMPLE CORNED BEEF

Nutrition: Cal 251 ;Fat 3 g; Carb 1g;Protein 7g
Serving 6; Cook time 75 min

Ingredients
- 4 pounds beef brisket
- 2 oranges, sliced
- 2 garlic cloves, minced
- 2 yellow onions, thinly sliced
- 11 ounces celery, thinly sliced
- 1 tbsp dill, dried
- 3 bay leaves
- 4 cinnamon sticks, cut into halves
- Salt and black pepper to taste
- 17 ounces water

Instructions
1. Put the beef in the bowl, add some water to hide, leave aside to soak for a few hours, drain and transfer for a instant pot.
2. Add celery, orange slices, onions, garlic, bay leaves, dill, cinnamon, dill, salt and pepper and 17 ounces water.
3. Stir, cover and cook on High for 50 minutes.
4. Release the pressure, leave beef aside to chill down for 5 minutes, transfer to a cutting board, slice and divide among plates.
5. Drizzle the juice and veggies through the pot over beef and serve.

BEEF BOURGUIGNON

Nutrition: Cal 442 ;Fat 17 g; Carb 16 g;Protein 39 g
Serving 6; Cook time 45 min

Ingredients
- 5 pounds round steak, cut into small cubes
- 2 carrots, sliced
- ½ cup beef stock
- 1 cup dry burgandy or merlot wine
- 3 bacon slices, chopped
- 8 ounces mushrooms, cut into quarters
- 2 tbsp white flour
- 12 pearl onions
- 2 garlic cloves, minced
- ¼ tsp basil, dried
- Salt and black pepper to taste

Instructions
1. Set your instant pot on Sauté mode, add bacon and brown it for 2 minutes.
2. Add beef pieces, stir and brown for 5 minutes.
3. Add flour and stir well.
4. Add salt, pepper, wine, stock, onions, garlic and basil, stir, cover and cook on High for 20 minutes.
5. Release pressure to succeed quickly, uncover your pot, add mushrooms and carrots, cover again and cook on High for 5 minutes more.
6. Release pressure to succeed again, spoon beef bourguignon onto plates and serve.

ASIAN BEEF CURRY

Nutrition: Cal 434 ;Fat 20 g; Carb 14 g;Protein 27 g
Serving 4; Cook time 30 min

Ingredients
- 2 pounds beef steak, cubed
- 2 tbsp extra virgin olive oil
- 3 potatoes, diced
- 1 tbsp wine mustard
- 2 and ½ tbsp curry powder
- 2 yellow onions, chopped
- 2 garlic cloves, minced
- 10 ounces canned coconut milk
- 2 tbsp tomato sauce
- Salt and black pepper to taste

Instructions
1. Set your instant pot on Sauté mode, add the oil and heat
2. Add onions and garlic, stir and cook for 4 minutes.
3. Add potatoes and mustard, stir and cook for 1 minute.
4. Add beef, stir and brown on the sides.
5. Add curry powder, salt and pepper, stir and cook for just two minutes.
6. Add coconut milk and tomato sauce, cover and cook on High for ten mins.
7. Release the pressure, serve and luxuriate in.

BORDEAUX POT ROAST

Nutrition: Cal 290 ;Fat 20 g; Carb 2 g;Protein 25 g
Serving 6; Cook time 70 min

Ingredients
- 3 pounds beef roast
- Salt and black pepper to taste
- 17 ounces beef stock
- 3 ounces red
- ½ tsp chicken salt
- ½ tsp smoked paprika
- 1 yellow onion, chopped
- 4 garlic cloves, minced
- 3 carrots, chopped
- 5 potatoes, chopped

Instructions
1. In a bowl, mix salt, pepper, chicken salt and paprika and stir.
2. Rub beef using this type of mixture and put roast inside your instant pot.
3. Add onion, garlic, stock and wine, toss to coat, cover and cook on High for 50 minutes.
4. Release the stress quickly, uncover, add carrots and potatoes, cover again and cook on High for ten minutes.
5. Release pressure again, uncover, transfer roast to some platter, drizzle cooking juices all over and serve with veggies privately.

BEEF HOT POT
Nutrition: Cal 221 ;Fat 5.3 g; Carb 13 g;Protein 23 g
Serving 4; Cook time 40 min

Ingredients
- 2 tbsp extra virgin olive oil
- 1 ½ pounds beef stew meat, cubed
- 4 tbsp white flour
- 1 yellow onion, chopped
- 2 tbsp red wine
- 2 garlic cloves, minced
- 2 cups water
- 2 cups beef stock
- Salt and black pepper to taste
- 1 bay leaf
- ½ tsp thyme, dried
- 2 celery stalks, chopped
- 2 carrots, chopped
- 4 potatoes, chopped
- ½ bunch parsley, chopped

Instructions
1. Season beef with salt and pepper and mix with half of the flour.
2. Set your instant pot on Sauté mode, add oil and heat
3. Add beef, brown for just two minutes and transfer to a bowl.
4. Add onion in your pot, stir and fry for 3 minutes.
5. Add garlic, stir and cook for 1 minute.
6. Add wine, stir well and cook for 15 seconds.
7. Add the others from the flour and stir well for two main minutes to stop lumps forming.
8. Return meat to pot, add stock, water, bay leaf and thyme, stir, cover and cook on High for 12 minutes.
9. Release pressure quickly, add carrots, celery and potatoes, stir and cover pot again and cook on High for 5 minutes.
10. Release the pressure naturally for 10 minutes and serve with parsley sprinkled ahead.

BEEF AND PASTA CASSEROLE
Nutrition: Cal 182 ;Fat 5.3 g; Carb 28 g;Protein 14 g
Serving 4; Cook time 30 min

Ingredients
- 17 ounces pasta
- 1 pound beef, ground
- 13 ounces mozzarella cheese, shredded
- 16 ounces tomato puree
- 1 celery stalk, chopped
- 1 yellow onion, chopped
- 1 carrot, chopped
- 1 tbsp dark wine
- 2 tbsp butter
- Salt and black pepper to taste

Instructions
1. Set your instant pot on Sauté mode, add the butter and melt.
2. Add carrot, onion and celery and fry for 5 minutes.

3. Add beef, salt and pepper and cook for 10 more minutes.
4. Add wine, while stirring and cook to get a further minute.
5. Add pasta, tomato puree and water to cover pasta, stir, cover and cook on High for 6 minutes.
6. Release the stress, uncover, add cheese, stir well to melt cheese and enjoy.

KOREAN HOT BEEF SALAD
Nutrition: Cal 310 ;Fat 9 g; Carb 18 g;Protein 35 g
Serving 4 Cook time 35 min

Ingredients
- ¼ cup Korean soybean paste
- 1 cup chicken stock
- 2 pounds beef steak, cut into thin strips
- ¼ tsp red pepper flakes
- Salt and black pepper to taste
- 1 yellow onion, thinly sliced
- 1 zucchini, cubed
- 1 ounce shiitake mushroom caps, cut into quarters
- 12 ounces extra firm tofu, cubed
- 1 chili pepper, sliced
- 1 scallion, chopped

Instructions
1. Set your instant pot on Sauté mode, add stock and soybean paste, stir and simmer for two minutes.
2. Add beef, salt, pepper and pepper flakes, stir, cover and cook on High for fifteen minutes.
3. Release pressure quickly, add tofu, onion, zucchini and mushrooms, stir, bring to your boil, cover and cook on High for 4 minutes more.
4. Release the stress again, increase the salt and pepper to taste, add chili and scallion, stir well and ladle into bowls and serve.

CHINESE BEEF AND BROCCOLI
Nutrition: Cal 310 ;Fat 9 g; Carb 18 g;Protein 35 g
Serving 4 Cook time 20 min

Ingredients
- 3 pounds chuck roast, cut into thin strips
- 1 tbsp peanut oil
- 1 yellow onion, chopped
- ½ cup beef stock
- 1 pound broccoli florets
- 2 tsp toasted sesame oil
- 2 tbsp potato starch

For the marinade:
- ½ cup soy sauce
- ½ cup black soy sauce
- 1 tbsp sesame oil
- 2 tbsp fish sauce
- 5 garlic cloves, minced
- 3 red peppers, dried and crushed
- ½ tsp Chinese five spice
- White rice, already cooked for servings
- Toasted sesame seeds for serving

Instructions
1. In a bowl, mix black soy sauce with soy sauce, fish sauce, 1 tbsp sesame oil, 5 garlic cloves, five spice and crushed red peppers and stir well.
2. Add beef strips, toss to coat and marinade for ten minutes.
3. Set your instant pot on Sauté mode, add peanut oil and also heat
4. Add onions, stir and fry for 4 minutes.
5. Add beef and marinade, stir and cook for 2 minutes.
6. Add stock, stir, cover and cook on High for 5 minutes.
7. Release the stress naturally for ten mins, uncover, add cornstarch after you've mixed it to a smooth paste with ¼ cup liquid from your pot, add broccoli on the steamer basket, cover pot again and cook for 3 minutes on High.
8. Release pressure again and dish up beef into bowls at the top of rice, add broccoli quietly, drizzle toasted sesame oil over items in bowls, sprinkle sesame seeds and enjoy this delicious Chinese meal.

BRISKET AND CABBAGE HODGEPODGE
Nutrition: Cal 340 ;Fat 24 g; Carb 14 g;Protein 26 g
Serving 6 Cook time 90 min

Ingredients
- 2 ½ pounds beef brisket
- 4 cups water
- 2 bay leaves
- 3 garlic cloves, chopped
- 4 carrots, chopped
- 1 cabbage heat, cut into 6 wedges
- 6 potatoes, cut into quarters
- Salt and black pepper to taste
- 3 turnips, cut into quarters
- Horseradish sauce for serving

Instructions
1. Put beef brisket and water with your instant pot, add salt, pepper, garlic and bay leaves, cover and cook on High for an hour and 15 minutes.
2. Release pressure quickly, uncover, add carrots, cabbage, potatoes and turnips, stir, cover again and cook on High for 6 minutes.
3. Release pressure naturally, uncover your pot and serve this delicious meal with horseradish sauce.

MERLOT LAMB SHANKS
Nutrition: Cal 430 ;Fat 17 g; Carb 11 g;Protein 50 g
Serving 4 Cook time 45 min

Ingredients
- 4 lamb shanks
- 2 tbsp extra virgin organic olive oil
- 2 tbsp white flour
- 1 yellow onion, finely chopped
- 3 carrots, roughly chopped
- 2 garlic cloves, minced
- 2 tbsp tomato paste
- 1 tsp oregano, dried
- 1 tomato, roughly chopped
- 2 tbsp water
- 4 ounces red Merlot wine
- Salt and black pepper to taste
- 1 beef bouillon cube

Instructions
1. In a bowl, mix flour with salt and pepper.
2. Add lamb shanks and toss to coat.
3. Set your instant pot on Sauté mode, add oil and warmth
4. Add lamb, brown on the sides and transfer with a bowl.
5. Add onion, oregano, carrots and garlic for the pot, stir and cook for 5 minutes.
6. Add tomato, tomato paste, water, wine and bouillon cube, stir and produce to your boil.
7. Return lamb to pot, cover and cook on High for 25 minutes.
8. Release pressure to succeed and set one shank on each plate, pour cooking sauce over and get with seasonal vegetables!

ROSEMARY LAMB RIBS
Nutrition: Cal 234 ;Fat 8.5 g; Carb 3 g;Protein 35 g
Serving 8 Cook time 35 min

Ingredients
- 8 lamb ribs
- 4 garlic cloves, minced
- 2 carrots, chopped
- 13 ounces veggie stock
- 4 rosemary springs
- 2 tbsp extra virgin organic olive oil
- Salt and black pepper to taste
- 3 tbsp white flour

Instructions
1. Set your instant pot on Sauté mode, add the oil as well as heat
2. Add lamb, garlic, salt and pepper and brown it on every side.
3. Add flour, stock, rosemary and carrots, stir well, cover and cook on High for 20 minutes.
4. Release pressure quickly and discard rosemary, divide lamb ribs onto plates and serve while using cooking liquid drizzled on the top.

MEDITERRANEAN LAMB
Nutrition: Cal 238 ;Fat 5 g; Carb 17 g;Protein 27 g
Serving 4 Cook time 75 min

Ingredients
- 6 pounds lamb leg, boneless
- 2 tbsp extra virgin organic olive oil
- Salt and black pepper to taste
- 1 bay leaf
- 1 tsp marjoram
- 1 tsp sage, dried
- 1 tsp ginger, grated
- 3 garlic cloves, minced
- 1 tsp thyme, dried
- 2 cups veggie stock

- •3 pounds potatoes, chopped
- •3 tbsp arrowroot powder blended with 1/3 cup water

Instructions
1. Set your instant pot on Sauté mode, add the oil and warmth
2. Add lamb leg and brown on all sides.
3. Add salt, pepper, bay leaf, marjoram, sage, ginger, garlic, thyme and stock, stir, cover and cook on High for 50 minutes.
4. Release pressure to succeed quickly and add potatoes, arrowroot mix, more salt and pepper if needed, stir, cover again and cook on High for ten minutes.
5. Release pressure to succeed again, uncover, divide Mediterranean lamb onto serving plates and revel in.

CREAMY LAMB CURRY
Nutrition: Cal 378 ;Fat 8 g; Carb 18 g;Protein 22 g
Serving 6 Cook time 35 min

Ingredients
- •1 ½ pounds lamb shoulder, cut into medium chunks
- •2 ounces coconut milk
- •3 ounces dry white wine
- •3 tbsp pure cream
- •3 tbsp curry powder
- •2 tbsp vegetable oil
- •3 tbsp water
- •1 yellow onion, chopped
- •1 tbsp parsley, chopped
- •Salt and black pepper to taste

Instructions
1. In a bowl, mix half with the curry powder with salt, pepper and coconut milk and stir well.
2. Set your instant pot on Sauté mode, add oil and also heat
3. Add onion, stir and fry for 4 minutes.
4. Add the remaining of the curry powder, stir and cook for 1 minute.
5. Add lamb pieces, brown them for 3 minutes and mix with water, salt, pepper and wine.
6. Stir, cover and cook on High for 20 mins.
7. Release the stress quickly, set pot to Simmer mode, add coconut milk mixture, stir and boil for 5 minutes.
8. Divide among serving plates, sprinkle parsley at the top and serve.

LAMB AND VEGETABLE HOT POT
Nutrition: Cal 435 ;Fat 31 g; Carb 6 g;Protein 22 g
Serving 6 Cook time 50 min

Ingredients
- •3 pounds lamb chops
- •Salt and black pepper to taste
- •2 tbsp flour
- •2 tbsp extra virgin olive oil
- •2 yellow onions, chopped
- •3 ounces red
- •2 garlic cloves, crushed
- •2 carrots, sliced

- •2 celery sticks, chopped
- •2 tbsp tomato sauce
- •2 bay leaves
- •1 cup green peas
- •14 ounces canned tomatoes, chopped
- •4 ounces green beans
- •2 tbsp parsley, finely chopped
- •Beef stock to the pot

Instructions
1. Put flour in a very bowl and mix with salt and pepper.
2. Add lamb chops and toss to coat.
3. Set your instant pot on Sauté mode, add the oil as well as heat
4. Add lamb, stir, brown for 3 minutes on the sides and transfer to a plate.
5. Add garlic and onion and stir for two main minutes.
6. Add wine and cook an extra 2 minutes.
7. Add bay leaves, carrots, celery and return lamb to pot.
8. Also add tomato sauce, tomatoes, green beans and peas and stir.
9. Add stock to hide
10. Ingredients, cover and cook on High for 20 mins.
11. Release pressure to succeed, uncover, add parsley, more salt and pepper if required.

MOROCCAN LAMB
Nutrition: Cal 434 ;Fat 21 g; Carb 41 g;Protein 20 g
Serving 6 Cook time 35 min

Ingredients
- •2 ½ pounds lamb shoulder, chopped
- •3 tbsp honey
- •3 ounces almonds, peeled and chopped
- •9 ounces prunes, pitted
- •8 ounces vegetable stock
- •2 yellow onions, chopped
- •2 garlic cloves, minced
- •1 bay leaf
- •Salt and black pepper to tastes
- •1 cinnamon stick
- •1 tsp cumin powder
- •1 tsp turmeric powder
- •1 tsp ginger powder
- •1 tsp cinnamon powder
- •Sesame seeds for servings
- •3 tbsp extra virgin organic olive oil

Instructions
1. In a bowl, mix cinnamon powder with ginger, cumin, turmeric, garlic and 2 tbsp extra virgin olive oil and stir well.
2. Add meat and toss to coat.
3. Put prunes in the bowl, cover them hot water and leave aside.
4. Set your instant pot on Sauté mode, add the remainder of the oil as well as heat
5. Add onions, stir, cook for 3 minutes, transfer to your bowl and then leave aside.
6. Add meat to your pot and brown it for 10 minutes.

7. Add stock, cinnamon stick, bay leaf and return onions, stir, cover and cook on High for 25 minutes.
8. Release pressure to succeed naturally, uncover, add drained prunes, salt, pepper, honey and stir.
9. Set the pot on Simmer mode, cook mixture for 5 minutes and discard bay leaf and cinnamon stick.
10. Divide among plates and scatter almonds and sesame seeds ahead.

LAMB RAGOUT
Nutrition: Cal 360 ;Fat 14 g; Carb 15 g;Protein 30 g
Serving 8 Cook time 75 min

Ingredients
• 1 ½ pounds mutton, bone-in
• 2 carrots, sliced
• ½ pound mushrooms, sliced
• 4 tomatoes, chopped
• 1 small yellow onion, chopped
• 6 garlic cloves, minced
• 2 tbsp tomato paste
• 1 tsp vegetable oil
• Salt and black pepper to taste
• 1 tsp oregano, dried
• A handful parsley, finely chopped

Instructions
1. Set your instant pot on Sauté mode, add oil and warmth
2. Add meat and brown it on the sides.
3. Add tomato paste, tomatoes, onion, garlic, mushrooms, oregano, carrots and water to pay for.
4. Add salt, pepper, stir, cover and cook on High for one hour.
5. Release the pressure, take meat out from the pot and discard bones before shredding.
6. Return meat to pot, add parsley and stir.
7. Add more salt and pepper as needed and serve right away.

LAMB AND BARLEY BOWLS
Nutrition: Cal 484 ;Fat 19 g; Carb 21 g;Protein 44 g
Serving 4 Cook time 60 min

Ingredients
• 6 ounces barley
• 5 ounces peas
• 1 lamb leg, already cooked, boneless and chopped
• 3 yellow onions, chopped
• 5 carrots, chopped
• 6 ounces beef stock
• 12 ounces water
• Salt and black pepper to taste

Instructions
1. In your instant pot, mix stock with water and barley, cover and cook on High for 20 minutes.
2. Release pressure to succeed, uncover, add onions, peas and carrots, stir, cover again and cook on High for ten mins.
3. Release pressure again, add meat, salt and pepper to taste, stir, dish into bowls and serve.

MEXICAN STYLE LAMB
Nutrition: Cal 324 ;Fat 9 g; Carb 19 g;Protein 15 g
Serving 4 Cook time 60 min

Ingredients
• 3 pounds lamb shoulder, cubed
• 19 ounces enchilada sauce
• 3 garlic cloves, minced
• 1 yellow onion, chopped
• 2 tbsp extra virgin olive oil
• Salt to taste
• ½ bunch cilantro, finely chopped
• Corn tortillas, warm for serving
• Lime wedges for serving
• Refried beans for serving

Instructions
1. Put enchilada sauce inside a bowl, add lamb meat and marinade for 24 hours.
2. Set your instant pot on Sauté mode, add the oil as well as heat
3. Add onions and garlic and fry for 5 minutes.
4. Add lamb, salt and its particular marinade, stir, bring to a boil, cover and cook on High for 45 minutes.
5. Release the stress, take meat and set on a cutting board and then leave for cooling down for a couple of minutes.
6. Shred meat and set inside a bowl.
7. Pour cooking sauce over it and stir.
8. Portion out meat onto tortillas, sprinkle cilantro on each, add beans, squeeze lime juice over, roll and serve.

GOAT AND TOMATO POT
Nutrition: Cal 340 ;Fat 4 g; Carb 12 g;Protein 12 g
Serving 4 Cook time 70 min

Ingredients
• 17 ounces goat meat, cubed
• 1 carrot, chopped
• 1 celery rib, chopped
• 4 ounces tomato paste
• 1 yellow onion, chopped
• 3 garlic cloves, crushed
• A dash of sherry wine
• ½ cup water
• Salt and black pepper to taste
• 1 cup chicken stock
• 2 tbsp extra virgin olive oil
• 1 tbsp cumin seeds, ground
• A pinch of rosemary, dried
• 2 roasted tomatoes, chopped

Instructions
1. Set your instant pot on Sauté mode, add 1 tbsp oil and also heat
2. Add goat meat, salt and pepper and brown for a few minutes on either side.
3. Add cumin seeds, rosemary, stir, cook for just two minutes and transfer to your bowl.
4. Add the remainder in the oil on the pot and warmth

5. Add onion, garlic, salt and pepper, stir and cook for 1 minute.
6. Add carrot and celery, stir and cook 2 minutes.
7. Add sherry wine, stock, water, goat meat, tomato paste, more salt and pepper, stir, cover and cook on High for 40 minutes.
8. Release pressure naturally, uncover, add tomatoes, stir, divide among plates and serve.

CORNED BEEF WITH VEGETABLE
Nutrition: Cal 434 ;Fat 22 g; Carb 21 g;Protein 28 g
Serving 8 Cook time 90 min

Ingredients
- 3 lbs corned beef brisket
- 10 peppercorns
- 4 garlic cloves, peeled
- 1 cup onion, minced
- 3 cups water
- 3 cups chicken broth
- 1 cabbage head, cut into wedges
- 4 carrots, peeled and cut into pieces
- 5 potatoes, cut into pieces
- 1/2 Tsp salt

Instructions
1. Place beef to the instant pot atart exercising . 1/2 cup onions, peppercorns, 2 garlic cloves, chicken stock, and water.
2. Seal pot with lid and select MANUAL and hang up the timer for one hour.
3. Once all pressure release its very own then open lid and take away corned beef from instant pot make on a dish.
4. Cover beef with foil and hang up aside.
5. Now add potatoes, salt, garlic, onions, carrots, and cabbage within the pot.
6. Seal pot with lid and select MANUAL button as well as set the timer for ten minutes.
7. Allow to releasing steam its very own then open.
8. Sliced cooked beef and serve with vegetables.

SPICY TACO MEAT
Nutrition: Cal 414 ;Fat 21 g; Carb 7 g;Protein 47 g
Serving 6 Cook time 45 min

Ingredients
- 2 lbs ground beef
- 1/2 tbsp chili powder
- 1/4 Tsp chipotle powder
- 1 tsp cayenne
- 1/2 Tsp cumin
- 1/2 Tsp smoked paprika
- 1/2 Tsp turmeric
- 2 tsp oregano
- 2 large sweet peppers, diced
- 1 large onion, diced
- 4 tbsp olive oil
- 3 garlic cloves, minced
- 1/4 Tsp black pepper

- 1 tsp salt
Instructions
1. Add all ingredients except meat in to the instant pot.
2. Select sauté and stir fry for 5 minutes.
3. Add ground beef and stir until lightly brown.
4. Seal pot with lid and cook on HIGH pressure for half an hour.
5. Allow to releasing steam its then open.
6. Select sauté function and stir for 10 mins.
7. Garnish with fresh chopped cilantro and serve.

BEEF BEAN RICE
Nutrition: Cal 506 ;Fat 17 g; Carb 28 g;Protein 38 g
Serving 6 Cook time 25 min

Ingredients
- 1 lb ground beef
- 1 1/2 cup cheese, shredded
- 3 tbsp fresh cilantro, chopped
- 1 cup fresh corn
- 14 oz can black beans, rinsed and drained
- 16 oz salsa
- 2 cups beef stock
- 1 cup rice, rinsed and drained
- 1/2 Tsp cumin
- 1 1/2 Tsp chili powder
- 1 onion, diced
- 1 tbsp extra virgin olive oil
- 1/2 Tsp salt

Instructions
1. Select sauté function with the instant pot.
2. Once the pot is hot then adds organic olive oil, ground beef, cumin, chili powder, onion, and salt and sauté for 5 minutes or until browned.
3. Add rice, corn, black beans, salsa, and stock in a very pot and stir well.
4. Seal pot with lid and select MANUAL HIGH pressure for 8 minutes.
5. Quick release steam then opens the lid and stir well.
6. Top with cilantro and cheese.
7. Serve and revel in.

BEEF STROGANOFF
Nutrition: Cal 317 ;Fat 19 g; Carb 8 g;Protein 29 g
Serving 4 Cook time 40 min

Ingredients
- Beef (1 pound, chopped in cubes)
- Bacon (2 slices, cut in cubes)
- Beef stock (250 ml)
- Mushrooms (9 oz.)
- Onion (1, chopped)
- Garlic (2 cloves, chopped)
- Tomato paste (3 tbsp)
- Smoked paprika (1 tbsp)
- Sour cream
Instructions

1. Add oil inside Pressure cooker dish, and hang up it to "Sauté"; add the onion, bacon, and garlic and cook shortly or before the onion is tender.
2. Put the beef and continue to cook prior to the meat is cooked on every side (it will get brown color).
3. Add the mushrooms, beef broth, tomato paste, and paprika and stir well; close the lid and set it to high-pressure cooking for 30 minutes.
4. Use the quick-release approach to release the stress.
5. Serve while hot and top it with sour cream.

Chile Lime Steak Fajitas
Nutrition: Cal 230;Fat 30 g; Carb 13 g;Protein 25 g
Serving 4; Cook time 15 min

Ingredients
Marinade
- 2 tablespoons olive oil
- 1/3 cup freshly squeezed lime juice
- 2 tablespoons fresh chopped cilantro
- 2 cloves garlic , crushed
- 1 teaspoon brown sugar
- ¾ teaspoon red chilli flakes (adjust to your preference of spice)
- ½ teaspoon ground cumin
- 1 teaspoon salt
- 1 pound (500 g) steak (rump, skirt, or flank steak)

Fajitas
- 3 bell peppers (capsicums) of different colors: red, yellow, and green, deseeded and sliced
- 1 onion, sliced
- 1 avocado sliced

Optional Serving Suggestion:
- Flour tortillas
- Lettuce leaves for low-carb option
- Extra cilantro leaves to garnish
- Sour cream to serve

Instructions
1. Whisk marinade ingredients together to combine. Pour out half of the marinade into a shallow dish to marinade the steak for 30 minutes, if time allows. Alternatively, refrigerate for 2 hours or overnight. Remove from the refrigerator 30 minute prior to cooking.
Refrigerate the reserved untouched marinade to use later

For Skillet
2. Heat about one teaspoon of oil in a grill pan or cast iron skillet over medium-high heat and grill steak on each side until desired doneness (about 4 minutes each side for medium-rare, depending on thickness). Set aside and allow to rest for 5 minutes.

For Grilling
3. Heat barbecue (or grill) on high heat. Remove steak from the marinade. Grill for 5-7 minutes per side, or until desired doneness is reached. Transfer to a plate and allow to rest for 5-10 minutes.

For Vegetables
4. Wipe pan or grill plates over with paper towel; drizzle (or brush) with another teaspoon of oil and fry peppers (capsicums) and onion strips. Add half of the reserved marinade, salt and pepper; continue cooking until done.

Assemble
5. To serve steak, slice against the grain into thin strips. Pack into warmed tortillas, extra cilantro leaves, sour cream, sliced avocado (or your desired fillings), and drizzle over the remaining reserved untouched marinade.

Keto Beef and Broccoli
Nutrition: Cal 294;Fat 14 g; Carb 13 g;Protein 29 g
Serving 4; Cook time 35 min

Ingredients
- 1 pound flank steak sliced into 1/4 inch thick strips
- 5 cups small broccoli florets about 7 ounces
- 1 tablespoon avocado oil
- For the sauce:
- 1 yellow onion sliced
- 1 Tbs butter
- ½ tbs olive oil
- 1/3 cup low-sodium soy sauce
- ⅓ cup beef stock
- 1 tablespoon fresh ginger minced
- 2 cloves garlic minced

Instructions
1. Heat avocado oil in a pan over medium heat for a few minutes or until hot.
2. Add sliced beef and cook until it browns, less than 5 minutes, don't stir too much, you want it to brown. Transfer to a plate and set aside.
3. Add onions to a skillet with butter and olive oil and cook 20 minutes until onions are caramelized and tender.
4. Add all other sauce ingredients into the skillet and stir the ingredients together over medium-low heat until it starts to simmer, about 5 minutes.
5. Use an immersion blender to blend sauce.
6. Keep the sauce warm over low heat, and add broccoli to the skillet.
7. Return beef to the pan and toss with broccoli and sauce top. Stir until everything is coated with the sauce.
8. Bring to a simmer and cook for another few minutes until broccoli is tender.
9. Season with salt and pepper to taste, if needed.
10. Serve immediately, optionally pairing with cooked cauliflower rice.

Meatloaf Recipe
Nutrition: Cal 575;Fat 44 g; Carb 10 g;Protein 35 g
Serving 4; Cook time 70 min

Ingredients
- 1 tablespoon tallow
- 1 small onion finely chopped
- 2 cloves garlic crushed
- 2 pounds ground beef
- 2 large eggs
- 2 tablespoons oregano dried
- 1 1/2 teaspoon salt
- 1/4 teaspoon pepper ground
- 1/3 cup low carb marinara sauce
- 1/3 cup almond flour

• 2 tablespoons low carb marinara sauce extra

Instructions

1. Preheat your oven to 160C/320F and prepare a loaf tin by lining with baking paper.
2. Place a non-stick frying pan over high heat and saute the onion and garlic in the tallow, until the onion is turning translucent. Set aside to cool slightly.
3. In a large mixing bowl add the warm onion mixture and all remaining ingredients, except the extra marinara sauce.
4. Using clean hands, or wearing disposable gloves, mix the ingredients very well.
5. Press into the base of your prepared loaf tin, ensuring there are no air bubbles, and smooth the top.
6. Bake for 50 minutes.
7. Drain off some of the juices and top the meatloaf with the extra marinara sauce.
8. Bake for another 10 minutes.
9. Leave to sit for 10 minutes to rest, before slicing and serving.

Moroccan Meatballs

Nutrition: Cal 363;Fat 27 g; Carb 6 g;Protein 22 g
Serving 8; Cook time 6 hours

Ingredients

• 2 pounds of Ground Beef
• 1 small Onion, grated
• 4 cloves of Garlic, crushed
• 1 large Egg
• 2 tablespoons of Cilantro, finely chopped
• 1 tablespoon of Cumin, ground
• 1 tablespoon of Coriander, ground
• 1 tablespoon of Smoked Paprika, ground
• 2 teaspoons of Ground Ginger
• 1 teaspoon of Cinnamon, ground
• 1 teaspoon of Salt
• 2 tablespoon of Olive Oil
• 2 tablespoons of Tomato Paste
• 1 ½ cups of Tomato Passata
• ½ cup of Beef Stock ro, to serve

Instructions

1. In a large bowl add the beef, half the grated onion, half the garlic, egg, cilantro, cumin, coriander, paprika, ginger, cinnamon, and salt. Mix well.
2. Roll into 2 tablespoon-sized meatballs and set aside. We got 40.
3. Place the oil, remaining onion, and garlic into a nonstick frying pan over high heat. Saute for 3-5 minutes, until fragrant.
4. Add the tomato paste and cook for another 3 minutes, then add to your slow cooker, followed by the passata and stock. Mix well.
5. Add the meatballs to the sauce.
6. Cook on low for 5 hours

Low Carb Beef Bolognese Sauce

Nutrition: Cal 279;Fat 21 g; Carb 5 g;Protein 17 g
Serving 6; Cook time 75 min

Ingredients

• 4 cups of Beef Stock or Broth
• 2 ounces of Tallow
• 1 medium Onion, diced
• 6 cloves of Garlic, crushed
• 1 tablespoon of Marjoram, dried
• 1 teaspoon of Salt
• 3 pounds of Ground Beef
• 24 ounces of Tomato Puree
• 1 teaspoon of Pepper
• 2 tablespoons of Basil, chopped
• 2 tablespoons of Oregano, chopped
• 1 tablespoon of Parsley, chopped

Instructions

1. Place the beef stock into a small saucepan and simmer over medium-high heat until it reduces into 1 cup of liquid.
2. In a large saucepan over high heat, place the tallow and allow to melt and heat.
3. Add the diced onion, garlic, marjoram, and salt. Saute for 5 minutes, until the onions have softened and turned translucent.
4. Add the ground beef and saute until browned. Reduce the heat to low.
5. Pour in the tomato puree and reduced beef stock and simmer, uncovered, and stirring occasionally for 30-60 minutes. Until the liquid is mostly absorbed, leaving a thick and rich sauce.
6. Add the remaining ingredients, check the seasoning, and add more salt or pepper if desired.
7. Remove from the heat, serve, and enjoy.

Keto Lamb Chops on the Grill

Nutrition: Cal 446;Fat 27 g; Carb 4 g;Protein 22 g
Serving 8; Cook time 30 min

Ingredients

• 3 lbs of lamb loin chops (I had 8 6oz chops)
• 1/4 cup of white wine vinegar
• 1/2 cup of olive oil
• 1 teaspoon of oregano
• 1/2 teaspoon of salt
• 1/4 teaspoon of pepper
• 2 cloves of garlic, crushed
• zest of 1 lemon
• juice of 2 lemons (approx. 6 tablespoons)

Instructions

1. Whisk together all of the marinade ingredinets. Add the chops to a large baggie and pour the marinade over top.
2. Seal the bag and use your hands to mix the marinade through the chops and then place in the refrigerator for 8 hours or overnight.
3. Take out the lamb chops when ready to eat and let them sit on the ccounter for 15 minutes. Place them on a plate and discard the marinade.

4. Grill the lamb chops for about 5-6 minutes per side. The time will depend on the size and thickness of the chops. Mine were about 1 - 1.5 inches thick and too 6 minutes on each side and came out medium rare.

Keto Lamb Curry
Nutrition: Cal 480;Fat 17 g; Carb 2 g;Protein 30 g
Serving 8; Cook time 2 hours35 min

Ingredients
Marinade
- 2 teaspoons of Ginger, crushed
- 3 cloves of Garlic, crushed
- 2 teaspoons of Cumin, ground
- 2 teaspoons of Coriander, ground
- 1 teaspoon of Onion Powder
- 1 teaspoon of Cardamon, ground
- 1 teaspoon of Paprika, ground
- 1 teaspoon of Turmeric, ground
- 1 teaspoon of Kashmiri Chili Powder
- 2 tablespoons of Olive Oil

Curry
- 4 pounds of Lamb Shoulder, diced
- 3 tablespoons of Ghee
- 1 medium Onion, diced
- 1 teaspoon of Cinnamon, ground
- 1 teaspoon of Kashmiri Chili Powder
- 2 teaspoons of Salt
- 1 teaspoon of Pepper
- 1 cup of Heavy Cream
- ½ cup of Flaked Almonds
- 3 tablespoons of Cilantro, roughly chopped

Instructions
1. The Marinade: In a mixing bowl combine all marinade ingredients.
2. Add the diced lamb and mix well.
3. Store in the fridge to marinate for at least 1 hour, or overnight.
4. The Curry: In a large saucepan add the ghee and place over medium heat.
5. Add the onion, cinnamon & chili powder and saute for 3 minutes.
6. Add the marinated lamb, salt, and pepper and stir to ensure that lamb is browning.
7. Allow the lamb to cook for 10 minutes before adding the cream and reducing the heat to low.
8. Simmer the curry, partially covered, for 1 hour. Check the lamb for tenderness. If the lamb is tough, continue cooking until tender.
9. Remove the lid and simmer for another 10 minutes.
10. Add the flaked almonds and stir well. Add any extra seasoning.
11. Remove from the heat, garnish with coriander and serve.

Rosemary Dijon Roasted Lamb Chops
Nutrition: Cal 446;Fat 40 g; Carb 2 g;Protein 18 g
Serving 4; Cook time 17 min

Ingredients

- 1 tbsp Dijon mustard
- 2 cloves garlic minced
- 3 tbsp olive oil
- 2 tsp fresh rosemary finely chopped
- 1/2 tsp salt
- 1/4 tsp pepper
- 4 lamb loin chops aprrox 2 lbs with bone-in

Instructions
1. Whisk together Dijon mustard, garlic, olive oil, rosemary, and salt and pepper in a bowl. Place lamb chops in a large zip-top bag or other airtight container. Coat lamb with Dijon mixture on both sides. Let marinate in the fridge for at least 30 minutes, but up to 24 hours.
2. Position an oven rack to the highest position in the oven and line a broiler pan with aluminum foil.
3. Take lamb chops out of the bag and place onto prepared pan. Set oven to broil on high and place pan into the oven.
4. Cook lamb chops for 8 minutes, until brown, and then flip and cook for an additional 3-5 minutes depending on the doneness you like your meat. (3 minutes for medium rare, 4 for medium, 5 for well done)

Keto Lamb Koftas
Nutrition: Cal 330;Fat 26 g; Carb 3 g;Protein 22 g
Serving 4; Cook time 20 min

Ingredients
- 500 g minced (ground) lamb (1.1 lb)
- 1 garlic clove, minced
- 1/2 medium yellow onion, diced (50 g/ 1.8 oz)
- 1 tsp dried oregano
- 2 tbsp chopped fresh parsley
- 1/2 tsp sea salt
- 1/4 tsp ground black pepper
- 1 tbsp extra virgin olive oil (15 ml)

Instructions
1. Place your skewers in cold water for half and hour prior to starting (ideally leave them to soak for at least 30 minutes). Alternatively, you can use stainless steel skewers that don't require soaking.
2. Add minced lamb, diced onions, chopped garlic, finely chopped parsley and the herbs and seasonings into a large mixing bowl. Retain the olive oil.
3. Mix well with your hands until thoroughly combined.
4. Portion out into eight portions and place each one around a skewer. You need to gently squeeze and press your mixture around the skewer until you're happy with the result. If your skewers will fit in a pan, heat it on the stove top. Mine were too big so I cooked them on our barbeque instead.
5. Brush the surface with the retained olive oil before placing the koftas onto the hot pan.
6. Store the koftas in the refrigerator, covered for 4 days.

Greek Lamb and Cabbage Bowls
Nutrition: Cal 334;Fat 10 g; Carb 15 g;Protein 34 g
Serving 4; Cook time 24 min

Ingredients

- 1 tablespoon olive oil
- 1 large clove garlic, minced
- 1 small onion, diced
- 1 lb grass-fed ground lamb
- ¼ cup tomato paste
- 1 teaspoon ground cinnamon
- ½ teaspoon dried oregano
- ¼ teaspoon ground nutmeg
- ½ cup water (or broth), more or less as needed
- ½ large head green cabbage (or 1 small), cored and sliced
- 1 teaspoon sea salt and ½ teaspoon black pepper, or to taste

Instructions
1. In a large pan, dutch oven or skillet, heat the olive oil over medium-high heat. Add the onion, garlic and ground lamb. Sauté until the lamb is cooked about 5-7 minutes.
2. Add in the tomato paste, cinnamon, oregano and nutmeg. Stir until well combined.
3. Add in the cabbage and continue to sauté. You want to cook until the cabbage is gently cooked with a little bite, not mushy.
4. Add a little water or broth, as needed if it's too dry.
5. Serve over cauli-rice or rice, zucchini noodles or pasta.

Lamb Meatballs with Mint Gremolata
Nutrition: Cal 306;Fat 17 g; Carb 4 g;Protein 34 g
Serving 4; Cook time 20 min

Ingredients
For the meatballs:
- 2 lbs ground lamb
- 2 eggs
- 1/2 cup superfine almond flour **
- 1/4 cup fresh parsley, chopped
- 1 clove garlic, minced
- 1 1/2 Tbsp Za'atar seasoning
- 1 tsp kosher salt
- 3 Tbsp water
- 2 Tbsp olive oil for frying
- **For the gremolata:**
- 2 Tbsp chopped fresh parsley
- 2 Tbsp chopped fresh mint
- 1 Tbsp lime zest
- 2 cloves garlic, minced

Instructions
For the meatballs:
1. Combine the meatball ingredients (except olive oil) in a medium bowl and mix well.
2. Form into 24 one and a half inch (approximately) meatballs.
3. Heat the olive oil in a nonstick saute pan over medium heat
4. Cook the meatballs in batches until brown on both sides and cooked through – about 2-3 minutes per side.
5. Remove cooked meatballs and place on a paper towel lined plate until ready to serve.
6. Serve warm, sprinkled generously with gremolata.

For the gremolata:
7. Combine the ingredients in a small bowl and mix well.

LAMB CASSOULET WITH BEANS
Nutrition: Cal 274;Fat 8 g; Carb 26 g;Protein 18 g
Serving 6; Cook time 5 hours

Ingredients
- 2 cups can great northern beans
- 1/2 tsp garlic, minced
- 1 tbsp fresh parsley
- 1/2 tsp thyme, crushed
- 2 tbsp organic olive oil
- 1 cup dry white wine
- 1 cup tomato sauce
- 2 bay leaves
- 8 ounces lean lamb, cut into 1/2-inch pieces
- 3/4 cup onion, chopped
- 1/4 cup water
- 2 tbsp flour

Instructions
1. In an immediate pot combine beans, wine, tomato sauce, bay leaves, garlic, parsley, and thyme.
2. Heat oil in a very saucepan over medium-high heat and cook lamb and onion until lamb is well browned on all sides, drain.
3. Stir lamb and onion into bean mixture in instant pot.
4. Cover and turn the steam release handle to the venting position.
5. Select the slow cooker setting and set to medium.
6. Cook for 5 hours.
7. Turn to high. Heat until bubbly (don't lift cover).
8. Slowly blend the cold water into flour, stir into meat-bean mixture.
9. Cover and cook until slightly thickened.
10. Before serving, remove bay leaves and discard.

ITALIAN RICE CASSEROLE
Nutrition: Cal 508;Fat 14 g; Carb 66 g;Protein 26 g
Serving 8; Cook time 6 hours

Ingredients
- 1 pound ground beef
- 3 cups rice, long grain and uncooked
- 3 cups tomato sauce
- 1 cup onion, chopped
- 1 tsp Italian seasoning
- 1/2 tsp garlic, minced
- 6 ounces mozzarella, shredded
- 1 cup cottage type cheese
- 4 cups water

Instructions
1. Place ground beef and chopped onion in the nonstick skillet.
2. Brown over medium-high heat and then drain.
3. Combine beef mixture and remaining
4. Ingredient in instant pot.
5. Cover and turn the steam release handle on the venting position.
6. Select the slow cooker setting and hang to high.

7. Cook for 6 hours.

SWISS CHEESE BEEF ZUCCHINI CASSEROLE
Nutrition: Cal 454;Fat 30 g; Carb 13 g;Protein 30 g
Serving 4; Cook time 2 hours

Ingredients
- 1 pound extra-lean ground beef
- 4 cups zucchini, sliced
- 10 ounces cream of mushroom soup
- 1/2 cup onion, chopped
- 1/4 tsp ground black pepper
- 1 cup Swiss cheese, shredded

Instructions
1. In a skillet over medium-high heat, brown ground beef with onions and pepper until don't pink. Drain.
2. Layer zucchini and beef mixture alternately in instant pot.
3. Top with soup. Sprinkle with cheese.
4. Cover and turn the steam release handle to the venting position.
5. Select the slow cooker setting and set to medium.
6. Cook for 120 minutes.

CHILI VERDE WITH POTATOES
Nutrition: Cal 414;Fat 20 g; Carb 40 g;Protein 21 g
Serving 8; Cook time 4 hours

Ingredients
- 1 pound extra-lean ground beef
- 1/2 pound ground pork
- 4 large potatoes, diced
- 10 ounces corn, frozen
- 3 cups chicken broth
- 2 cups water
- 8 ounces green chilies, diced
- 2 tbsp essential olive oil
- 1 cup onion, diced
- 1 tsp garlic, minced
- 1 tsp ground black pepper
- 1/2 tsp oregano
- 1 tsp cumin
- 1/2 tsp salt

Instructions
1. Heat oil inside a skillet over medium-high heat and after that brown onion, garlic, beef, and pork.
2. Cook until meat is no longer pink.
3. Combine meat mixture and remaining
4. Ingredients in instant pot.
5. Cover and turn the steam release handle for the venting position.
6. Select the slow cooker setting and hang up to medium.
7. Cook for 4 hours.

SIMPLE & CLASSIC GOULASH
Nutrition: Cal 167;Fat 10 g; Carb 8 g;Protein 11 g
Serving 8; Cook time 5 hours

Ingredients
- 1 pound ground beef, browned
- 1/2 cup ketchup

- 2 tbsp Worcestershire sauce
- 1 tbsp brown sugar
- 1 cup onion, chopped
- 1/2 tsp garlic, minced
- 2 tsp paprika
- 1/2 tsp dry mustard
- 1 cup water

Instructions
1. Place meat in instant pot. Cover with onions.
2. Combine remaining
3. Ingredients and pour over meat.
4. Cover and turn the steam release handle for the venting position.
5. Select the slow cooker setting and hang up to medium.
6. Cook for 5 hours.
Serve over rice or noodles.

BEEF AND BROCCOLI STIR-FRY
Nutrition: Cal 588;Fat 38 g; Carb 6 g;Protein 54 g
Serving 4; Cook time 25 min

Ingredients
- 6 tablespoons coconut aminos
- ¼ cup avocado oil
- 2 tablespoons toasted sesame oil
- 1 teaspoon garlic powder
- 1 teaspoon onion powder
- Salt
- Freshly ground black pepper
- 1½ pounds sirloin steak, cut into ¼-inch-thick slices

FOR THE BEEF AND BROCCOLI
- 1 teaspoon salt, plus more for seasoning
- 2 broccoli crowns, florets separated and trimmed
- 2 tablespoons avocado oil
- 3 garlic cloves, minced
- 1 tablespoon finely minced ginger or ½ tablespoon ground ginger
- ¼ cup coconut aminos
- ¼ cup toasted sesame oil
- Freshly ground black pepper

Instructions
TO MAKE THE MARINADE
In a bowl, combine the coconut aminos, avocado oil, sesame oil, garlic powder, onion powder, salt, and pepper. Add the steak and toss to coat. Marinate for at least 30 minutes or up to 24 hours in the refrigerator.

TO MAKE THE BEEF AND BROCCOLI
1. Fill a large pot halfway with water and add 1 teaspoon of salt. Bring to a boil.
2. Add the broccoli and blanch for 1 to 3 minutes; drain in a colander. Rinse with cold water to prevent further cooking. Set aside.
3. Heat a large skillet over medium-high heat and combine the avocado oil, garlic, and ginger and cook for 30 seconds.

4. Add the sliced beef, discarding the marinade, and cook, stirring constantly, for 2 to 3 minutes. Add the broccoli, coconut aminos, and sesame oil to the skillet and season with salt and pepper. Continue to cook until the beef has reached your desired doneness (about 5 to 7 minutes for medium).
5. Divide the stir-fry evenly between 4 storage containers.

Cheddar-Stuffed Burgers with Zucchini
Nutrition: Cal 470;Fat 30 g; Carb 4,5 g;Protein 47 g
Serving 4; Cook time 25 min

Ingredients
- 1 pound ground beef (80% lean)
- 2 large eggs
- ¼ cup almond flour
- 1 cup shredded cheddar cheese
- Salt and pepper
- 2 tablespoons olive oil
- 1 large zucchini, halved and sliced

Instructions
1. Combine the beef, egg, almond flour, cheese, salt, and pepper in a bowl.
2. Mix well, then shape into four even-sized patties.
3. Heat the oil in a large skillet over medium-high heat.
4. Add the burger patties and cook for 5 minutes until browned.
5. Flip the patties and add the zucchini to the skillet, tossing to coat with oil.
6. Season with salt and pepper and cook for 5 minutes, stirring the zucchini occasionally.
7. Serve the burgers with your favorite toppings and the zucchini on the side.

Beef and Broccoli Stir-Fry
Nutrition: Cal 350;Fat 19.5g; Carb 6,5 g;Protein 37 g
Serving 4; Cook time 35 min

Ingredients
- ¼ cup soy sauce
- 1 tablespoon sesame oil
- 1 teaspoon garlic chili paste
- 1 pound beef sirloin
- 2 tablespoons almond flour
- 2 tablespoons coconut oil
- 2 cups chopped broccoli florets
- 1 tablespoon grated ginger
- 3 cloves garlic, minced

Instructions
1. Whisk together the soy sauce, sesame oil, and chili paste in a small bowl.
2. Slice the beef and toss with almond flour, then place in a plastic freezer bag.
3. Pour in the sauce and toss to coat, then let rest for 20 minutes.
4. Heat the oil in a large skillet over medium high heat.
5. Pour the beef and sauce into the skillet and cook until the beef is browned.
6. Push the beef to the sides of the skillet and add the broccoli, ginger, and garlic.

7. Sauté until the broccoli is tender-crisp, then toss it all together and serve hot.

Hearty Beef and Bacon Casserole
Nutrition: Cal 410;Fat 26 g; Carb 8 g;Protein 37 g
Serving 8; Cook time 55 min

Ingredients
- 8 slices uncooked bacon
- 1 medium head cauliflower, chopped
- ¼ cup canned coconut milk
- Salt and pepper
- 2 pounds ground beef (80% lean)
- 8 ounces mushrooms, sliced
- 1 large yellow onion, chopped
- 2 cloves garlic, minced

Instructions
1. Preheat the oven to 375°F.
2. Cook the bacon in a skillet until crisp, then drain on paper towels and chop.
3. Bring a pot of salted water to boil, then add the cauliflower.
4. Boil for 6 to 8 minutes until tender, then drain and add to a food processor with the coconut milk.
5. Blend the mixture until smooth, then season with salt and pepper.
6. Cook the beef in a skillet until browned, then drain the fat.
7. Stir in the mushrooms, onion, and garlic, then transfer to a baking dish.
8. Spread the cauliflower mixture over top and bake for 30 minutes.

Broil on high heat for 5 minutes, then sprinkle with bacon to serve.

Slow Cooker Beef Bourguignon
Nutrition: Cal 335;Fat 12,5 g; Carb 6,5 g;Protein 37.5 g
Serving 8; Cook time 4 hours 55 min

Ingredients
- 2 tablespoons olive oil
- 2 pounds boneless beef chuck roast, cut into chunks
- Salt and pepper
- ¼ cup almond flour
- ½ cup beef broth
- 2 cups red wine (dry)
- 2 tablespoons tomato paste
- 1 pound mushrooms, sliced
- 1 large yellow onion, cut into chunks

Instructions
1. Heat the oil in a large skillet over medium-high heat.
2. Season the beef with salt and pepper, then toss with almond flour.
3. Add the beef to the skillet and cook until browned on all sides then transfer to a slow cooker.
4. Reheat the skillet over medium high heat, then pour in the broth.
5. Scrape up the browned bits, then whisk in the wine and tomato paste.
6. Bring to a boil, then pour into the slow cooker.

7. Add the mushrooms and onion, then stir everything together.
8. Cover and cook on low heat for 4 hours until the meat is very tender. Serve hot.

Pepper Grilled Ribeye with Asparagus
Nutrition: Cal 380;Fat 25 g; Carb 4,5 g;Protein 35 g
Serving 4; Cook time 20 min

Ingredients
- 1 pound asparagus, trimmed
- 2 tablespoons olive oil
- Salt and pepper
- 1 pound ribeye steak
- 1 tablespoon coconut oil

Instructions
1. Preheat the oven to 400°F and line a small baking sheet with foil.
2. Toss the asparagus with olive oil and spread on the baking sheet.
3. Season with salt and pepper then place in the oven.
4. Rub the steak with the pepper and season with salt.
5. Melt the coconut oil in a cast-iron skillet and heat over high heat.
6. Add the steak and cook for 2 minutes then turn it.
7. Transfer the skillet to the oven and cook for 5 minutes or until the steak is done to the desired level.
8. Slice the steak and serve with the roasted asparagus.

Steak Kebabs with Peppers and Onions
Nutrition: Cal 350;Fat 20 g; Carb 6,5 g;Protein 35 g
Serving 4; Cook time 40 min

Ingredients
- 1 pound beef sirloin, cut into 1-inch cubes
- ¼ cup olive oil
- 2 tablespoons balsamic vinegar
- Salt and pepper
- 1 medium yellow onion, cut into chunks
- 1 medium red pepper, cut into chunks
- 1 medium green pepper, cut into chunks

Instructions
1. Toss the steak cubes with the olive oil, balsamic vinegar, salt, and pepper.
2. Slide the cubes onto skewers with the peppers and onions.
3. Preheat a grill to high heat and oil the grates.
4. Grill the kebabs for 2 to 3 minutes on each side until done to your liking.

Seared Lamb Chops with Asparagus
Nutrition: Cal 380;Fat 18.5 g; Carb 4,5 g;Protein 48 g
Serving 4; Cook time 20 min

Ingredients
- 8 bone-in lamb chops
- Salt and pepper
- 1 tablespoon fresh chopped rosemary
- 1 tablespoon olive oil
- 1 tablespoon butter
- 16 spears asparagus, cut into 2-inch chunks

Instructions
1. Season the lamb with salt and pepper then sprinkle with rosemary.
2. Heat the oil in a large skillet over medium-high heat.
3. Add the lamb chops and cook for 2 to 3 minutes on each side until seared.
4. Remove the lamb chops to rest and reheat the skillet with the butter.
5. Add the asparagus and turn to coat then cover the skillet.
Cook for 4 to 6 minutes until tender-crisp and serve with the lamb.

Lamb Chops with Kalamata Tapenade
Nutrition: Cal 348;Fat 28 g; Carb 2 g;Protein 21 g
Serving 4; Cook time 40 min

Ingredients
FOR THE TAPENADE
- 1 cup pitted Kalamata olives
- 2 tablespoons chopped
- fresh parsley
- 2 tablespoons extra-virgin
- olive oil
- 2 teaspoons minced garlic
- 2 teaspoons freshly squeezed
- lemon juice

FOR THE LAMB CHOPS
- 2 (1-pound) racks French-cut
- lamb chops (8 bones each)
- Sea salt
- Freshly ground black pepper
- 1 tablespoon olive oil

Instructions
TO MAKE THE TAPENADE
1. Place the olives, parsley, olive oil, garlic, and lemon juice in a food processor and process until the mixture is puréed but still slightly chunky.
2. Transfer the tapenade to a container and store sealed in the refrigerator until needed.

TO MAKE THE LAMB CHOPS
1. Preheat the oven to 450°F.
2. Season the lamb racks with salt and pepper.
3. Place a large ovenproof skillet over medium-high heat and add the olive oil.
4. Pan sear the lamb racks on all sides until browned, about 5 minutes in total.
5. Arrange the racks upright in the skillet, with the bones interlaced, and roast them in the oven until they reach your desired doneness, about 20 minutes for medium-rare or until the internal temperature reaches 125°F.
6. Let the lamb rest for 10 minutes and then cut the lamb racks into chops. Arrange 4 chops per person on the plate and top with the Kalamata tapenade

Rosemary-Garlic Lamb Racks
Nutrition: Cal 354;Fat 30 g; Carb 1 g;Protein 21 g
Serving 4; Cook time 1 hours 35 min

Ingredients
- 4 tablespoons extra-virgin olive oil
- 2 tablespoons finely chopped
- fresh rosemary
- 2 teaspoons minced garlic
- Pinch sea salt
- 2 (1-pound) racks French-cut
- lamb chops (8 bones each)

Instructions
1. In a small bowl, whisk together the olive oil, rosemary, garlic, and salt.
2. Place the racks in a sealable freezer bag and pour the olive oil mixture into the bag. Massage the meat through the bag so it is coated with the marinade. Press the air out of the bag and seal it.
3. Marinate the lamb racks in the refrigerator for 1 to 2 hours.
4. Preheat the oven to 450°F.
5. Place a large ovenproof skillet over medium-high heat. Take the lamb racks out of the bag and sear them in the skillet on all sides, about 5 minutes in total.
6. Arrange the racks upright in the skillet, with the bones interlaced, and roast them in the oven until they reach your desired doneness, about 20 minutes for medium-rare or until the internal temperature reaches 125°F.
7. Let the lamb rest for 10 minutes and then cut the racks into chops.
8. Serve 4 chops per person.

Lamb Leg with Sun-dried Tomato Pesto
Nutrition: Cal 352;Fat 29 g; Carb 5 g;Protein 17 g
Serving 8; Cook time 85 min

Ingredients
FOR THE PESTO
- 1 cup sun-dried tomatoes packed
- in oil, drained
- ¼ cup pine nuts
- 2 tablespoons extra-virgin olive oil
- 2 tablespoons chopped fresh basil
- 2 teaspoons minced garlic

FOR THE LAMB LEG
- 1 (2-pound) lamb leg
- Sea salt
- Freshly ground black pepper
- 2 tablespoons olive oil

Instructions
TO MAKE THE PESTO
1. Place the sun-dried tomatoes, pine nuts, olive oil, basil, and garlic in a blender or food processor; process until smooth.
2. Set aside until needed.

TO MAKE THE LAMB LEG
1. Preheat the oven to 400°F.
2. Season the lamb leg all over with salt and pepper.
3. Place a large ovenproof skillet over medium-high heat and add the olive oil.
4. Sear the lamb on all sides until nicely browned, about 6 minutes in total.
5. Spread the sun-dried tomato pesto all over the lamb and place the lamb on a baking sheet. Roast until the meat reaches your desired doneness, about 1 hour for medium.
6. Let the lamb rest for 10 minutes before slicing and serving.

Sirloin with Blue CheEse Compound ButTer
Nutrition: Cal 544;Fat 44 g; Carb 1 g;Protein 35 g
Serving 4; Cook time 1 hours 22 min

Ingredients
- 6 tablespoons butter, at room
- temperature
- 4 ounces blue cheese, such
- as Stilton or Roquefort
- 4 (5-ounce) beef sirloin steaks
- 1 tablespoon olive oil
- Sea salt
- Freshly ground black pepper

Instructions
1. Place the buter in a blender and pulse until the buter is whipped, about 2 minutes.
2. Add the cheese and pulse until just incorporated.
3. Spoon the buter mixture onto a sheet of plastic wrap and roll it into a log about 1½ inches in diameter by twisting both ends of the plastic wrap in opposite directions.
4. Refrigerate the buter until completely set, about 1 hour.
5. Slice the buter into ½-inch disks and set them on aplate in the refrigerator until you are ready to serve the steaks. Store lefover buter in the refrigerator for up to 1 week.
6. Preheat a barbecue to medium-high heat.
7. Let the steaks come to room temperature.
8. Rub the steaks all over with the olive oil and season them with salt and pepper.
9. Grill the steaks until they reach your desired doneness, about 6 minutes per side for medium.
10. If you do not have a barbecue, broil the steaks in a preheated oven for 7 minutes per side for medium.
11. Let the steaks rest for 10 minutes. Serve each topped with a disk of the compound buter.

Garlic-Braised Short Ribs
Nutrition: Cal 481;Fat 38 g; Carb 5 g;Protein 29 g
Serving 4; Cook time 2 hours 30 min

Ingredients
- 4 (4-ounce) beef short ribs
- Sea salt
- Freshly ground black pepper
- 1 tablespoon olive oil
- 2 teaspoons minced garlic
- ½ cup dry red wine
- 3 cups Beef Stock

Instructions

1. Preheat the oven to 325°F.
2. Season the beef ribs on all sides with salt and pepper.
3. Place a deep ovenproof skillet over medium-high heat and add the olive oil.
4. Sear the ribs on all sides until browned, about 6 minutes in total. Transfer the ribs to a plate.
5. Add the garlic to the skillet and sauté until translucent, about 3 minutes.
6. Whisk in the red wine to deglaze the pan. Be sure to scrape all the browned bits from the meat from the botom of the pan. Simmer the wine until it is slightly reduced, about 2 minutes.
7. Add the beef stock, ribs, and any accumulated juices on the plate back to the skillet and bring the liquid to a boil.
8. Cover the skillet and place it in the oven to braise the ribs until the meat is fall-of-the-bone tender, about 2 hours.
9. Serve the ribs with a spoonful of the cooking liquid drizzled over each serving.

Bacon-WrapPed BeEf Tenderloin
Nutrition: Cal 565;Fat 49 g; Carb 2g;Protein 28 g
Serving 4; Cook time 25 min

Ingredients
- 4 (4-ounce) beef tenderloin steaks
- Sea salt
- Freshly ground black pepper
- 8 bacon slices
- 1 tablespoon extra-virgin olive oil

Instructions
1. Preheat the oven to 450°F.
2. Season the steaks with salt and pepper.
3. Wrap each steak snugly around the edges with 2 slices of bacon and secure the bacon with toothpicks.
4. Place a large skillet over medium-high heat and add the olive oil.
5. Pan sear the steaks for 4 minutes per side and transfer them to a baking sheet.
6. Roast the steaks until they reach your desired doneness, about 6 minutes for medium.
7. Remove the steaks from the oven and let them rest for 10 minutes.
8. Remove the toothpicks and serve.

CheEseburger CasSerole
Nutrition: Cal 410;Fat 33 g; Carb 3g;Protein 20 g
Serving 6; Cook time 40 min

Ingredients
- 1 pound 75% lean ground beef
- ½ cup chopped sweet onion
- 2 teaspoons minced garlic
- 1&½ cups shredded aged Cheddar, divided
- ½ cup heavy (whipping) cream
- 1 large tomato, chopped
- 1 teaspoon minced fresh basil
- ¼ teaspoon sea salt
- ⅛ teaspoon freshly ground black pepper

Instructions

1. Preheat the oven to 350°F.
2. Place a large skillet over medium-high heat and add the ground beef.
3. Brown the beef until cooked through, about 6 minutes, and spoon of any excess fat.
4. Stir in the onion and garlic and cook until the vegetables are tender, about 4 minutes.
5. Transfer the beef and vegetables to an 8-by-8-inch casserole dish.
6. In medium bowl, stir together 1 cup of shredded cheese and the heavy cream, tomato, basil, salt, and pepper until well combined.
7. Pour the cream mixture over the beef mixture and top the casserole with the remaining ½ cup of shredded cheese.
8. Bake until the casserole is bubbly and the cheese is melted and lightly browned, about 30 minutes.

Italian BeEf Burgers
Nutrition: Cal 440;Fat 37 g; Carb 4g;Protein 22 g
Serving 4; Cook time 22 min

Ingredients
- 1 pound 75% lean ground beef
- ¼ cup ground almonds
- 2 tablespoons chopped fresh basil
- 1 teaspoon minced garlic
- ¼ teaspoon sea salt
- 1 tablespoon olive oil
- 1 tomato, cut into 4 thick slices
- ¼ sweet onion, sliced thinly

Instructions
1. In a medium bowl, mix together the ground beef, ground almonds, basil, garlic, and salt until well mixed.
2. Form the beef mixture into four equal paties and flaten them to about ½ inch thick.
3. Place a large skillet on medium-high heat and add the olive oil.
4. Panfry the burgers until cooked through, flipping them once, about 12 minutes in total.
5. Pat away any excess grease with paper towels and serve the burgers with a slice of tomato and onion

Pork and Ham

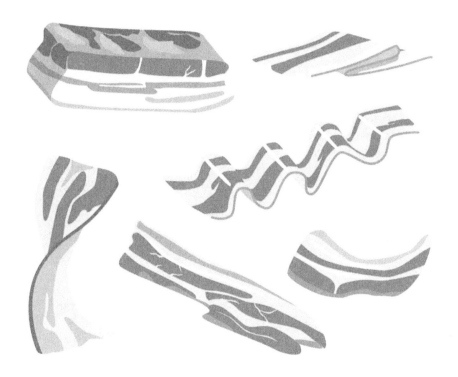

Ham and Provolone Sandwich

Nutrition: Cal 425;Fat 31 g;Carb 5 g;Protein 31 g
Serving 1; Cook time 35 min

Ingredients:
- 1 large egg, separated
- Pinch cream of tartar
- Pinch salt
- 1 ounce cream cheese, softened
- ¼ cup shredded provolone cheese
- 3 ounces sliced ham

Instructions:
1. For the bread, preheat the oven to 300°F and line a baking sheet with parchment.
2. Beat the egg whites with the cream of tartar and salt until soft peaks form.
3. Whisk the cream cheese and egg yolk until smooth and pale yellow.
4. Fold in the egg whites a little at a time until smooth and well combined.
5. Spoon the batter onto the baking sheet into two even circles.
6. Bake for 25 minutes until firm and lightly browned.
7. Spread the butter on one side of each bread circle then place one in a preheated skillet over medium heat.
8. Sprinkle with cheese and add the sliced ham then top with the other bread circle, butter-side-up.
9. Cook the sandwich for a minute or two then carefully flip it over.
10. Let it cook until the cheese is melted then serve.

Spring Salad with Shaved Parmesan

Nutrition: Cal 295;Fat 25.5 g;Carb 3 g;Protein 6.5 g
Serving 2; Cook time 15 min

Ingredients:
- 3 slices uncooked bacon
- 2 tablespoons red wine vinegar
- 1 tablespoon Dijon mustard
- Salt and pepper
- Liquid stevia extract, to taste
- 4 ounces mixed spring greens
- ½ small red onion, sliced thinly
- ⅓ cup roasted pine nuts
- ¼ cup shaved parmesan

Instructions:
1. Cook the bacon in a skillet until crisp then remove to paper towels.
2. Reserve ¼ cup of bacon fat in the skillet, discarding the rest, then chop the bacon.
3. Whisk the red wine vinegar and mustard into the bacon fat in the skillet.
4. Season with salt and pepper, then sweeten with stevia to taste and let cool slightly.
5. Combine the spring greens, red onion, pine nuts, and parmesan in a salad bowl.
6. Toss with the dressing, then top with chopped bacon to serve.

Three Meat and Cheese Sandwich

Nutrition: Cal 610;Fat 48 g;Carb 3 g;Protein 40 g
Serving 1; Cook time 35 min

Ingredients:
- 1 large egg, separated
- Pinch cream of tartar
- Pinch salt
- 1 ounce cream cheese, softened
- 1 ounce sliced ham
- 1 ounce sliced hard salami
- 1 ounce sliced turkey
- 2 slices cheddar cheese

Instructions:
1. For the bread, preheat the oven to 300°F and line a baking sheet with parchment.
2. Beat the egg whites with the cream of tartar and salt until soft peaks form.
3. Whisk the cream cheese and egg yolk until smooth and pale yellow.
4. Fold in the egg whites a little at a time until smooth and well combined.
5. Spoon the batter onto the baking sheet into two even circles.
6. Bake for 25 minutes until firm and lightly browned.
7. To complete the sandwich, layer the sliced meats and cheeses between the two bread circles.
8. Grease a skillet with cooking spray and heat over medium heat.
9. Add the sandwich and cook until browned underneath, then flip and cook until the cheese is just melted.

Ham, Egg, and Cheese Sandwich

Nutrition: Cal 365;Fat 21 g;Carb 6.5 g;Protein 35.5 g
Serving 1; Cook time 35 min

Ingredients:
- 1 large egg, separated
- Pinch cream of tartar
- Pinch salt
- 1 ounce cream cheese, softened
- 1 large egg
- 1 teaspoon butter
- 3 ounces sliced ham
- 1 slice cheddar cheese

Instructions:
1. For the bread, preheat the oven to 300°F and line a baking sheet with parchment.
2. Beat the egg whites with the cream of tartar and salt until soft peaks form.
3. Whisk the cream cheese and egg yolk until smooth and pale yellow.
4. Fold in the egg whites a little at a time until smooth and well combined.
5. Spoon the batter onto the baking sheet into two even circles.
6. Bake for 25 minutes until firm and lightly browned.
7. To complete the sandwich, fry the egg in butter until done to your preference.
8. Arrange the sliced ham on top of one bread circle.

9. Top with the fried egg and the sliced cheese then the second bread circle.
10. Serve immediately or cook in a greased skillet to melt the cheese first.

Chopped Kale Salad with Bacon Dressing
Nutrition: Cal 230;Fat 12 g;Carb 14 g;Protein 16 g
Serving 2; Cook time 15 min

Ingredients:
- 6 slices uncooked bacon
- 2 tablespoons apple cider vinegar
- 1 teaspoon Dijon mustard
- Liquid stevia, to taste
- Salt and pepper
- 4 cups fresh chopped kale
- ¼ cup thinly sliced red onion

Instructions:
1. Cook the bacon in a skillet until crisp then remove to paper towels and chop.
2. Reserve ¼ cup of the bacon grease in the skillet and warm over low heat.
3. Whisk in the apple cider vinegar, mustard, and stevia then season with salt and pepper.
4. Toss in the kale and cook for 1 minute then divide between two plates.
5. Top the salads with red onion and chopped bacon to serve.

CREAMY HONEY & MUSTARD PORK RIBS
Nutrition: Cal 385 ;Fat 17 g; Carb 16 g;Protein 39 g
Serving 6 Cook time 4 hours

Ingredients
- 3 1/2 pounds country style pork ribs
- 1/2 cup honey mustard
- 1 cup BBQ sauce
- 2 tsp Salt-Free Seasoning Blend

Instructions
1. Place ribs in instant pot.
2. In a tiny bowl, stir together barbecue sauce, honey mustard, and seasoning blend.
3. Pour over ribs in instant pot, stir to coat.
4. Cover and turn the steam release handle on the venting position.
5. Select the slow cooker setting and set to high. Cook for 4 hours.
6. Transfer ribs to a serving platter.
7. Strain sauce into a bowl, skim fat from sauce.
8. Drizzle some in the sauce in the ribs and pass the rest of the sauce in the table.

TENDER AND JUICY SHREDDED PORK
Nutrition: Cal 550 ;Fat41 g; Carb 2 g;Protein 38 g
Serving 8 Cook time 8 hours

Ingredients
- 4 pounds pork shoulder roast
- 4 ounces green chilies, diced
- 1 cup using apple cider vinegar

- 1 1/2 tsp garlic, minced
- 1 cup onion, finely chopped
- 1 tsp ground black pepper
- 1 tsp salt

Instructions
1. Place roast in instant pot.
2. Combine remaining ingredients and pour over roast.
3. Cover and turn the steam release handle towards the venting position.
4. Select the slow cooker setting and hang to medium.
5. Cook for 8 hours.
6. Remove to some chopping board and shred with two forks, discarding fat and bones.

Keto Prosciutto Spinach Salad
Nutrition: Cal 420 ;Fat 16 g; Carb 8 g;Protein 25 g
Serving 2 Cook time 10 min

Ingredients
- 2 cups baby spinach
- 1/3 lb. prosciutto
- 1 cantaloupe
- 1 avocado
- 1/4 cup diced red onion
- Handful of raw, unsalted walnuts

Instructions
1. lace a cup of spinach on each plate.
2. Top with diced prosciutto, cubes of balls of melon, slices of avocado, a sprinkling of red onion, and a few walnuts.
3. Add some freshly ground pepper, if you like.

Bright Salsa Pork Chops
Nutrition: Cal 460 ;Fat 22 g; Carb 8 g;Protein 25 g
Serving 2 Cook time 8 hours 20 min

Ingredients
- 2 x Pork Loins
- 75g Salsa
- 3 Tablespoon Lime Juice
- ½ tsp. Ground Cumin
- ½ tsp. Garlic Powder
- ½ tsp. Salt
- ½ tsp. Ground Black Pepper
- Calorie Free Cooking Spray

Instructions
1. In a small bowl combine cumin, garlic powder, salt and pepper and rub the spice mixture into pork chops.
2. Brown chops 5 minutes each side on a medium heat.
3. Spray the insides of your slow cooker cooking spray and add the pork chops.
4. Add the salsa and lime mixture.
5. Slow cook on low for 8 hours.

Loaded Cauliflower

Nutrition: Cal 200;Fat 17 g; Carb 8 g;Protein 12 g
Serving 6; Cook time 20 min

Ingredients
- 1 pound cauliflower florettes
- 4 ounces sour cream
- 1 cup grated cheddar cheese
- 2 slices cooked bacon, crumbled
- 2 tablespoons snipped chives
- 3 tablespoons butter
- 1/4 teaspoon garlic powder
- Salt and pepper, to taste

Instructions
1. Cut the cauliflower into florettes and add them to a microwave-safe bowl. Add 2 tablespoons of water and cover with cling film. Microwave for 5-8 minutes, depending on your microwave, until completely cooked and tender. Drain the excess water and let sit uncovered for a minute or two. (alternately, steam your cauliflower the conventional way. You may need to squeeze a little water out of the cauliflower after cooking).
2. Add the cauliflower to a food processor and process until fluffy. Add the butter, garlic powder, and sour cream and process until it resembles the consistency of mashed potatoes. Remove the mashed cauliflower to a bowl and add most of the chives, saving some to add to the top later. Add half of the cheddar cheese and mix by hand. Season with salt and pepper.
3. Top the loaded cauliflower with the remaining cheese, remaining chives and bacon. Put back into the microwave to melt the cheese or place the cauliflower under the broiler for a few minutes.
4. I visually divide the cauliflower into sixths. Serving size is approximately 1/3-1/2 cup.

Pan-Seared Pork Tenderloin Medallions

Nutrition: Cal 150;Fat 7 g; Carb 3 g;Protein 18 g
Serving 4; Cook time 18 min

Ingredients
- 1 tablespoon canola oil 1 (1-lb.)
- pork tenderloin, trimmed and cut crosswise into 12 medallions
- 1/2 teaspoon kosher salt
- 1/4 teaspoon garlic powder
- 1/4 teaspoon black pepper Fresh thyme leaves (optional)

Instructions
1. Heat oil in a 12-inch skillet over medium-high. Arrange pork medallions in a single layer on a work surface, and press each with the palm of your hand to flatten to an even thickness.
2. Combine salt, garlic powder, and pepper; sprinkle evenly over pork. Add pork to skillet in a single layer; cook just until done, about 3 minutes per side
3. Remove from heat; let stand 5 minutes before serving. Garnish with thyme leaves, if desired.

Coconut Pork Curry

Nutrition: Cal 260;Fat 16 g; Carb 10 g;Protein 18 g
Serving 4; Cook time 60 min

Ingredients
- 1 teaspoon ground cumin
- 1 teaspoon ground coriander
- 1/2 teaspoon ground cinnamon
- 1/4 teaspoon ground chilli powder
- 800g diced pork
- 1 tablespoon vegetable oil
- 1 large (200g) brown onion, chopped
- 2 cloves garlic, chopped
- 4cm piece (20g) fresh ginger, grated
- 1 tablespoon water
- 400ml can coconut cream or coconut milk
- 2 tablespoons brown sugar
- 1 teaspoon salt
- 1 tablespoon lemon juice
- 1/4 cup fresh coriander leaves

Instructions
1. Combine the spices in a medium bowl; add pork, toss to coat.
2. Heat half the oil in a large frying pan. Cook the pork in 2 batches, using the remaining oil, until browned all over. Remove from pan.
3. Add onion to same pan with garlic, ginger and water; cook, stirring, over medium heat until softened. Return the pork to the pan with coconut cream, sugar and salt. Simmer, covered, stirring occasionally, for about 1 hour to 1 hour 30 minutes or until the pork is tender and the sauce is thickened.
4. Stir in juice; season to taste with salt and pepper. Sprinkle with coriander.

The Best Baked Garlic Pork Tenderloin

Nutrition: Cal 449;Fat 13 g; Carb 6 g;Protein 32 g
Serving 4; Cook time 60 min

Ingredients
- 2 tbsp extra virgin olive oil
- 1 tbsp celtic sea salt and fresh cracked pepper
- 2 lb pork tenderloin, optional: pre-marinate pork before cooking
- 4 tbsp butter, sliced into 4-6 pats
- 2 tbsp diced garlic
- 1 tsp dried basil*
- 1 tsp dried oregano*
- 1 tsp dried thyme*
- 1 tsp dried parsley*
- ½ tsp dried sage*
- 2 tbsp Italian Herb Seasoning Blend

Instructions
1. Preheat oven to 350 degrees.
2. Line baking sheet with aluminum foil.
3. In a small bowl, combine garlic, basil, oregano, thyme, parsley, and sage. Set aside.
4. Generously season meat with salt and pepper.
5. In a large pan, heat oil until shimmery.
6. Add to pan, and cook on all sides until dark golden brown.
7. Transfer to baking sheet.

8. Generously coat with herb mix.
9. Place pats of butter on top of the pork.
10. Wrap in foil, bake until meat is 150 degrees internally at the widest, thickest part of the tenderloin (about 25 minutes.)
11. When pork has come to temperature, remove and let rest, tented with foil, for at least five minutes to lock in juices.
12. Slice against the grain and serve immediately.
13. To store leftovers, place in an airtight container and keep in refrigerator for up to three days.
14. To freeze leftovers, place in a plastic bag or wrap in plastic wrap and keep in freezer for up to three months.
15. To reheat, let thaw naturally in the refrigerator overnight, and bake at 350, wrapped in foil, until piping hot when ready to serve.

Pork Skewers with Chimichurri
Nutrition: Cal 450;Fat 36 g; Carb 6 g;Protein 30 g
Serving 2; Cook time 20 min

Ingredients
- 1/2 pound boneless pork shoulder
- 1/4 teaspoon ground cumin
- 1/4 teaspoon paprika
- 1 tablespoon coconut oil
- 1/4 cup olive oil
- 1/4 cup diced green peppers
- 3 tablespoons fresh chopped parsley
- 1 tablespoon fresh chopped cilantro
- 1 1/2 tablespoons fresh lemon juice
- 1 garlic clove (minced)
- salt and pepper

Instructions
1. Cut the pork into slices about 1-inch thick.
2. Season the pork with salt, pepper, cumin and paprika.
3. Slide the pork slices onto wooden skewers and heat the coconut oil in a skillet.
4. Fry the skewers until both sides are browned and the meat is cooked through.
5. Combine the remaining ingredients in a food processor.
6. Pulse several times to chop then blend until smooth.
7. Serve the pork skewers with the chimichurri spooned over them.

APRICOT GLAZED PORK
Nutrition: Cal 315;Fat 10 g; Carb 20 g;Protein 35 g
Serving 12; Cook time 4 hours

Ingredients
- 4 pounds boneless pork loin roast
- 1 cup onion, chopped
- 2 tbsp Dijon mustard
- 2 cups beef broth
- 1 cup apricot preserves

Instructions
1. Mix broth, preserves, onion, and mustard in instant pot.
2. Cut pork to match. Add to instant pot.
3. Cover and turn the steam release handle towards the venting position.

4. Select the slow cooker setting and set to high.
5. Cook for 4 hours.

EASY BBQ HAM
Nutrition: Cal 315;Fat 15 g; Carb 2 g;Protein 35 g
Serving 24; Cook time 14 hours

Ingredients
- 3 pounds ham, boneless
- 2 cups water
- 2 cups onions, sliced
- 6 whole cloves
- 2 cups BBQ sauce

Instructions
1. Place half in the onions in bottom in the instant pot.
2. Stick cloves in ham and set it on top of onions in instant pot.
3. Put the others in the onions on top. Pour water.
4. Cover and turn the steam release handle for the venting position.
5. Select the slow cooker setting and hang up to medium.
6. Cook for 10 hours.
7. Shred or cut up meat and onion.
8. Put back to the instant pot.
9. Add barbecue sauce and cook 4 hours more.

CHEESY SCALLOPED POTATOES WITH HAM
Nutrition: Cal 435;Fat 15 g; Carb 23 g;Protein 23 g
Serving 24; Cook time 14 hours

Ingredients
- 1 pound ham, sliced
- 8 medium potatoes, peeled and sliced
- 2 cups onions, sliced
- 1 cup Cheddar cheese, grated
- ½ tsp cream of tartar
- 1 cup water
- 10 ounces cream of mushroom soup
- Paprika

Instructions
1. Toss sliced potatoes in cream of tartar and water. Drain.
2. Put half ham, potatoes, and onions in instant pot.
3. Sprinkle with grated cheese.
4. Repeat with remaining half ham, potatoes, and onions.
5. Spoon undiluted soup over top.
6. Sprinkle with paprika.
7. Cover and turn the steam release handle to the venting position.
8. Select the slow cooker setting and hang to high.
9. Cook for 4 hours.

SALAD WITH BROCCOLI, CAULIFLOWER AND BACON
Nutrition: Cal 164;Fat 14 g; Carb 8 g;Protein 5 g
Serving 4; Cook time 15 min

Ingredients
- Broccoli (3/4 cups, chopped)
- Cauliflower (3/4 cups, chopped)
- Bacon (3 slices, chopped)
- Onion (1, chopped)

- Vinegar (1 teaspoon)
- Sour cream (3/4 cups)
- Salt and Pepper

Instructions

1. Put the cauliflower and broccoli inside the pressure cooker as well as set it to "Steam" for the matter of minutes (they shouldn't be too tender).Take out your vegetables in the boiling water and hang up them aside.
2. Fry the bacon till it turns brown, set it up aside and allow it cool.
3. Mix the onion (you can use spring onion also) using the vinegar, salt, pepper, and sour cream.
4. Mix the sauce while using broccoli and cauliflower, serve with many more bacon pieces for decoration.

ASPARAGUS WRAPPED IN PROSCIUTTO

Nutrition: Cal 555;Fat 45 g; Carb 6.7 g;Protein 33 g
Serving 3; Cook time 25 min

Ingredients

- Mushrooms (3 cups)
- Rice (1 ½ cups)
- Chicken stock (4 cups)
- Olive oil (1/4 cup)
- Onion (1 cup, chopped)
- Butter (unsalted, ¼ cup)
- White wine (3/4 cup)
- Rosemary
- Parmesan (half cup, grated)
- Salt and pepper

Instructions

1. Set the Pressure cooker to "Sauté"; add the olive oil and butter and let it melt for any matter of minutes. Add the mushrooms and cook them about 3 minutes).
2. Put within the onion, stir and cook to get a couple of more minutes. Add the rosemary and cook it to get a minute.
3. Add the rice and stir until it coats inside the butter and olive oil mix; stir for a couple of minutes and after that pour the wine. Let it simmer for three more minutes.
4. Pour inside the chicken stock, stir for any minute.
5. Now close and secure the lid and select to "High pressure" as well as set the timer for 6 minutes.
6. Let the stress out naturally for 5 minutes.
7. Open the lid and stir the risotto (it ought to turn creamy); remove the rosemary (if you are using spring, if it's chopped, then get forced out as it really is).
8. Sprinkle salt, pepper, and parmesan, and stir till the cheese melts.

Serve while it's hot.

BRATWURSTS AND SAUERKRAUT

Nutrition: Cal 525;Fat 42 g; Carb 12 g;Protein 24 g
Serving 4; Cook time 50 min

Ingredients

- 2 tablespoons avocado oil
- 1 yellow onion, thinly sliced

- 1 pound bratwurst
- 1 (16-ounce) jar sauerkraut, drained
- 1½ cups chicken broth
- 1 teaspoon garlic powder
- Salt
- Freshly ground black pepper

Instructions

1. In large cast-iron skillet over medium heat, add the oil, onion, and bratwurst and cook for 6 to 8 minutes, or until they get some color.
2. Add the sauerkraut, broth, garlic powder, salt, and pepper and simmer for 30 to 40 minutes, or until the sausages are cooked through.
3. In each of 4 storage containers, place 1 cup of sauerkraut and 1 bratwurst.

Rosemary Roasted Pork with Cauliflower

Nutrition: Cal 300;Fat 17 g; Carb 3 g;Protein 37 g
Serving 4; Cook time 30 min

Ingredients

- 1 ½ pounds boneless pork tenderloin
- 1 tablespoon coconut oil
- 1 tablespoon fresh chopped rosemary
- Salt and pepper
- 1 tablespoon olive oil
- 2 cups cauliflower florets

Instructions

1. Rub the pork with coconut oil, then season with rosemary, salt, and pepper.
2. Heat the olive oil in a large skillet over medium-high heat.
3. Add the pork and cook for 2 to 3 minutes on each side until browned.
4. Sprinkle the cauliflower in the skillet around the pork.
5. Reduce the heat to low, then cover the skillet and cook for 8 to 10 minutes until the pork is cooked through.

Slice the pork and serve with the cauliflower.

Sausage Stuffed Bell Peppers

Nutrition: Cal 355;Fat 23,5 g; Carb 16,5 g;Protein 19 g
Serving 4; Cook time 55 min

Ingredients

- 1 medium head cauliflower, chopped
- 1 tablespoon olive oil
- 12 ounces ground Italian sausage
- 1 small yellow onion, chopped
- 1 teaspoon dried oregano
- Salt and pepper
- 4 medium bell peppers

Instructions

1. Preheat the oven to 350°F.
2. Pulse the cauliflower in a food processor into rice-like grains.
3. Heat the oil in a skillet over medium heat then add the cauliflower – cook for 6 to 8 minutes until tender.
4. Spoon the cauliflower rice into a bowl, then reheat the skillet.

5. Add the sausage and cook until browned, then drain the fat.
6. Stir the sausage into the cauliflower, then add the onion, oregano, salt andpepper.
7. Slice the tops off the peppers, remove the seeds and pith, then spoon the sausage mixture into them.
8. Place the peppers upright in a baking dish, then cover the dish with foil.
9. Bake for 30 minutes, then uncover and bake 15 minutes more. Serve hot.

Cheddar, Sausage, and Mushroom Casserole
Nutrition: Cal 450;Fat 34 g; Carb 6 g;Protein 28 g
Serving 6; Cook time 45 min

Ingredients
- 1 pound ground Italian sausage
- 8 ounces mushrooms, diced
- 1 large yellow onion, chopped
- 1 cup shredded cheddar cheese
- 8 large eggs
- ½ cup heavy cream
- Salt and pepper

Instructions
1. Preheat the oven to 375°F and grease a baking dish.
2. Heat the sausage in a large skillet over medium-high heat.
3. Cook the sausage until browned then stir in the mushrooms and onions.
4. Cook for 4 to 5 minutes then spread in the baking dish.
5. Sprinkle the dish with cheese then whisk together the remaining ingredients in a separate bowl.
6. Pour the mixture into the dish then bake for 35 minutes until bubbling.

Cauliflower Crust Meat Lover's Pizza
Nutrition: Cal 560;Fat 40 g; Carb 11 g;Protein 41 g
Serving 2; Cook time 40 min

Ingredients
- 1 tablespoon butter
- 2 cups riced cauliflower
- Salt and pepper
- 1 ½ cups shredded mozzarella cheese, divided into 1 cup and ½ cup
- 1 cup fresh grated parmesan
- 1 teaspoon garlic powder
- 1 large egg white
- 1 teaspoon dried Italian seasoning
- ¼ cup low-carb tomato sauce
- 2 ounces sliced pepperoni
- 1 ounce diced ham
- 2 slices bacon, cooked and crumbled

Instructions
1. Preheat the oven to 400°F and line a baking sheet with parchment.
2. Heat the butter in a skillet over medium-high heat and add the cauliflower.
3. Season with salt and pepper, then cover and cook for 15 minutes, stirring occasionally, until very tender.

4. Spoon the cauliflower into a bowl and stir in ½ cup mozzarella along with the parmesan and garlic powder.
5. Stir in the egg white and Italian seasoning, then pour onto the baking sheet.
6. Shape the dough into a circle about ½-inch thick, then bake for 15 minutes.
7. Top with tomato sauce, along with the remaining mozzarella and the pepperoni, bacon, and ham.
8. Broil until the cheese is browned, then slice to serve.

Bacon-Wrapped Pork Tenderloin with Cauliflower
Nutrition: Cal 330;Fat 18,5 g; Carb 3 g;Protein 38 g
Serving 4; Cook time 35 min

Ingredients
- 1 ¼ pounds boneless pork tenderloin
- Salt and pepper
- 8 slices uncooked bacon
- 1 tablespoon olive oil
- 2 cups cauliflower florets

Instructions
1. Preheat the oven to 425°F and season the pork with salt and pepper.
2. Wrap the pork in bacon and place on a foil-lined roasting pan.
3. Roast for 25 minutes until the internal temperature reaches 155°F.
4. Meanwhile, heat the oil in a skillet over medium heat.
5. Add the cauliflower and sauté until tender-crisp – about 8 to 10 minutes.
6. Turn on the broiler and place the pork under it to crisp the bacon.
7. Slice the pork to serve with the sautéed cauliflower

Roasted Pork Loin with Grainy Mustard Sauce
Nutrition: Cal 368;Fat 29 g; Carb 2 g;Protein 25 g
Serving 8; Cook time 80 min

Ingredients
- 1 (2-pound) boneless pork loin roast
- Sea salt
- Freshly ground black pepper
- 3 tablespoons olive oil
- 1&½ cups heavy (whipping) cream
- 3 tablespoons grainy mustard, such as Pommery

Instructions
1. Preheat the oven to 375°F.
2. Season the pork roast all over with sea salt and pepper.
3. Place a large skillet over medium-high heat and add the olive oil.
4. Brown the roast on all sides in the skillet, about 6 minutes in total, and place the roast in a baking dish.
5. Roast until a meat thermometer inserted in the thickest part of the roast reads 155°F, about 1 hour.
6. When there is approximately 15 minutes of roasting time lef, place a small saucepan over medium heat and add the heavy cream and mustard.

7. Stir the sauce until it simmers, then reduce the heat to low. Simmer the sauce until it is very rich and thick, about 5 minutes. Remove the pan from the heat and set aside.
8. Let the pork rest for 10 minutes before slicing and serve with the sauce

FISH and SEAFOOD

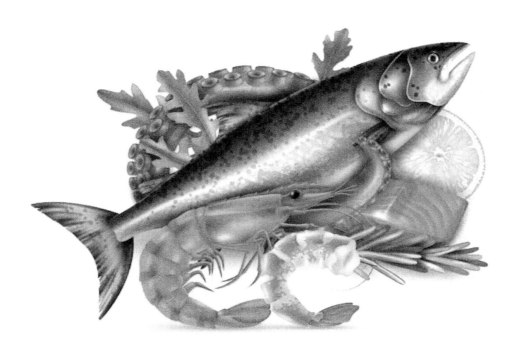

Quick & Easy Keto Tuna Fish Salad
Nutrition: Cal 430;Fat 3 g;Carb 22 g;Protein 18 g
Serving 2; Cook time 15 min

Ingredients
2 cups mixed greens
1 large tomato, diced
¼ cup fresh parsley, chopped
¼ cup fresh mint, chopped
10 large kalamata olives, pitted
1 small zucchini, sliced lengthwise
½ avocado, diced
1 green onion, sliced
1 can chunk light tuna in water, drained
1 tablespoon extra-virgin olive oil
1 tablespoon balsamic vinegar
¼ teaspoon Himalayan or fine sea salt
¾ teaspoon freshly cracked black peper

Instructions
1. In a sizzling hot cast iron skillet grill pan, grill the zucchini slices on both sides (or on a very hot grill).
2. Remove from pan and let cool for a few minutes.
3. Slice into bite size pieces.
4. Add all the ingredients in a large mixing bowl and mix until well combined

Simple Tuna Salad on Lettuce
Nutrition: Cal 550;Fat 35 g;Carb 8 g;Protein 38 g
Serving 2; Cook time 10 min

Ingredients:
- ¼ cup mayonnaise
- 1 tablespoon fresh lemon juice
- 1 tablespoon pickle relish
- 2 (6-ounce) cans tuna in oil, drained and flaked
- ½ cup cherry tomatoes, halved
- ¼ cup diced cucumber
- Salt and pepper
- 4 cups chopped romaine lettuce

Instructions:
1. Whisk together the mayonnaise, lemon juice, and relish in a bowl.
2. Toss in the flaked tuna, tomatoes, and cucumber – season with salt and pepper.
3. Spoon over chopped lettuce to serve.

Fried Tuna Avocado Balls
Nutrition: Cal 455;Fat 38 g;Carb 8 g;Protein 23 g
Serving 4; Cook time 20 min

Ingredients:
- ¼ cup canned coconut milk
- 1 teaspoon onion powder
- 1 clove garlic, minced
- Salt and pepper
- 10 ounces canned tuna, drained
- 1 medium avocado, diced finely
- ½ cup almond flour
- ¼ cup olive oil

Instructions:
1. Whisk together the coconut milk, onion powder, garlic, salt and pepper in a bowl.
2. Flake the tuna into the bowl and stir in the avocado.

3. Divide the mixture into 10 to 12 balls and roll in the almond flour.
4. Heat the oil in a large skillet over medium-high heat.
5. Add the tuna avocado balls and fry until golden brown then drain on paper towels.

Thai Coconut Shrimp Soup
Nutrition: Cal 375;Fat 29 g; Carb 13 g;Protein 18 g
Serving 4; Cook time 40 min

Ingredients:
- 1 tablespoon coconut oil
- 1 small yellow onion, diced
- 4 cups chicken broth
- 1 (14-ounce) can coconut milk
- 1 cup fresh chopped cilantro
- 1 jalapeno, seeded and chopped
- 1 tablespoon grated ginger
- 2 cloves garlic, minced
- 1 lime, zested and juiced
- 6 ounces uncooked shrimp, peeled and deveined
- 1 cup sliced mushrooms
- 1 small red onion, sliced thinly
- 1 tablespoon fish sauce

Instructions:
1. Heat the coconut oil in a saucepan over medium heat.
2. Add the yellow onions and sauté until translucent, about 6 to 7 minutes.
3. Stir in the chicken broth, coconut milk, cilantro, and jalapeno.
4. Add the ginger, garlic, and lime zest then bring to boil.
5. Reduce heat and simmer for 20 minutes - strain the mixture and discard the solids.
6. Return the remaining liquid to the saucepan and add the shrimp, mushrooms, and red onion.
7. Stir in the lime juice and fish sauce then simmer for 10 minutes. Serve hot.

Shrimp Avocado Salad
Nutrition: Cal 340;Fat 33 g; Carb 12 g;Protein 24 g
Serving 2; Cook time 10 min

Ingredients
- 8 ounces shrimp peeled, deveined, patted dry
- 1 large avocado, diced
- 1 small beefsteak tomato, diced and drained
- 1/3 cup crumbled feta cheese
- 1/3 cup freshly chopped cilantro or parsley
- 2 tablespoons salted butter, melted
- 1 tablespoon lemon juice
- 1 tablespoon olive oil
- 1/4 teaspoon salt
- 1/4 teaspoon black pepper

Instructions
1. Toss shrimp with melted butter in a bowl until well-coated.
2. Heat a pan over medium-high heat for a few minutes until hot. Add shrimp to the pan in a single layer, searing for a minute or until it starts to become pink around the edges, then flip and cook until shrimp are cooked through, less than a minute.

3. Transfer the shrimp to a plate as they finish cooking. Let them cool while you prepare the other ingredients.
4. Add all other ingredients to a large mixing bowl -- diced avocado, diced tomato, feta cheese, cilantro, lemon juice, olive oil, salt, and pepper -- and toss to mix.
5. Add shrimp and stir to mix together. Add additional salt and pepper, to taste.

Caprese Tuna Salad Stuffed Tomatoes
Nutrition: Cal 196;Fat 5 g; Carb 5 g;Protein 30 g
Serving 2; Cook time 10 min

Ingredients
- 1 medium tomato
- 1 (5 ounce) can tuna, very well drained
- 2 teaspoons balsamic vinegar
- 1 tablespoon chopped mozzarella (1/4 ounce)
- 1 tablespoon chopped fresh basil
- 1 tablespoon chopped green onion

Instructions
1. Cut the top 1/4-inch off the tomato. Use a spoon to scoop out the insides of the tomato. Set aside while you make the tuna salad.
2. Stir together the drained tuna, balsamic vinegar, mozzarella, basil, and green onion. Put the tuna salad in the hollowed out tomato, and enjoy!

Spicy Kimchi Ahi Poke
Nutrition: Cal 300;Fat 18 g; Carb 5 g;Protein 5 g
Serving 4; Cook time 10 min

Ingredients
- 1 lb sushi-grade ahi tuna, diced to roughly 1 inch
- 1 tablespoon soy sauce (or coconut aminos for paleo)
- 1/2 teaspoon sesame oil
- 1/4 cup mayo
- 2 tablespoons Sriracha
- 1 ripe avocado, diced
- 1/2 cup kimchi
- Chopped green onion
- Sesame seeds

Instructions
1. In a medium mixing bowl, add diced tuna.
2. Add soy sauce, sesame oil, mayo, Sriracha to the bowl and toss to combine.
3. Add diced avocado and kimchi to the bowl and gently combine.
4. Serve on top of salad greens, cauli rice, or traditional rice and top with a sprinkle of chopped green onion and sesame seeds if desired.

Prosciutto Blackberry Shrimp
Nutrition: Cal220;Fat 11 g; Carb 6 g;Protein 21 g
Serving 2; Cook time 20 min

Ingredients
- 10 Oz Pre-Cooked Shrimp
- 11 Slices Prosciutto
- 1/3 cup Blackberries, Ground
- 1/3 cup Red Wine
- 2 tbsp. Olive Oil
- 1 tbsp. Mint Leaves, Chopped
- 1-2 Tbsp. Erythritol (to taste)

Instructions
1. Preheat oven to 425 degrees.
2. Slice each piece of prosciutto in half depending on size of shrimp.
3. Wrap prosciutto around shrimp starting from tale up.
4. Place on baking sheet and drizzle with olive oil.
5. Bake for 15 minutes.
6. In a pan, add ground blackberries, mint leaves and erythritol.
7. Cook for 2-3 minutes.
8. Mix in red wine and reduce while shrimp cooks.
9. Strain if desired.

Spicy Shrimp Taco Lettuce Wraps
Nutrition: Cal 186;Fat 17 g; Carb 8 g;Protein 2 g
Serving 4; Cook time 20 min

Ingredients
- 20 medium shrimp peeled and deveined (about 1 pound)
- 1 tablespoon oil of choice
- 1 clove garlic minced
- 1/2 teaspoon
- 1/2 teaspoon ground cumin
- 1/4 teaspoon kosher salt
- 1 tablespoon olive oil
- squeeze of lime optional

Avocado Salsa
- 1 avocado cut into chunks
- 1 tomato, chopped
- 1/4 cup loosely packed fresh cilantro leaves coarsely chopped
- 1 tablespoon fresh lime juice from half a lime
- 1/2 teaspoon salt
- 1/4 teaspoon black pepper

Cilantro Sauce
- 1/4 cup sour cream
- 1/4 cup cilantro
- 1 clove garlic
- 1 tablespoon fresh lime juice
- salt and pepper, to taste
- 8-12 lettuce leaves

Instructions
To cook the shrimp
1. In a medium bowl whisk together olive oil, garlic, cumin, chili, and salt. Add shrimp and mix until shrimp is covered in seasoning. Heat a large heavy-duty or cast iron skillet on high heat for 2 minutes. Add the olive oil and shrimp. Cook 2-3 minutes per side or until shrimp is cooked through. Turn off heat and finish with a squeeze of lime (optional).

To make avocado tomato salsa
2. In a medium bowl, gently combine tomato, avocado, cilantro, lime juice and a sprinkle of salt and pepper and mixed through. Set aside.

To make the Jalapeno Cilantro Sauce

3. Add the sour cream, jalapeno, garlic, cilantro, lime and salt and pepper to a food processor. Blend for 30 seconds or until creamy.

To assemble:

Plac two romaine or butter lettuce leaves on top of eachother for each lettuce wraps. Top with 4-5 pieces of shrimp, a few tablespoons of avocado salsa and a genros drizzle of the spicy jalapeno cilantro sauce. Enjoy hot or cold!

Keto Shrimp Thai Salad

Nutrition: Cal 380 ;Fat 9 g; Carb 14 g;Protein 25 g
Serving 4 Cook time 15 min

Ingredients

- 6 Tablespoon extra-virgin olive oil, divided
- 2 Tablespoon. soy sauce
- 1 teaspoon fish sauce
- 1 teaspoon sambal oelek
- 1 Tablespoon brown sugar
- 3 Tablespoon lime juice
- 1 Tablespoon minced red pepper
- 1/2 pound shrimp, peeled and deveined
- 1 cup sugar snap peas, blanched and cooled in an ice bath
- 2 bundles vermicelli noodles, boiled and rinsed under cool water (you can use the same water you boiled the snap peas in)
- 4 cups shredded romaine lettuce
- 1/2 cup cherry tomatoes, halved
- 1/2 cup thinly sliced sweet peppers
- cilantro, mint leaves and crushed peanuts for garnish
- coarse salt and freshly ground peanuts to taste

Instructions

1. In a medium bowl, beat together 4 tablespoons of oil, soy sauce, fish sauce, sambal oelek, sugar, lime juice and the minced red pepper.
2. Heat the remaining oil in a large skillet over medium-high.
3. Add the shrimp, season with salt and pepper and sear on one side for 2 minutes.
4. Flip and sear another minute.
5. Salad Assembly:
6. In 2 bowls add romaine lettuce
7. Add some vermicelli noodles, the snow peas, peppers, tomatoes, shrimp, cilantro, mint, and some good crushed peanuts.
8. Shake up (or whisk) your dressing and then drizzle it over the salads.

Shrimp and Nori Rolls

Nutrition: Cal 340 ;Fat 12 g; Carb 8 g;Protein 25 g
Serving 1 Cook time 10 min

Ingredients

- 1 cup shrimp
- 1 tbsp. Mayonnaise
- 1 thinly sliced green onion
- 2 sheets Nori
- ¼ cucumber diced and seeded
- 1 tbsp. toasted Sesame seeds

Instructions

1. Wash and drain shrimp.
2. Add together shrimp with Mayonnaise and green onions.
3. Place Nori on flat surface and spoon on the shrimp and green onion mixture.
4. Dust with cucumber and sesame seeds.

Roll tightly and cut into bite size pieces.

Crispy Fish Sticks with Caper Dill Sauce

Nutrition: Cal 360 ;Fat 14 g; Carb 12 g;Protein 25 g
Serving 1 Cook time 30 min

Ingredients

- 1 lb. white fish fillets
- 1 cup grated parmesan
- 1 cup almond meal/flour
- 1/4 tsp. chili powder
- 1/2 tsp. dried parsley
- 1/4 tsp. salt
- pinch of pepper
- 2 tbsp. mayo
- 1 egg
- coconut oil for frying

Caper Dill Tartar Sauce

- 1/2 cup mayo
- 1/2 cup sour cream
- 1 1/2 tbsp. capers (including the caper juice)
- 2 medium dill/garlic pickles, diced
- 2 tbsp. chopped fresh dill
- 2 tsp. lemon juice

Instructions

1. Combine the dry ingredients, put in shallow dish and set aside.
2. Whisk together the egg and mayo.
3. Prepare tartar sauce by combining all ingredients cover and refrigerate until the fish is ready.
4. Cut the fillets to desired size. Dip the fish into the egg mixture and dredge in the breading mixture.
5. Heat 1/2-inch oil in a medium skillet and drop 2 fish sticks at a time for consistent cooking.
6. Cook for 1-2 minutes on each side, until golden.
7. Remove and drain on paper-towel.

Serve with tartar sauce.

Creamy shrimp and mushroom skillet

Nutrition: Cal 400 ;Fat 12 g; Carb 6 g;Protein 20 g
Serving 2 Cook time 15 min

Ingredients

- 4 slices organic uncured bacon
- 1 cup sliced mushrooms
- 4 oz. smoked salmon
- 4 oz. raw shelled shrimp (I used TJ's Argentinian wild)
- ½ cup heavy whipping cream OR coconut cream for a dairy free option

•1 pinch Celtic Sea Salt
•freshly ground black pepper

Instructions

1. Cut the bacon in 1 inch pieces and cook over medium heat.
2. Add sliced mushrooms and cook for 5 minutes.
3. Add strips of smoked salmon and cook for 2 to 3 minutes.
4. Add the shrimp and sauté on a high for 2 minutes.
5. Stir in cream and salt.

Lower heat and let cook for 1 minute until thick and creamy.

Buttered Cod in Skillet

Nutrition: Cal 294;Fat 18 g; Carb 2 g;Protein 30 g
Serving 4; Cook time 15 min

Ingredients

•1 1/2 lbs cod fillets
•6 tablespoons unsalted butter, sliced
Seasoning
•¼ teaspoon garlic powder
•½ teaspoon table salt
•¼ teaspoon ground pepper
•¾ teaspoon ground paprika
•Few lemon slices
•Herbs, parsley, or cilantro

Instructions

1. Stir together ingredients for seasoning in a small bowl.
2. Cut cod into smaller pieces, if desired. Season all sides of the cod with the seasoning.
3. Heat 2 tablespoons butter in a large skillet over medium-high heat. Once butter melts, add cod to skillet. Cook 2 minutes.
4. Turn heat down to medium. Turn cod over, top with remaining butter and cook another 3-4 minutes.
5. Butter will completely melt and the fish will cook. (Don't overcook the cod, it will become mushy and completely fall apart.)
6. Drizzle cod with fresh lemon juice. Top with fresh herbs, if desired. Serve immediately.

Avocado Lime Salmon

Nutrition: Cal 570;Fat 44 g; Carb 12 g;Protein 26 g
Serving 16; Cook time 20 min

Ingredients

•100 grams chopped cauliflower
•1 large avocado
•1 tablespoon fresh lime juice
•2 tablespoons diced red onion
•2 tablespoons olive oil
•2 (6-ounce) boneless salmon fillets
•Salt and pepper

Instructions

1. Melt your butter in a pan and fry 2-3 eggs until the whites are set and yolk is to desired doneness. Season Place the cauliflower in a food processor and pulse into rice-like grains.
2. Grease a skillet with cooking spray and heat over medium heat.

3. Add the cauliflower rice and cook, covered, for 8 minutes until tender. Set aside.
4. Combine the avocado, lime juice, and red onion in a food processor and blend smooth.
5. Heat the oil in a large skillet over medium-high heat.
6. Season the salmon with salt and pepper, then add to the skillet skin-side down.
7. Cook for 4 to 5 minutes until seared, then flip and cook for another 4 to 5 minutes.
8. Serve the salmon over a bed of cauliflower rice topped with the avocado cream.

Broccoli and Shrimp Sautéed in Butter

Nutrition: Cal 277;Fat 14 g; Carb 5 g;Protein 30 g
Serving 2; Cook time 15 min

Ingredients

•1 cup broccoli, cut into small pieces
•1 clove garlic, crushed
•300 g shrimp, cleaned
•2 tbsp butter
•1 tsp lemon juice
•Salt, to taste

Instructions

1. Chop the broccoli into small portions or whichever size you prefer, but smaller pieces cook faster.
2. Melt the butter in a preheated pan. Gently toss in the chopped broccoli and crushed garlic when the butter becomes hot (but not smoking). Stir to cook.
3. Leave over the heat for 3-4 minutes. Stir from time to time.
4. Clean the shrimp before adding them to the pan. Let it cook for around 3-4 minutes.
5. Once the shrimp turns pink and opaque, drizzle the lemon juice all over.

Keto Calamari

Nutrition: Cal 286;Fat 15 g; Carb 11 g;Protein 22 g
Serving 4; Cook time 30 min

Ingredients

•1 lb fresh squid cleaned
•
•1 egg beaten
•1/2 cup coconut flour
•1 teaspoon salt
•1 teaspoon paprika
•1/2 teaspoon garlic powder
•1/2 teaspoon onion powder
•Coconut oil for frying (about 1/4 cup)
•Minced cilantro optional
•Sliced Fresno chili optional
•Squeeze of lime optional
•Harissa Mayo
•1/4 cup mayonnaise
•1 tablespoon prepared hariss

Instructions

1. In a small bowl beat the egg. In another bowl combine the coconut flour and spices.
2. Pat the squid dry and dip into the beaten egg then dredge through the flour mixture.

3.Heat the oil in a 10" or larger cast-iron skillet over medium-high heat.

4.Frying in batches making sure to not overcrowd the skillet, fry 2 minutes per side until golden and crisp. Drain on paper towels

5.Either serve as is or toss with cilantro, chilis, and lime and serve with the harissa mayo

Calamari Stuffed with Pancetta and Vegetables
Nutrition: Cal 456;Fat 35 g; Carb 10 g;Protein 24 g
Serving 4; Cook time 20 min

Ingredients
- 500 g (8 large or 12 16 smaller) squid cleaned
- 82 g (1/2 cup) keto bun center only diced into very small pieces
- Stuffing
- 70 g (3 oz) pancetta or pork belly chopped into very small pieces
- 42 g (3 tbsp) of olive oil for grilling
- 68 g (5 tbsp) olive oil for stuffing
- 40 g (1/4 cup) carrots grated
- 8 g (1 tbsp) garlic grated
- 80 g (3/4 cup) celery diced into very small pieces
- 100 g (1 cup, or one bulb) fennel bulb diced into very small pieces
- 1/2 g (1/2 tsp) thyme powder
- 1-2 bunches fresh rosemary
- 6 g (1 tsp) salt
- 2 g (1 tsp) black pepper
- 14 g (1 tbsp) olive oil drizzling over prepared stuffed squid
- 15 g (1 tbsp) lemon juice freshly squeezed

Instructions
1.Clean your squid or purchase cleaned squid with tentacles. Rinse under cold running water and set aside

2.Prepare and weigh your vegetables: grate the carrots, onion and garlic. Chop the celery and fennel bulb into very small pieces

3.Cut the pancetta or pork belly and the squid arms into thin strips and then chop into very small pieces

4.Heat a grilling pan and add 3 tbsp of olive oil. When oil is sizzling add the pancetta/pork belly and squid arms, carrots, celery, fennel, onion and garlic. Place the fresh bunch of rosemary into the pan. Season with salt. Stir and cook on low heat until the vegetables are translucent, and the pancetta/pork belly is done (but not crispy). Remove the rosemary and discard

5.When stuffing is done, place into a mixing bowl and add 2 tbsp of olive oil and the pepper. Toss to combine

6.Use a teaspoon to insert the stuffing into each squid. Quantity of stuffing needed per squid will depend on the size of your squid. Do not overstuff as the squid will shrink as it cooks. Use a toothpick to seal the opening

7.Heat up the grill pan, and add the olive oil. Reduce heat to low and lay your stuffed squid perpendicular to the grill ridges. Cook for 5-6 minutes on the first side then flip and cook 5-6 minutes on the other side. Remove from heat and place on a platter

8.Finish by drizzling the tablespoon of fresh lemon juice on top and then the tablespoon of olive oil. Garnish with the fennel leaves and a wedge of lemon.

Low Carb Almond Crusted Cod
Nutrition: Cal 219;Fat 13 g; Carb 4 g;Protein 22 g
Serving 4; Cook time 25 min

Ingredients
- 1 4 filets cod or other white fish
- 1 med lemon zested and juiced
- 1/2 cup crushed almonds can use a food processor or blender to crush
- 1 Tbsp dill either fresh
- 1 Tbsp olive oil
- salt & pepper to taste
- 1 tsp mild to med. chili spice optional
- 4 tsp Dijon mustard more if you like mustard

Instructions
1.Preheat oven to 400 degrees F. Prepare a baking sheet with either parchment paper laid on top or spray with cooking spray

2.Place cod filets on paper towels to drain of water and pat dry. Place on baking sheet.

3.In a small bowl, combine the lemon zest, lemon juice, crushed almonds, dill, oil, salt and pepper and chili spice if using.

4.Spread each cod filet with a tsp or so of Dijon mustard,smoothing it over the entire top of the filet. Divide the almond mixture among the 4 filets, pressing it evely into the mustard with your hands.

5.Bake the fish until opaue at the thickest part, about 7 minutes for most.cod filets (less time for thin filets).

6.Serve with a green vegetable and lemon slices for a great low carb or keto fish dinner.

Mexican Fish Stew
Nutrition: Cal 196;Fat 7 g; Carb 8 g;Protein 19 g
Serving 6; Cook time 30 min

Ingredients
- 2 Tbsp olive oil
- 1 med onion chopped
- 1 large carrot sliced thinly
- 3 med celery stalks sliced thinly
- 3-6 cloves garlic smashed or minced
- 1 tsp smoky pepper blend
- 1/2 tsp dried thyme
- 1 cup white wine
- 4 cups chicken broth
- 1/2 cup chopped cilantro
- 2 14 oz cans Rotel diced tomatoes
- 1/2 tsp salt
- 3 leaves bay
- 6 oz scallops
- 7 oz walleye, coarsely chopped
- 1 lb mussels
- 3 oz white fish, coarsely chopped
- 2 med limes, cut into wedges optional
- 1 med lemon, sliced for garnish

Instructions

1.Heat oil over med-high heat in a dutch oven or large pot. Saute onion, carrot and celery in oil for 3-5 minutes until translucent. Add smashed garlic and cook for 1 more minute

2.Add spices and stir in to the onion mixture to coat. Add wine, broth, cilantro, and tomatoes to pot and simmer together for 15-20 minutes over medium heat. Add salt to taste.

3.Add all fish to the pot and cook, covered for about 5 minutes or until mussels open and white fish is opaque.

4.Add sliced lemons to the pot and serve.

5.Optional: serve with lime wedges that people can squeeze into the soup.

Creamy Keto Fish Casserole
Nutrition: Cal 221;Fat 15 g; Carb 9 g;Protein 27 g
Serving 4; Cook time 30 min

Ingredients
- 1 tbsp butter, for greasing baking dish
- 3 tbsp olive oil
- 1 lb broccoli, small florets
- 1 tsp salt
- ½ tsp ground black pepper
- 4 oz. (1¼ cups) scallions, finely chopped
- 2 tbsp small capers (non-pareils)
- 1½ lbs white fish (see tip), cut into serving-sized pieces
- 1 tbsp dried parsley
- 1¼ cups heavy whipping cream
- 1 tbsp Dijon mustard
- 3 oz. butter, cut into thin, equal slices

Instructions
1.Preheat oven to 400°F (200°C). Grease a 13" x 9" (33 x 23 cm) baking dish, set aside.

2.Heat the oil in a large frying pan, over medium-high heat. Add the broccoli, and stir-fry for 5 minutes, or until lightly browned and tender. Season with salt and pepper.

3.Add the scallions and capers, stir together, and fry for a couple of minutes. Spoon the broccoli mixture into the baking dish.

4.Place the fish amongst the vegetables.

5.In a medium-sized bowl, whisk together the parsley, whipping cream, and mustard. Pour over the fish and vegetables. Top with the sliced butter.

6.Bake on the middle rack, uncovered, for 20 minutes or until the fish is cooked through, and flakes easily with a fork.

7.Serve as is, or with leafy greens on the side

Grilled Salmon with Avocado Salsa
Nutrition: Cal 528;Fat 43 g; Carb 13 g;Protein 25 g
Serving 2; Cook time 22 min

Ingredients
- 2 4-6 oz salmon fillets
- 2 tablespoons olive oil
- 1 clove garlic minced or crushed
- 1/2 teaspoon
- 1/2 teaspoon
- 1/2 teaspoon onion powder
- 1/4 teaspoon black pepper
- 1/4 teaspoon salt

- For the avocado salsa
- 1 ripe avocado pitted and diced
- 1/2 cup tomato diced (any type of tomato)
- 2 tablespoons onion diced
- 2 tablespoons cilantro minced
- 1 tablespoon olive oil
- 1 tablespoon lime juice
- salt and pepper to taste

Instructions
1.Stir the olive oil, garlic, and spices in a small bowl. Brush or rub salmon with the spice mixture.

2.Heat a large heavy-duty (preferably non-stick) pan or grill medium-high heat. Add salmon to the pan and cook for 5-6 minutes per side. Remove from pan, top with avocado salsa and serve immediately.

3.To make the avocado salsa: Add the avocado, tomato, onion, and cilantro to a large mixing bowl. Drizzle with olive oil, fresh lime juice and a pinch of salt and pepper. Gently mix with a spoon until fully combined. Cover with plastic wrap until ready to serve.

(Instant Pot) Coconut Curry Mussels with Zucchini Noodles
Nutrition: Cal 269;Fat 20 g; Carb 11 g;Protein 10 g
Serving 4; Cook time 25 min

Ingredients
- tablespoons avocado oil
- 1 (10- to 12-ounce) package zucchini noodles or 2 large zucchini, zoodled
- ⅓ cup diced onion
- 2 tablespoons minced fresh ginger
- 4 cloves garlic, minced
- 1 tablespoon red curry paste
- 1 cup coconut milk
- 1 cup chicken broth
- ¾ pound (15 to 18) mussels, scrubbed, beards removed
- ½ medium red bell pepper, cut into strips
- 1 tablespoon fish sauce
- ½ teaspoon fine Himalayan pink salt
- ¼ teaspoon black pepper
- Juice of ½ lime
- ¼ cup chopped fresh cilantro, for serving

Instructions
1.Select SAUTÉ on the Instant Pot. When the pot is hot, add 1 table- spoon of the avocado oil. Add the zucchini noodles to the hot oil and cook, stirring frequently, until just tender, 3 to 4 minutes. Select CANCEL. Transfer the zoodles to a dish and cover to keep warm.

2.Select SAUTÉ again. Add the remaining 2 tablespoons avocado oil to the pot. When the oil is hot, add the onion, ginger, garlic, and curry paste. Cook, stirring frequently, until fragrant, about 1 minute. Select CANCEL. Add the coconut milk, broth, mussels, and bell pep-per to the pot.

3.Secure the lid and close the pressure-release valve. Set the pot to HIGH pressure for 3 minutes. At the end of the cooking time, quick- release the pressure. Discard any mussels that have not opened.

4.Divide the zucchini noodles and mussels among four shallow serving bowls. Stir the fish sauce, pink salt, pepper, and lime juice into the curry sauce, then pour over the mussels. Sprinkle with cilantro before serving

CREAMY CHILE SHRIMP
Nutrition: Cal 103;Fat 6 g; Carb 5g;Protein 7g
Serving 4; Cook time 30 min

Ingredients
•1 lb. shrimp
•1 chile pepper, cut into thin strips
•½ cup bell pepper, cut into thin strips
•½ cup white cabbage
•½ tsp. cayenne powder
•½ cup chicken stock
•½ tsp. black pepper
•½ cup heavy cream
•½ tsp. hot sauce
•1 tbsp. garlic, minced
•½ tsp. lime juice
•¼ cup canola oil

Instructions
1.Deseed and cut the green chile into thin strips lengthwise.
2.In the Instant Pot, sauté the bell pepper, cabbage and green chili with half oil for 3-4 minutes. Remove and warm by covering with foil.
3.Sauté ginger and garlic inside the Instant Pot with the rest in the oil and add shrimp. Turn off "Sauté" function. Add the spices, hot sauce, and lime juice.
4.Add chicken stock and cook on high pressure for 4 minutes. Quick pressure release, add the sautéed vegetables and mix well.
5.Add cream and sauté before sauce thickens slightly. Serve.

LEMON KALAMATA OLIVE SALMON
Nutrition: Cal 440;Fat 34 g; Carb 3g;Protein 30g
Serving 3; Cook time 25 min

Ingredients
•4 x 0.3 lb. salmon filets
•2 tbsps. fresh lemon juice
•¼ tsp. black pepper
•½ cup red onion, sliced
•1 tsp. herbs de Provence
•1 can pitted kalamata olives
•1tsp. sea salt
•½ lemon, thinly sliced
•1 cup fish broth
•½ tsp. cumin
•½ cup essential olive oil

Instructions
1.Generously season salmon fillets with cumin, pepper, and salt; set your Instant Pot on "Sauté" mode as well as heat the essential olive oil; add fish and brown each side.
2.Stir the remainder

3.Ingredients to the pot and provide to your simmer; lock lid. Set your pot on manual high for ten minutes; when done, quick release pressure then serve.

SEAFOOD MEDLEY STEW
Nutrition: Cal 535;Fat 44 g; Carb 8g;Protein 27g
Serving 3; Cook time 25 min

Ingredients
•2 cups chicken broth
•2 tbsps. lemon juice
•½ lb. shrimp
•½ lb. mussels
•2 cloves garlic, crushed
•½ cup coconut cream
•½ tsp. black pepper
•100 g. halibut
•1 dried whole star anise
•1 bay leaf
•1 cup light cream
•3 tbsps. coconut oil

Instructions
1.In the Instant Pot, sauté the bay leaves, and star anise in coconut oil approximately 30 seconds.
2.Add garlic and attempt to sauté.
3.Add broth. Rub fresh lemon juice, salt, and pepper on fish fillets and put inside pot. Add shrimp and mussels too.
4.Cook for 10 mins. Release pressure naturally.
5.Add both creams and permit to simmer.
6.Remove bay leaves and star anise before serving.

FLAVORED OCTOPUS
Nutrition: Cal 180;Fat 3 g; Carb 1.5 g;Protein 30 g
Serving 4; Cook time 25 min

Ingredients
•1 tsp chopped cilantro
•2 tbsps. extra virgin olive oil
•0.6 pounds octopus
•2 tsps. garlic powder
•3 tbsps. lime juice
•salt and pepper, to taste

Instructions
1.Place the octopus within the steaming basket. Season with garlic powder, salt, and pepper. Drizzle with olive and lime juice.
2.Pour water in the Instant Pot and lower the steaming basket. Close the lid and cook for 8 minutes on high.
3.Do a simple pressure release.

CARAMELIZED TILAPIA
Nutrition: Cal 150;Fat 4 g; Carb 3 g;Protein 21 g
Serving 4; Cook time 50 min

Ingredients
•1-pound tilapia fillets
•1 red chili, minced
•3 tsp. minced garlic
•¼ cup granulated sweetener
•1 spring onion, minced

- ¾ cup coconut water
- 1/3 cup water
- 3 tbsp. fish sauce
- salt and pepper, to taste

Instructions

1. In a bowl, combine the fish sauce, garlic, salt, and pepper. Place the tilapia inside and mix to coat. Cover and let sit within the fridge for half an hour.
2. Meanwhile, combine the lake and sweetener inside Instant Pot. Cook on "Sauté" until caramelized.
3. Add fish and pour the coconut water over. Close the lid and cook on high for 10 minutes.
4. Do a fast pressure release. Top the fish with spring onion and chili.
5. Serve and enjoy!

CRUNCHY ALMOND TUNA
Nutrition: Cal 150;Fat 4 g; Carb 3 g;Protein 21 g
Serving 4; Cook time 15 min

Ingredients
- 2 cans of tuna, drained
- 1 cup shaved almond
- 2 tbsps. butter
- 1 tsp garlic powder
- 1 cup grated cheddar cheese

Instructions

1. Melt the butter in your Instant Pot on "Sauté." Add tuna, almonds, garlic powder, and cheddar. Cook on "Sauté" for 3 minutes.
2. Serve immediately over cauliflower, rice or on its own.
Side Dishes and Vegetables

ARUGULA AND SALMON SALAD
Nutrition: Cal 390;Fat 31 g; Carb 6 g;Protein 26 g
Serving 3; Cook time 25 min

Ingredients
- 3 (4-ounce) salmon fillets
- 5 tablespoons extra-virgin olive oil, divided
- 1 teaspoon garlic salt
- Juice of 1 lemon
- 4½ cups arugula

Instructions

1. Preheat the oven to 450°F. Line a baking sheet with aluminum foil.
2. Rub the fillets with 2 tablespoons of oil and the garlic salt. Place them on the prepared sheet and drizzle the lemon juice over the top of the fillets.
3. Bake until the salmon is cooked through and flaky, 8 to 12 minutes. Let the fillets rest for 10 minutes.
Into each of 3 storage containers, place 1 cups of arugula and season with salt and pepper. Top the arugula with the salmon fillets.To serve, drizzle the arugula in each container with 1 tablespoon of oil and toss.

Grilled Pesto Salmon with Asparagus
Nutrition: Cal 300;Fat 18 g; Carb 2.5 g;Protein 34 g
Serving 4; Cook time 20 min

Ingredients
- 4 (6-ounce) boneless salmon fillets
- Salt and pepper
- 1 bunch asparagus, ends trimmed
- 2 tablespoons olive oil
- ¼ cup basil pesto

Instructions

1. Preheat a grill to high heat and oil the grates.
2. Season the salmon with salt and pepper, then spray with cooking spray.
3. Grill the salmon for 4 to 5 minutes on each side until cooked through.
4. Toss the asparagus with oil and grill until tender, about 10 minutes.
5. Spoon the pesto over the salmon and serve with the asparagus

Grilled Salmon and Zucchini with Mango Sauce
Nutrition: Cal 485;Fat 32 g; Carb 6,5 g;Protein 43 g
Serving 6; Cook time 6 hours 10 min

Ingredients
- 4 (6-ounce) boneless salmon fillets
- 1 tablespoon olive oil
- Salt and pepper
- 1 large zucchini, sliced in coins
- 2 tablespoons fresh lemon juice
- ½ cup chopped mango
- ¼ cup fresh chopped cilantro
- 1 teaspoon lemon zest
- ½ cup canned coconut milk

Instructions

1. Preheat a grill pan to high heat and spray liberally with cooking spray.
2. Brush the salmon with olive oil and season with salt and pepper.Toss the zucchini with lemon juice and season with salt and pepper.
3. Place the salmon fillets and zucchini on the grill pan.
4. Cook for 5 minutes then turn everything and cook 5 minutes more.
5. Combine the remaining ingredients in a blender and blend into a sauce.
6. Serve the salmon fillets drizzled with the mango sauce and zucchini on the side.

Slow-Cooker Pot Roast with Green Beans
Nutrition: Cal 375;Fat 13.5g; Carb 6 g;Protein 53 g
Serving 8; Cook time 8 hours 10 min

Ingredients
- 4 (6-ounce) boneless salmon fillets
- 1 tablespoon olive oil
- Salt and pepper
- 1 large zucchini, sliced in coins
- 2 tablespoons fresh lemon juice
- ½ cup chopped mango
- ¼ cup fresh chopped cilantro
- 1 teaspoon lemon zest
- ½ cup canned coconut milk

Instructions

1. Combine the celery and onion in a slow cooker.

2. Place the roast on top and season liberally with salt and pepper.
3. Whisk together the beef broth and Worcestershire sauce then pour it in.
4. Cover and cook on low heat for 8 hours until the beef is very tender.
5. Remove the beef to a cutting board and cut into chunks.
6. Return the beef to the slow cooker and add the beans and chopped butter.

Fried Coconut Shrimp with Asparagus
Nutrition: Cal 535;Fat 38,5 g; Carb 18 g;Protein 31 g
Serving 6; Cook time 25 min

Ingredients
- 1 ½ cups shredded unsweetened coconut
- 2 large eggs
- Salt and pepper
- 1 ½ pounds large shrimp, peeled and deveined
- ½ cup canned coconut milk
- 1 pound asparagus, cut into 2-inch pieces

Instructions
1. Pour the coconut into a shallow dish.
2. Beat the eggs with some salt and pepper in a bowl.
3. Dip the shrimp first in the egg, then dredge with coconut.
4. Heat the coconut oil in a large skillet over medium-high heat.
5. Add the shrimp and fry for 1 to 2 minutes on each side until browned.
6. Remove the shrimp to paper towels and reheat the skillet.

Add the asparagus and season with salt and pepper – sauté until tender-crisp, then serve with the shrimp

Balsamic Salmon with Green Beans
Nutrition: Cal 320;Fat 18 g; Carb 6 g;Protein 35 g
Serving 4; Cook time 25 min

Ingredients
- ½ cup balsamic vinegar
- ¼ cup chicken broth
- 1 tablespoon Dijon mustard
- 2 cloves garlic, minced
- 2 tablespoons coconut oil
- 4 (6-ounce) salmon fillets
- Salt and pepper
- 2 cups trimmed green beans

Instructions
1. Combine the balsamic vinegar, chicken broth, mustard, and garlic in a small saucepan over medium-high heat.
2. Bring to a boil then reduce heat and simmer for 15 minutes to reduce by half.
3. Heat the coconut oil in a large skillet over medium-high heat.
4. Season the salmon with salt and pepper then add to the skillet.
5. Cook for 4 minutes until seared, then flip and add the green beans.

6. Pour the glaze into the skillet and simmer for 2 to 3 minutes until done.

Shrimp and Sausage "Bake"
Nutrition: Cal 323;Fat 24 g; Carb 8 g;Protein 20 g
Serving 4; Cook time 35 min

Ingredients
- 2 tablespoons olive oil
- 6 ounces chorizo sausage, diced
- ½ pound (16 to 20 count) shrimp, peeled and deveined
- 1 red bell pepper, chopped
- ½ small sweet onion, chopped
- 2 teaspoons minced garlic
- ¼ cup chicken stock
- Pinch red pepper flakes

Instructions
1. Place a large skillet over medium-high heat and add the olive oil.
2. Sauté the sausage until it is warmed through, about 6 minutes.
3. Add the shrimp and sauté until it is opaque and just cooked through, about 4 minutes.
4. Remove the sausage and shrimp to a bowl and set aside.
5. Add the red pepper, onion, and garlic to the skillet and sauté until tender, about 4 minutes.
6. Add the chicken stock to the skillet along with the cooked sausage and shrimp.
7. Bring the liquid to a simmer and simmer for 3 minutes.
8. Stir in the red pepper flakes and serve.

Herb ButTer ScalLops
Nutrition: Cal 306;Fat 24 g; Carb 4,5 g;Protein 20 g
Serving 4; Cook time 20 min

Ingredients
- 1 pound sea scallops, cleaned
- Freshly ground black pepper
- 8 tablespoons butter, divided
- 2 teaspoons minced garlic
- Juice of 1 lemon
- 2 teaspoons chopped fresh basil
- 1 teaspoon chopped fresh thyme

Instructions
1. Pat the scallops dry with paper towels and season them lightly with pepper.
2. Place a large skillet over medium heat and add 2 tablespoons of buter.
3. Arrange the scallops in the skillet, evenly spaced but not too close together, and sear each side until they are golden brown, about 2½ minutes per side.
4. Remove the scallops to a plate and set aside.
5. Add the remaining 6 tablespoons of buter to the skillet and sauté the garlic until translucent, about 3 minutes.
6. Stir in the lemon juice, basil, and thyme and return the scallops to the skillet, turning to coat them in the sauce.
7. Serve immediately

Pan-Seared Halibut with Citrus ButTer Sauce
Nutrition: Cal 320;Fat 26 g; Carb 2 g;Protein 22 g
Serving 4; Cook time 25 min

Ingredients
- 4 (5-ounce) halibut fillets, each about 1 inch thick
- Sea salt
- Freshly ground black pepper
- ¼ cup butter
- 2 teaspoons minced garlic
- 1 shallot, minced
- 3 tablespoons dry white wine
- 1 tablespoon freshly squeezed lemon juice
- 1 tablespoon freshly squeezed orange juice
- 2 teaspoons chopped fresh parsley
- 2 tablespoons olive oil

Instructions
1. Pat the fish dry with paper towels and then lightly season the fillets with salt and pepper. Set aside on a paper towel–lined plate.
2. Place a small saucepan over medium heat and melt the buter.
3. Sauté the garlic and shallot until tender, about 3 minutes.
4. Whisk in the white wine, lemon juice, and orange juice and bring the sauce to a simmer, cooking until it thickens slightly, about 2 minutes.
5. Remove the sauce from the heat and stir in the parsley; set aside.
6. Place a large skillet over medium-high heat and add the olive oil.
7. Panfry the fish until lightly browned and just cooked through, turning them over once, about 10 minutes in total.
8. Serve the fish immediately with a spoonful of sauce for each.

Fish CurRy
Nutrition: Cal 416;Fat 31 g; Carb 5 g;Protein 26 g
Serving 4; Cook time 35 min

Ingredients
- 2 tablespoons coconut oil
- 1&½ tablespoons grated fresh ginger
- 2 teaspoons minced garlic
- 1 tablespoon curry powder
- ½ teaspoon ground cumin
- 2 cups coconut milk
- 16 ounces firm white fish, cut into 1-inch chunks
- 1 cup shredded kale
- 2 tablespoons chopped cilantro

Instructions
1. Place a large saucepan over medium heat and melt the coconut oil.
2. Sauté the ginger and garlic until lightly browned, about 2 minutes.
3. Stir in the curry powder and cumin and sauté until very fragrant,
4. about 2 minutes.
5. Stir in the coconut milk and bring the liquid to a boil.
6. Reduce the heat to low and simmer for about 5 minutes to infuse the milk with the spices.
7. Add the fish and cook until the fish is cooked through, about 10 minutes.
8. Stir in the kale and cilantro and simmer until wilted, about 2 minutes.

Roasted Salmon with Avocado Salsa
Nutrition: Cal 320;Fat 26 g; Carb 2 g;Protein 22 g
Serving 4; Cook time 25 min

Ingredients
FOR THE SALSA
- 1 avocado, peeled, pitted,
- and diced
- 1 scallion, white and green parts,
- chopped
- ½ cup halved cherry tomatoes
- Juice of 1 lemon
- Zest of 1 lemon

FOR THE FISH
- 1 teaspoon ground cumin
- ½ teaspoon ground coriander
- ½ teaspoon onion powder
- ¼ teaspoon sea salt
- Pinch freshly ground black pepper
- Pinch cayenne pepper
- 4 (4-ounce) boneless, skinless
- salmon fillets
- 2 tablespoons olive oil

Instructions
TO MAKE THE SALSA
1. In a small bowl, stir together the avocado, scallion, tomatoes, lemon juice, and lemon zest until mixed.
2. Set aside.

TO MAKE THE FISH
1. Preheat the oven to 400°F. Line a baking sheet with aluminum foil and set aside.
2. In a small bowl, stir together the cumin, coriander, onion powder, salt, black pepper, and cayenne until well mixed.
3. Rub the salmon fillets with the spice mix and place them on the baking sheet.
4. Drizzle the fillets with the olive oil and roast the fish until it is just cooked through, about 15 minutes.
5. Serve the salmon topped with the avocado salsa

Sole Asiago
Nutrition: Cal 300;Fat 24 g; Carb 4 g;Protein 20 g
Serving 4; Cook time 20 min

Ingredients
- 4 (4-ounce) sole fillets
- ¾ cup ground almonds
- ¼ cup Asiago cheese
- 2 eggs, beaten
- 2&½ tablespoons melted coconut oil

Instructions
1. Preheat the oven to 350°F. Line a baking sheet with parchment paper and set aside.

2. Pat the fish dry with paper towels.

3. Stir together the ground almonds and cheese in a small bowl.

4. Place the bowl with the beaten eggs in it next to the almond mixture.

5. Dredge a sole fillet in the beaten egg and then press the fish into the almond mixture so it is completely coated. Place on the baking sheet and repeat until all the fillets are breaded.

6. Brush both sides of each piece of fish with the coconut oil.

7. Bake the sole until it is cooked through, about 8 minutes in total.

8. Serve immediately

Baked Coconut HadDock

Nutrition: Cal 406;Fat 31 g; Carb 6 g;Protein 29 g
Serving 4; Cook time 22 min

Ingredients

- 4 (5-ounce) boneless haddock fillets
- Sea salt
- Freshly ground black pepper
- 1 cup shredded unsweetened coconut
- ¼ cup ground hazelnuts
- 2 tablespoons coconut oil, melted

Instructions

1. Preheat the oven to 400°F. Line a baking sheet with parchment paper and set aside.

2. Pat the fillets very dry with paper towels and lightly season them with salt and pepper.

3. Stir together the shredded coconut and hazelnuts in a small bowl.

4. Dredge the fish fillets in the coconut mixture so that both sides of each piece are thickly coated.

5. Place the fish on the baking sheet and lightly brush both sides of each piece with the coconut oil.

6. Bake the haddock until the topping is golden and the fish flakes easily with a fork, about 12 minutes total.

CheEsy Garlic Salmon

Nutrition: Cal 356;Fat 28 g; Carb 2 g;Protein 24 g
Serving 4; Cook time 30 min

Ingredients

- ½ cup Asiago cheese
- 2 tablespoons freshly squeezed
- lemon juice
- 2 tablespoons butter, at room
- temperature
- 2 teaspoons minced garlic
- 1 teaspoon chopped fresh basil
- 1 teaspoon chopped fresh oregano
- 4 (5-ounce) salmon fillets
- 1 tablespoon olive oil

Instructions

1. Preheat the oven to 350°F. Line a baking sheet with parchment paper and set aside.

2. In a small bowl, stir together the Asiago cheese, lemon juice, buter, garlic, basil, and oregano.

3. Pat the salmon dry with paper towels and place the fillets on the baking sheet skin-side down. Divide the topping evenly between the fillets and spread it across the fish using a knife or the back of a spoon.

4. Drizzle the fish with the olive oil and bake until the topping is golden and the fish is just cooked through, about 12 minutes.

VEGETABLE DISHES

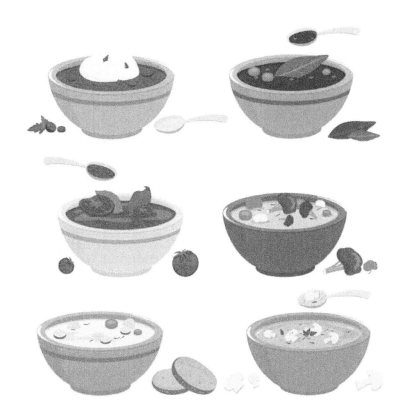

Snap Pea Salad

Nutrition: Cal 212;Fat 20 g; Carb 6 g;Protein 4 g
Serving 4; Cook time 40 min

Ingredients
- 8 ounces cauliflower riced
- 1/4 cup lemon juice
- 1/4 cup olive oil
- 1 clove garlic crushed
- 1/2 teaspoon coarse grain dijon mustard
- 1 teaspoon granulated stevia/erythritol blend
- 1/4 teaspoon pepper
- 1/2 teaspoon sea salt
- 1/2 cup sugar snap peas ends removed and each pod cut into three pieces
- 1/4 cup chives
- 1/2 cup sliced almonds
- 1/4 cup red onions minced

Instructions
1. Pour 1 to 2 inches of water in a pot fitted with a steamer. Bring water to a simmer.
2. Place riced cauliflower in the steamer basket, sprinkle lightly with sea salt, cover, and place over the simmering water in the bottom of the steamer. Steam until tender, about 10-12 minutes.
3. When cauliflower is tender, remove the top of the steamer from the simmering water and place it over a bowl, so any excess water can drain out. Allow to cool, uncovered for about 10 minutes, then cover and place the steamer and the bowl in the refrigerator. Chill for at least 1/2 hour or until cool to the touch.
4. While cauliflower is cooling, make the dressing. Pour olive oil in a small mixing bowl. Gradually stream in the lemon juice while vigorously whisking. Whisk in the garlic, mustard, sweetener, pepper, and salt.
5. In a medium mixing bowl, combine chilled cauliflower, peas, chives, almonds, and red onions. Pour dressing over and stir to mix. Transfer to an airtight container and refrigerate until serving. This salad is best if it is allowed to sit for a few hours in the refrigerator so the flavors mingle.

Garlic & Chive Cauliflower Mash

Nutrition: Cal 178;Fat 18 g; Carb 3 g;Protein 2 g
Serving 2; Cook time 20 min

Ingredients
- 4 cups cauliflower florets
- 1/3 cup mayonnaise
- 1 clove garlic, peeled
- 1 Tbsp water
- 1/2 tsp Kosher salt
- 1/8 tsp black pepper
- 1/4 tsp lemon juice
- 1/2 tsp lemon (or lime) zest
- 1 Tbsp fresh chives, chopped

Instructions

1. Combine the cauliflower, mayonnaise, garlic, water, salt and pepper in a large microwave safe bowl, stirring to coat.
2. Microwave on high for 12-15 minutes (or longer), until completely softened.
3. Add the cooked mixture to a magic bullet or food processor and puree until smooth.
4. Add the lemon juice, zest and chives and pulse until combined.
5. Serve warm.

Creamy Cilantro Lime Coleslaw

Nutrition: Cal 119;Fat 9 g; Carb 9 g;Protein 3 g
Serving 5; Cook time 10 min

Ingredients
- 14 oz coleslaw, bagged
- 1 1/2 avocados
- 1/4 cup cilantro leaves
- 2 limes, juiced
- 1 garlic clove
- 1/4 cup water
- 1/2 teaspoon salt
- cilantro to garnish

Instructions
1. In a food processor add the garlic and cilantro and process until chopped.
2. Add the lime juice, avocados and water. Pulse until nice and creamy.
3. Take out the avocado mixture and in a large bowl mix it with the coleslaw. It will be a bit thick but it will cover the slaw nicely.
4. For best results, refrigerate for a few hours before eating to soften the cabbage.

Cauliflower Hummus

Nutrition: Cal 119;Fat 14 g; Carb 4 g;Protein 2 g
Serving 1; Cook time 20 min

Ingredients
- 3 cups raw cauliflower florets
- 2 Tbsp water
- 2 Tbsp avocado or olive oil
- 1/2 tsp salt
- 3 whole garlic cloves
- Tbsp Tahini paste
- 3 Tbsp lemon juice
- 2 raw garlic cloves, crushed (in addition to above)
- 3 Tbsp extra virgin olive oil
- 3/4 tsp kosher salt
- smoked paprika and extra olive oil for serving

Instructions
1. Combine the cauliflower, water, 2 Tbsp avocado or olive oil, 1/2 tsp kosher salt, and 3 whole garlic cloves to a microwave safe dish. Microwave for about 15 minutes – or until softened and darkened in color.

2. Put the cauliflower mixture into a magic bullet, blender, or food processor and blend. Add the tahini paste, lemon juice, 2 raw garlic cloves, 3 Tbsp olive oil, and 3/4 tsp kosher salt. Blend until mostly smooth. Taste and adjust seasoning as necessary.
3. To serve, place the hummus in a bowl and drizzle with extra virgin olive oil and a sprinkle of paprika. Use thinly sliced tart apples, celery sticks, raw radish chips, or other vegges to dip with.

Crispy Tofu and Bok Choy Salad
Nutrition: Cal 398;Fat 6 g; Carb 9 g;Protein 24 g
Serving 3; Cook time 40 min

Ingredients
Oven Baked Tofu
- 15 ounces extra firm tofu
- 1 tablespoon soy sauce
- 1 tablespoon sesame oil
- 1 tablespoon water
- 2 teaspoons minced garlic
- 1 tablespoon rice wine vinegar
- Juice ½ lemon

Bok Choy Salad
- 9 ounces bok choy
- 1 stalk green onion
- 2 tablespoons chopped cilantro
- 3 tablespoons coconut oil
- 2 tablespoons soy sauce
- 1 tablespoon sambal olek
- 1 tablespoon peanut butter
- Juice ½ lime
- 7 drops liquid stevia

Instructions
1. Start by pressing the tofu. Lay the tofu in a kitchen towel and put something heavy over the top (like a cast iron skillet). It takes about 4-6 hours to dry out, and you may need to replace the kitchen towel half-way through.
2. Once the tofu is pressed, work on your marinade. Combine all of the ingredients for the marinade (soy sauce, sesame oil, water, garlic, vinegar, and lemon).
3. Chop the tofu into squares and place in a plastic bag along with the marinade. Let this marinate for at least 30 minutes, but preferably over night.
4. Pre-heat oven to 350°F. Place tofu on a baking sheet lined with parchment paper (or a silpat) and bake for 30-35 minutes.
5. As the tofu is cooked, get started on the bok choy salad. Chop cilantro and spring onion.
6. Mix all of the other ingredients together (except lime juice and bok choy) in a bowl. Then add cilantro and spring onion. Note: You can microwave coconut oil for 10-15 seconds to allow it it to melt.
7. Once the tofu is almost cooked, add lime juice into the salad dressing and mix together.
8. Chop the bok choy into small slices, like you would cabbage.

9. Remove the tofu from the oven and assemble your salad with tofu, bok choy, and sauce.

Vegan Kale and Spinach Soup
Nutrition: Cal 110;Fat 12 g; Carb 6 g;Protein 4 g
Serving 4; Cook time 15 min

Ingredients
- ½ cup coconut oil, melted
- 8 oz. kale
- 8 oz. (7½ cups) fresh spinach
- 2 (14 oz.) avocados
- 3½ cups coconut milk or coconut cream
- 1 cup water
- fresh mint or dried mint (optional)
- 1 tsp salt
- ¼ tsp ground black pepper
- 1 tbsp lime juice

Fried kale
- 3 oz. kale
- 2 garlic cloves, chopped
- 2 tbsp coconut oil
- ½ tsp ground cardamom (green)
- salt and pepper

Instructions
1. Melt the coconut oil in a hot thick-bottomed pot or pan.
2. Sauté the spinach and kale briefly. The vegetable should just shrink and get a little color, but no more. Remove from the heat.
3. Add water, coconut milk, avocado and spices. Blend with a hand blender until creamy.
4. Add lime juice. Add more spices if you want.
5. Fry kale and garlic on high heat until the garlic turns golden. Garnish the soup and serve.

Carrot Salad
Nutrition: Cal 110;Fat 12 g; Carb 6 g;Protein 4 g
Serving 5; Cook time 10 min

Ingredients
- 1 pound carrots, julienned
- 3 Medjool dates, pitted and diced
- ¼ cup chopped pistachios
- ⅓ cup finely chopped cilantro
- ¼ cup mint leaves, optional

Dressing
- 2 tablespoons extra-virgin olive oil
- 2 tablespoons fresh lemon juice
- 1 tablespoon tahini
- 1 tablespoon honey
- 1 small garlic clove, grated
- ¼ teaspoon cumin
- ¼ teaspoon sea salt

Instructions
1. Place the julienned carrots in a large bowl and sprinkle the dates on top.

2.Make the dressing: In a small bowl, whisk together the olive oil, lemon juice, tahini, honey, garlic, cumin, and salt.
3.Drizzle the dressing over the carrots and toss to coat. Sprinkle on the pistachios and cilantro and toss again. Sprinkle the mint leaves and serve.

Cabbage Soup
Nutrition: Cal 112;Fat 8 g; Carb 16 g;Protein 8g
Serving 6; Cook time 35 min

Ingredients
•2 tablespoons extra-virgin olive oil
•2 carrots, chopped
•1 medium yellow onion, diced
•1 celery rib, diced
•2 tablespoons white wine vinegar
•2 (14.5-ounce) cans fire roasted diced tomatoes
•4 cups vegetable broth
•1 (15.5-ounce) can cooked white beans, drained and rinsed
•4 garlic cloves, grated
•2 Yukon gold potatoes, diced
•1 small green cabbage, about 1 pound (9 cups chopped)
•1 teaspoon dried thyme
•¾ teaspoon sea salt
•Freshly ground black pepper
•Fresh parsley, for garnish

Instructions
1.Heat the oil in a large pot over medium heat. Add the carrots, onion, celery, salt, and several grinds of fresh pepper, and cook, stirring occasionally, for 8 minutes.
2.Add the vinegar, stir, and then add the tomatoes, broth, beans, garlic, potatoes, cabbage and thyme. Cover and simmer for 20 to 30 minutes, or until the potatoes and cabbage are tender.
3.Season to taste, garnish with fresh parsley, and serve.

Creamy Dairy Free Avocado Sauce
Nutrition: Cal 180;Fat 16 g; Carb 8 g;Protein 6 g
Serving 5; Cook time 10 min

Ingredients
•1 Avocado
•1 Tbspn lemon juice
•1 garlic clove
•3 Tbspn olive oil
•2 Tbspn fresh parsley
•3 Tbspn water
•Sea Salt and freshly ground black pepper to taste

Instructions
1.Add all ingredients into food processor or blender.
2.Blend until smooth.
3.Add more water to reach a thinner consistency if desired.
4.Taste and adjust seasoning if necessary.

Easy No-Churn Avocado Ice Cream
Nutrition: Cal 274;Fat 17 g; Carb 29 g;Protein3 g
Serving 4; Cook time 5 hours

Ingredients
•1/4 cup hardened coconut cream (from 1 14-oz can full-fat coconut milk, refrigerated overnight — only the cream)
•2 ripe avocados, halved, pitted and peeled
•2 very ripe bananas, sliced and frozen
•3 tbsp pure maple syrup, plus more, to taste
•1 tbsp freshly squeezed lemon juice

Instructions
1.Add sliced, peeled fresh avocado to a food processor or high-speed blender, and blend until smooth.
2.Add hardened coconut cream from canned coconut milk, along with sliced frozen bananas, pure maple syrup, and lemon juice, and blend until smooth and creamy. If bananas are not fully ripe, you may need to add in additional maple syrup.
3.Taste, and add any more pure maple syrup, as needed, to reach the desired sweetness.
4.Transfer the mixture into a freezer-safe container, and place in freezer for at least 3-4 hours or overnight.
5.When ready to serve, let soften for 10-15 minutes at room temperature before scooping.

PortobelLo MushroOm PizZa
Nutrition: Cal 274;Fat 17 g; Carb 29 g;Protein 3 g
Serving 4; Cook time 20 min

Ingredients
•4 large portobello mushrooms, stems removed
•¼ cup olive oil
•1 teaspoon minced garlic
•1 medium tomato, cut into 4 slices
•2 teaspoons chopped fresh basil
•1 cup shredded mozzarella cheese

Instructions
1.Preheat the oven to broil. Line a baking sheet with aluminum foil and set aside.
2.In a small bowl, toss the mushroom caps with the olive oil until well coated. Use your fingertips to rub the oil in withou breaking the mushrooms.
3.Place the mushrooms on the baking sheet gill-side down and broil the mushrooms until they are tender on the tops,about 2 minutes.
4.Flip the mushrooms over and broil 1 minute more.
5.Take the baking sheet out and spread the garlic over each mushroom, top each with a tomato slice, sprinkle with the basil,and top with the cheese.
6.Broil the mushrooms until the cheese is melted and bubbly, about 1 minute.

Arugula Avocado Tomato Salad
Nutrition: Cal 112;Fat 9 g; Carb 12 g;Protein 3 g
Serving 5; Cook time 10 min

Ingredients
•5 oz baby arugula roughly chopped
•6 large basil leaves thinly sliced

- 1 pint yellow grape tomatoes sliced in half
- 1 pint red grape tomatoes sliced in half
- 2 large avocados cut into chunks
- ½ cup red onion minced

Balsamic Vinaigrette
- 2 tbsp balsamic vinegar
- 1 tbsp olive oil
- 1 tbsp maple syrup
- 1 tbsp lemon juice
- 1 small garlic clove minced
- ¼ tsp himalayan pink sea salt
- ¼ tsp black pepper

Instructions
1. Put the roughly chopped arugula and sliced basil leaves into a large mixing bowl. Add the sliced grape tomatoes, avocado chunks, and minced red onion to the bowl. Toss to combine.
2. In a small bowl, whisk together 2 tbsp balsamic vinegar, 1 tbsp olive oil, 1 tbsp maple syrup, 1 tbsp lemon juice, 1 garlic clove, ¼ tsp salt, and ¼ tsp black pepper until well combined.
3. Pour the balsamic dressing over the salad. Gently mix the salad until the dressing has been evenly distributed and then transfer the salad to a large platter.

Red Curry Cauliflower Soup
Nutrition: Cal 274;Fat 16 g; Carb 18 g;Protein 6 g
Serving 6; Cook time 45 min

Ingredients
- 1 medium yellow onion sliced
- 3 medium garlic cloves sliced
- 4 ounces thai red curry paste (about 4 tbsp)
- 1 medium cauliflower (about 1 lb cauliflower florets)
- ½ cup red lentils
- 1 ½ cups water
- 4 cups low-sodium vegetable broth
- ½ tsp Himalayan pink sea salt
- ½ tsp black pepper
- 14 ounce can unsweetened coconut milk
- 3 tbsp lemon juice (1 large lemon)
- 1 tbsp chives sliced

Instructions
1. In a large pot, saute the sliced onions in 3-4 tbsp vegetable broth until soft. Add the sliced garlic and cook for 1-2 minutes until fragrant.
2. Add 4 tbsp red curry paste, cauliflower florets, ½ cup red lentils, 1 ½ cups water, 4 cups vegetable broth, ½ tsp salt, and ½ tsp black pepper to the pot. Bring the soup to a low simmer and then reduce the heat to medium. Let it cook for 15-20 minutes or until the cauliflower and red lentils are tender, stirring occasionally.
3. Transfer the soup to a large high-powered blender cup and then blend it on high until the soup is completely smooth. You may need to work in batches depending on how large your blender cup is.

4. Pour the blended soup back into the pot and stir in the coconut milk over medium heat. Add 3 tbsp lemon juice and stir it in. Garnish with chives before serving.

Keto Oven Roasted Vegetables
Nutrition: Cal 113;Fat 7 g; Carb 11 g;Protein 2 g
Serving 8; Cook time 40 min

Ingredients
- 2 cups Broccoli (cut into florets)
- 2 cups Cauliflower (cut into florets)
- 2 cups Zucchini (sliced into 1/4 inch thick circles)
- 2 cups Bell peppers (cut into 1.5 inch pieces)
- 2 cups Red onion (cut into 1.5 inch pieces)
- 1/4 cup Olive oil
- 2 tbsp Balsamic vinegar
- 1 tsp Garlic powder
- 1 tsp Italian seasoning
- 1 tsp Sea salt
- 1/2 tsp Black pepper

Instructions
1. Preheat the oven to 425 degrees F. Line an extra-large baking sheet with foil, if desired.
2. Combine the vegetables in a large bowl.
3. In a small bowl, whisk together the olive oil, balsamic vinegar, garlic powder, Italian seasoning, sea salt, and black pepper. Pour the mixture over the vegetables.
4. Arrange the vegetables in a single layer on the prepared baking sheet, making sure each piece is touching the pan. Do not overcrowd the pan - use multiple pans if needed.
5. Roast the vegetables in the oven for about 30 minutes, until they are golden brown.

Vegan Keto Coconut Curry
Nutrition: Cal 425;Fat 33 g; Carb 10 g;Protein 18 g
Serving 4; Cook time 35 min

Ingredients
- ¼ cup vegan butter
- ½ green bell pepper, thinly sliced
- 2 scallions, thinly sliced, white and green parts kept separate
- 2 garlic cloves, thinly sliced
- 2½ tablespoons vegan red curry paste
- 1 medium zucchini, diced
- 1 medium carrot, diced
- 1½ cups unsweetened full-fat coconut milk
- 1 cup vegetable stock
- 2 tablespoons unflavored vegan protein powder
- 2 tablespoons natural unsweetened peanut butter
- 4 drops liquid stevia
- 1 teaspoon sea salt
- Freshly ground black pepper
- 16 ounces extra-firm tofu, cut into medium dice
- 1 cup baby spinach
- ¼ cup chopped fresh cilantro, plus more for serving
- 4 tablespoons coconut oil, melted

Instructions

1. In a large pot, melt the butter over medium heat. Add the bell pepper, scallion whites and garlic; cook until fragrant, about 1 minute. Add the curry paste and cook, stirring constantly, until fragrant, about 1 minute.
2. Stir in the zucchini, carrot, coconut milk, vegetable stock, protein powder, peanut butter, stevia, salt and black pepper. Bring to a boil, then reduce the heat to medium-low and simmer uncovered until the vegetables are tender, 8 to 10 minutes. Taste and adjust the seasoning if necessary.
3. Add the tofu and simmer for 5 minutes to warm through. Add the spinach and cilantro to wilt. Taste and adjust the seasoning if necessary.
4. Divide the curry among four bowls. Drizzle 1 tablespoon melted coconut oil over each portion. Sprinkle with the scallion greens and more cilantro.

STUFFED BELL PEPPERS
Nutrition: Cal 202;Fat 16 g; Carb 7 g;Protein 8 g
Serving 3; Cook time 50 min

Ingredients
- 2 medium-sized yellow bell peppers, halved
- ½ cup mozzarella cheese
- ½ cup tomatoes, diced
- 2 medium-sized green bell pepper, halved
- 2 cups button mushrooms, diced
- 1 cup feta cheese, crumbled
- 2 tbsps. celery leaves, finely chopped
- 2 tbsps. extra virgin olive oil
- ½ tsp. black pepper, ground
- ½ tsp. smoked paprika, ground
- ¼ tsp. red pepper cayenne, ground
- ½ tsp. salt

Instructions
1. Cut the peppers in half and take away the stem and seeds. Set aside.
2. In a large mixing bowl, combine button mushrooms, feta cheese, mozzarella cheese, tomatoes, celery, and olive oil. Add all spices and mix until well incorporated. Stuff the bell pepper halves with this particular mixture. Use some additional oil to brush the peppers externally.
3. Line some parchment paper over a fitting springform pan and hang aside
4. Plug inside instant pot and pour 1 cup of water in the stainless insert. Set the trivet around the bottom and set the stuffed peppers on the top.
5. Close the lid and hang up the steam release handle. Press the "Manual" button and set the timer for a half-hour. Cook on underhand.
6. When done, perform a quick pressure release and open the pot.
7. Transfer the peppers to a serving plate and sprinkle by incorporating dried oregano or dried rosemary before serving. Optionally, top with Greek yogurt.

Garlicky GreEn Beans
Nutrition: Cal 104;Fat 9 g; Carb 2 g;Protein 4 g
Serving 4; Cook time 20 min

Ingredients
- 1 pound green beans, stemmed
- 2 tablespoons olive oil
- 1 teaspoon minced garlic
- Sea salt
- Freshly ground black pepper
- ¼ cup freshly grated Parmesan Cheese

Instructions
1. Preheat the oven to 425°F. Line a baking sheet with aluminum foil and set aside.
2. In a large bowl, toss together the green beans, olive oil, and garlic until well mixed.
3. Season the beans lightly with salt and pepper.
4. Spread the beans on the baking sheet and roast them until they are tender and lightly browned, stirring them once, about 10 minutes.
5. Serve topped with the Parmesan cheese

Sautéed Asparagus with Walnuts
Nutrition: Cal 124;Fat 12 g; Carb 4 g;Protein 3 g
Serving 4; Cook time 20 min

Ingredients
- 1&½ tablespoons olive oil
- ¾ pound asparagus, woody ends trimmed
- Sea salt
- Freshly ground pepper
- ¼ cup chopped walnuts

Instructions
1. Place a large skillet over medium-high heat and add the olive oil.
2. Sauté the asparagus until the spears are tender and lightly browned, about 5 minutes.
3. Season the asparagus with salt and pepper.
4. Remove the skillet from the heat and toss the asparagus with the walnuts.

WHITE BEAN & SPINACH QUESADILLAS
Nutrition: Cal 500;Fat 20 g; Carb 35 g;Protein 19 g
Serving 5; Cook time 30 min

Ingredients
- 19 oz can of white beans navy, cannellini or white kidney beans are all fine, drained and rinsed
- 3 oz spinach chopped (roughly 3 cups chopped fresh spinach or 1 1/2cups frozen spinach)
- 1 teaspoon ground cumin
- 1 teaspoon ground coriander
- 1 1/8 teaspoon salt
- 3/4 cup feta cheese crumbled
- 1 1/4 cups shredded cheese
- 5 large 12 inch tortillas

Instructions
1. If spinach is frozen, thaw and press out extra moisture.

2. In a large bowl, mash the white beans using a fork or potato masher.
3. Stir in the spinach, cumin, coriander and salt. Stir/mash until the spinach is slightly wilted and fold in the feta cheese.
4. Heat a large pan over medium heat. Spray with oil, then assemble quesadillas in the pan (cooking 2 at a time).
5. Spoon out ½ cup of white bean/spinach filling, then sprinkle with ¼ cup cheese. Fold the tortilla over, then press down firmly.
6. Cook for 3 or so minutes per side, until golden and crispy.

BrusSels Sprouts CasSerole
Nutrition: Cal 217;Fat 14 g; Carb 11 g;Protein 10 g
Serving 8; Cook time 45 min

Ingredients
- 8 bacon slices
- 1 pound Brussels sprouts, blanched for 10 minutes and cut into quarters
- 1 cup shredded Swiss cheese, divided
- ¾ cup heavy (whipping) cream

Instructions
1. Preheat the oven to 400°F.
2. Place a skillet over medium-high heat and cook the bacon until it is crispy, about 6 minutes.
3. Reserve 1 tablespoon of bacon fat to grease the casserole dish and roughly chop the cooked bacon.
4. Lightly oil a casserole dish with the reserved bacon fat and set aside.
5. In a medium bowl, toss the Brussels sprouts with the chopped bacon and ½ cup of cheese and transfer the mixture to the caserole dish.
6. Pour the heavy cream over the Brussels sprouts and top the casserole with the remaining ½ cup of cheese.
7. Bake until the cheese is melted and lightly browned and the vegetables are heated through, about 20 minutes

SAUTÉED VEGETABLES
Nutrition: Cal 171;Fat 12 g; Carb 9 g;Protein 5.3g
Serving 5; Cook time 10 min

Ingredients
- 1 red bell pepper, sliced
- 1 small onion, sliced
- 1 small zucchini, cut into cubes
- 1 green bell pepper, sliced
- ¼ cup dried porcini mushrooms
- ¼ cup Feta cheese
- ½ cup sour cream
- 2 tbsps. tamari sauce
- 2 tbsps. sesame oil
- ½ tsp. dried thyme
- ¼ tsp. dried oregano
- 1 tsp. pink Himalayan salt

Instructions
1. Plug in the instant pot and press the "Sauté" button. Heat up the sesame oil and add zucchini. Sprinkle with many salt and cook for 5 - 6 minutes, stirring constantly.
2. Now add bell peppers and onions. Sprinkle with tamari sauce and provides it a good stir. Optionally, drizzle with a few rice vinegar.
3. Season by incorporating more salt, thyme, and oregano. Continue in order to cook for two - 3 minutes and atart exercising . Feta cheese and mushrooms. Pour in about three tablespoons of water and cook for three or four minutes.
4. When done, press the "Cancel" button and stir inside sour cream. To enjoy, serve it immediately.

STEAMED BROCCOLI WITH BASIL
Nutrition: Cal 181;Fat 10 g; Carb 10 g;Protein 10 g
Serving 3; Cook time 20 min

Ingredients
- 1 lb. broccoli, chopped
- 2 garlic cloves, peeled
- ½ cup fresh basil, chopped
- ½ cup some kinds of cheese
- ½ cup avocado, chopped
- 1 tbsp. extra virgin olive oil
- 1 tbsp. fresh lemon juice, freshly squeezed
- ¼ tsp. dried oregano, ground
- ½ tsp. red pepper, ground
- ¼ tsp. dried parsley, ground
- 1 tsp. salt

Instructions
1. Plug in the Instant Pot and pour in 1 cup of water inside the stainless insert.
2. Place the trivet about the bottom of the pot as well as set the steam basket at the top. Place broccoli inside the steam basket and sprinkle with salt and pepper. Close the lid and set the steam release handle by moving the valve on the "Sealing" position. Press the "Steam" button as well as set the timer for ten mins.
3. Meanwhile, combine basil, cottage type cheese, avocado, garlic, olive oil, fresh lemon juice, red pepper, parsley, and oregano in a mixer. Pulse until smooth and totally incorporated.
4. When you hear the cooker's end signal, release pressure to succeed naturally. Open the pot and transfer the broccoli to a serving plate. Top with basil cream and serve immediately!

ONION CAULIFLOWER HASH
Nutrition: Cal 217;Fat 14 g; Carb 11 g;Protein 10 g
Serving 3; Cook time 20 min

Ingredients
- 1 lb. cauliflower, chopped
- 1 cup green cabbage, shredded
- 2 medium-sized onions, sliced
- ¼ cup parmesan cheese
- 1 cup vegetable stock
- 2 tbsps. olive oil

- •¼ tsp. black pepper, ground
- •½ tsp. dried thyme, ground
- •½ tsp. smoked paprika, ground
- •1 tsp. salt

Instructions

1. Plug in the Instant Pot and grease the stainless steel insert with essential olive oil. Press the "Sauté" button and add cauliflower and onions. Sprinkle with salt, pepper, and thyme. Stir well and cook for 5 minutes.
2. Add cabbage and pour inside vegetables stock. Stir again and securely lock the lid. Set the steam release handle and press the "Manual" button. Set the timer for 8 minutes and cook on questionable.
3. When you hear the cooker's end signal, perform a quick release of the pressure by moving the valve for the "Venting" position. Open the pot and stir inside thyme and smoked paprika.
4. Transfer all to a serving plate and sprinkle with parmesan cheese before serving.

Pesto ZucChini NoOdles
Nutrition: Cal 93;Fat 8 g; Carb 2 g;Protein 4 g
Serving 4; Cook time 15 min

Ingredients
- •4 small zucchini, ends trimmed
- •¾ cup Herb Kale Pesto (page 133)
- •¼ cup grated or shredded
- •Parmesan cheese

Instructions

1. Use a spiralizer or peeler to cut the zucchini into "noodles" and place them in a medium bowl.
2. Add the pesto and the Parmesan cheese and toss to coat.

TASTY CREAMY COLLARD GREENS
Nutrition: Cal 217;Fat 17 g; Carb 25 g;Protein 5.7 g
Serving 4; Cook time 25 min

Ingredients
- •1 lb. collard greens, chopped
- •1 medium-sized onion, chopped
- •½ cup bacon, cut into bite-sized pieces
- •2 garlic cloves, finely chopped
- •1 cup sour cream
- •½ tsp. balsamic vinegar
- •1 tbsp. essential olive oil
- •¼ tsp. black pepper, ground
- •½ tsp. Italian seasoning
- •1 tsp. red pepper flakes
- •1 tsp. sea salt

Instructions

1. Plug with your Instant Pot and add the bacon for the stainless-steel insert. Press the "Sauté" button and cook for three to four minutes, or until crisp. Remove the bacon through the pot and add olive oil. When hot, add onions and garlic. Stir-fry for 3 - 4 minutes, or until the onions translucent.

2. Add collard greens and cook for two main minutes. Sprinkle with salt, pepper, Italian seasoning, and red pepper flakes. Pour in 1 cup of water and securely lock the lid. Adjust the steam release handle and press the "Manual" button. Set the timer for 5 minutes and cook on underhand.
3. When done, perform a quick pressure release and open the pot.
4. Stir in the sour cream, balsamic vinegar, and bacon. Press the "Sauté" button and cook for 2 - 3 minutes more, or until heated through. Turn over pot and transfer all to a serving plate.

Golden Rosti
Nutrition: Cal 171;Fat 15 g; Carb 3 g;Protein 5 g
Serving 8; Cook time 30 min

Ingredients
- •8 bacon slices, chopped
- •1 cup shredded acorn squash
- •1 cup shredded raw celeriac
- •2 tablespoons grated or shredded
- •Parmesan cheese
- •2 teaspoons minced garlic
- •1 teaspoon chopped fresh thyme
- •Sea salt
- •Freshly ground black pepper
- •2 tablespoons butter

Instructions

1. In a large skillet over medium-high heat, cook the bacon until crispy, about 5 minutes.
2. While the bacon is cooking, in a large bowl, mix together the squash, celeriac, Parmesan cheese, garlic, and thyme. Season the mixture generously with salt and pepper, and set aside.
3. Remove the cooked bacon with a sloted spoon to the rosti mixture and stir to incorporate.
4. Remove all but 2 tablespoons of bacon fat from the skillet and add the buter.
5. Reduce the heat to medium-low and transfer the rosti mixture to the skillet and spread it out evenly to form a large round paty about 1 inch thick.
6. Cook until the botom of the rosti is golden brown and crisp, about 5 minutes.
7. Flip the rosti over and cook until the other side is crispy and the middle is cooked through, about 5 minutes more.
8. Remove the skillet from the heat and cut the rosti into 8 pieces.

Creamed Spinach
Nutrition: Cal 195;Fat 20 g; Carb 3 g;Protein 3 g
Serving 4; Cook time 40 min

Ingredients
- •1 tablespoon butter
- •½ sweet onion, very thinly sliced
- •4 cups spinach, stemmed and thoroughly washed
- •¾ cup heavy (whipping) cream

•¼ cup Chicken Stock
•Pinch sea salt
•Pinch freshly ground black pepper
•Pinch ground nutmeg
Instructions
1. In a large skillet over medium heat, add the buter.
2. Sauté the onion until it is lightly caramelized, about 5 minutes.
3. Stir in the spinach, heavy cream, chicken stock, salt, pepper, and nutmeg.
4. Sauté until the spinach is wilted, about 5 minutes.
5. Continue cooking the spinach until it is tender and the sauce is thickened, about 15 minutes.

CELERY SPINACH STEW
Nutrition: Cal 280;Fat 28 g; Carb 5 g;Protein 2.5 g
Serving 4; Cook time 25 min

Ingredients
•2 cups fresh spinach, chopped
•1 small onion, chopped
•1 cup celery leaves, chopped
•2 cups heavy cream
•1 tbsp. fresh lemon juice
•2 tbsps. butter
•1 cup celery stalks, chopped
•2 garlic cloves, minced
•1/2 tsp. black pepper, ground
•1 tbsp. fresh mint, torn
•1 tsp. salt
Instructions
1. In a large colander, combine spinach and celery. Rinse well under running water and drain. Transfer to a cutting board cut into bite-sized pieces. Set aside.
2. Plug with your instant pot and press the "Sauté" button. Add butter and stir constantly until melts.
3. Add celery stalks, garlic, and onions. Cook for just two minutes and add celery leaves and spinach. Sprinkle with salt and pepper. Cook for 2 - 3 minutes and pour inside the heavy cream.
4. Securely lock the lid and press the "Manual" button. Adjust the steam release handle and hang up the timer for 5 minutes. Cook on high pressure.
5. When you hear the cooker's end signal, perform a quick release with the pressure and open the pot.
6. Stir within the mint and lemon juice. Let it chill for 5 minutes before serving.

SIMPLE BASIL PESTO ZUCCHINI
Nutrition: Cal 215;Fat 17 g; Carb 8 g;Protein 5 g
Serving 4; Cook time 15 min

Ingredients
•1 cup mozzarella cheese
•1 large red bell pepper, cut into strips
•2 medium-sized zucchinis, thinly sliced
•2 tbsps. organic olive oil
•1 medium-sized eggplant, thinly sliced
•1 tsp. Italian seasoning

•1 cup vegetable stock
FOR THE BASIL PESTO:
•½ tsp garlic powder
•2 tsps. balsamic vinegar
•½ tsp. black pepper, freshly ground
•2 tbsps. fresh basil, finely chopped
•2 tbsps. sour cream
•3 tbsps. organic olive oil
•¼ tsp. mustard seeds
Instructions
1. Combine sliced zucchinis, stripped red bell pepper, and sliced eggplant in a large bowl. Drizzle with olive oil and Italian seasoning. Optionally, add a pinch of salt and mix well using your hands. Set aside.
2. Combine all pesto
3. Ingredients in a blender and blend until smooth and creamy. Then schedule.
4. Plug inside the Instant Pot add vegetables within the stainless-steel insert. Pour within the vegetable stock and close the lid. Adjust the steam release handle and press the "Manual" button. Set the timer for 8 minutes and cook on high pressure.
5. When done; perform a quick pressure release by moving the valve on the "Venting" position.
6. Open the pot and transfer the vegetables to a serving plate. Top with basil pesto and serve immediately.
7. Optionally, garnish with some fresh basil leaves and get!

CheEsy Mashed Cauliflower
Nutrition: Cal 183;Fat 15 g; Carb 6 g;Protein 8 g
Serving 4; Cook time 20 min

Ingredients
•1 head cauliflower, chopped roughly
•½ cup shredded Cheddar cheese
•¼ cup heavy (whipping) cream
•2 tablespoons butter, at room temperature
•Sea salt
•Freshly ground black pepper
Instructions
1. Place a large saucepan filled three-quarters full with water over high heat and bring to a boil.
2. Blanch the cauliflower until tender, about 5 minutes, and drain.
3. Transfer the cauliflower to a food processor and add the cheese, heavy cream, and buter. Purée until very creamy and whipped.
4. Season with salt and pepper.

VEGETABLES À LA GRECQUE
Nutrition: Cal 326;Fat 25 g; Carb 8 g;Protein 15 g
Serving 4; Cook time 15 min

Ingredients
•2 tablespoons organic olive oil
•2 garlic cloves, minced
•1 red onion, chopped
•0.6 pounds button mushrooms, thinly sliced
•1 eggplant, sliced

- ½ teaspoon dried basil
- 1 teaspoon dried oregano
- 1 thyme sprig, leaves picked
- 2 rosemary sprigs, leaves picked
- ½ cup tomato sauce
- ¼ cup dry Greek wine
- ¼ cup water
- 0.5 pounds Halloumi cheese, cubed
- 4 tablespoons Kalamata olives, pitted and halved

Instructions

1. Press the "Sauté" button to heat your Instant Pot; now, heat the extra virgin olive oil. Cook the garlic and red onions for one to two minutes, stirring periodically.
2. Stir in the mushrooms and then sauté a different 2 to 3 minutes.
3. Add the eggplant, basil, oregano, thyme, rosemary, tomato sauce, Greek wine, and water.
4. Secure the lid. Choose "Manual" mode and low pressure; cook for 3 minutes. Once cooking is complete, use a quick pressure release; carefully remove the lid.
5. Top with cheese and olives.

Sautéed Crispy ZucChini
Nutrition: Cal 94;Fat 8 g; Carb 1 g;Protein 4 g
Serving 4; Cook time 25 min

Ingredients
- 2 tablespoons butter
- 4 zucchini, cut into
- ¼-inch-thick rounds
- ½ cup freshly grated Parmesan cheese
- Freshly ground black peppe

Instructions

1. Place a large skillet over medium-high heat and melt the buter.
2. Add the zucchini and sauté until tender and lightly browned, about 5 minutes.
3. Spread the zucchini evenly in the skillet and sprinkle the Parmesan cheese over the vegetables.
4. Cook without stirring until the Parmesan cheese is melted and crispy where it touches the skillet, about 5 minutes

MushroOms with Camembert
Nutrition: Cal 161;Fat 13 g; Carb 4 g;Protein 9 g
Serving 4; Cook time 20 min

Ingredients
- 2 tablespoons butter
- 2 teaspoons minced garlic
- 1 pound button mushrooms, halved
- 4 ounces Camembert cheese, diced
- Freshly ground black pepper

Instructions

1. Place a large skillet over medium-high heat and melt the buter.
2. Sauté the garlic until translucent, about 3 minutes.
3. Sauté the mushrooms until tender, about 10 minutes.

4. Stir in the cheese and sauté until melted, about 2 minutes.
5. Season with pepper and serve

MEXICAN-STYLE ZUCCHINI AND POBLANOS
Nutrition: Cal 250;Fat 20 g; Carb 2 g;Protein 14 g
Serving 6; Cook time 15 min

Ingredients
- 1 tablespoon vegetable oil
- 2 poblano peppers, seeded and cut lengthwise into ½-inch strips
- 2 teaspoons unsalted butter
- ½ onion, thinly sliced
- 1 tablespoon minced garlic
- 1-pound ground pork
- 1 zucchini, cut into thick rounds
- 1 yellow crookneck squash, cut into thick rounds
- ½ cup chicken broth
- ½ teaspoon ground cumin
- 1 teaspoon salt
- 1 tablespoon Mexican crema or sour cream

Instructions

1. Select "Sauté" to preheat the Instant Pot and adapt to high heat. When the hot, add the oil and invite it to shimmer. Add the poblano strips in a single layer, working in batches if necessary, and char on each side, flipping only occasionally, for around 10 minutes.
2. Add the butter for the pot. Once melted, add the onion and garlic, and sauté until soft, 2 to 3 minutes.
3. Add the soil pork and break it into chunks, mixing it well using the vegetables. Cook before lumps are finished in the meat, and it's half-way cooked, about four or five minutes.
4. Add the zucchini, squash, broth, cumin, and salt on the pot.
5. Lock the lid. Select "Pressure Cook" or "Manual" as well as set pressure to low. Cook for two main minutes. When the cooking is complete, quick-release pressure. Unlock the lid.
6. Stir inside cream, therefore it fully incorporates in the sauce.

ASPARAGUS WITH COLBY CHEESE
Nutrition: Cal 170;Fat 12 g; Carb 8 g;Protein 8 g
Serving 4; Cook time 10 min

Ingredients
- 1 ½ pounds fresh asparagus
- 2 tablespoons organic olive oil
- 4 garlic cloves, minced
- sea salt, to taste
- ¼ teaspoon ground black pepper
- ½ cup Colby cheese, shredded

Instructions

1. Add 1 cup of water as well as a steamer basket in your Instant Pot.

2. Now, put the asparagus around the steamer basket; drizzle your asparagus with olive oil. Scatter garlic in the top in the asparagus. Season with salt and black pepper.
3. Secure the lid. Choose "Manual" mode and questionable; cook for 1 minute. Once cooking is complete, work with a quick pressure release; carefully eliminate the lid.
4. Transfer the prepared asparagus to some nice serving platter and scatter shredded cheese in the top.

VEGGIE SCRAMBLE
Nutrition: Cal 200;Fat 5 g; Carb 9 g;Protein 20 g
Serving 4; Cook time 30 min

Ingredients
- 4 egg whites
- 1 egg yolk
- 2 tbsps. almond milk
- 1 cup spinach
- 1 tomato, chopped
- ½ white onion, chopped
- 3 fresh basil leaves, chopped
- salt and pepper, to taste
- ghee

Instructions
1. In a bowl, whisk the egg yolk and whites while using milk. Stir well.
2. Heat the ghee in the pan over medium heat. Add the onions and sauté until fragrant.
3. Add inside tomato to the pan with all the spinach and cook prior to the spinach is almost wilted.
4. Pour the egg mixture within the spinach and cook until firm (or before the egg sets). Stir constantly. Season with salt and pepper.

PRESSURE COOKER QUINOA AND RICE
Nutrition: Cal 100;Fat 0,6 g; Carb 0,7 g;Protein 3 g
Serving 4; Cook time 15 min

Ingredients
- Rice (white, freckled or brow, 1 ¾ cups)
- Quinoa (5 tbsp)
- Water (3 cups)

Instructions
1. Add the rinsed rice and quinoa and water inside Pressure cooker; close the top's and set to "High pressure" for 3 minutes.
2. Once the timer signalizes, the cooking ends, release pressure to succeed naturally for 10 minutes.
3. Open the lid, stir the rice and quinoa somewhat bit and serve while it's hot.

CHICKPEA CURRY AND RICE
Nutrition: Cal 200;Fat 5,6 g; Carb 50 g;Protein 0 g
Serving 4; Cook time 20 min

Ingredients
- Chickpeas (1 cup, make sure these were soaked in water overnight)
- Oil (by choice, 1 tbsp)
- Water (1 cup)
- Tomatoes pure or sauce (about 2 cups)
- Onion (1, chopped)
- Spice mix Chana Masala (2 tbsp)
- Ginger (1 tbsp, chopped)
- Garlic (1 tbsp, chopped)
- Salt (1 teaspoon)

Instructions
1. Pour water and add the rice in a very pot that's heat-proof and cover it which has a foil.
2. The pressure cooker should be pre-heated if you add inside oil and also the onion. Set it to "Sauté" and cook the onion till it glazes and softens up a bit bit.
3. Add the garlic, ginger and chana masala spice mix to pressure cooker and cook for half one minute.
4. Now add the chickpeas, water, and tomatoes and mix the ingredients.
5. Place the trivet inside pressure cooker (on the
6. ingredients) and on the top than it add the heatproof pot or container (make certain they can fit inside). Close and secure the coverage and hang to "High pressure" for twenty minutes.
7. Release pressure naturally for 10 mins once it's cooked; open the lid and serve the rice as well as the chickpeas in bowls.

VEGIES, LENTILS AND MILLET PRESSURE COOKER MIX
Nutrition: Cal 300;Fat 13 g; Carb 58 g;Protein 20 g
Serving 4; Cook time 30 min

Ingredients
- Leek (1 cup)
- Asparagus (1 cup)
- Sugar snap peas (1 cup)
- Bok Choy (half cup, chopped)
- Lentils (half cup)
- Mushrooms (any kind, half cup)
- Millet (1 cup)
- Garlic (2 cloves, chopped)
- Parsley, garlic chives and onion chives mix (1/4 cup)
- Lemon juice
- Salt

Instructions
1. Set the pressure cooker to "Sauté" and add inside the mushrooms and garlic and sauté to get a short while. Then add the lentils and millet and cook for one more minute. Then add the vegetable stock.
2. Close and secure the cover and hang it to "High pressure"; allow it to go cook for 10 mins and after that release pressure naturally.
3. Open the lid and add the peas, asparagus, and bok choy (you might be free to utilize some other vegetable by choice, obviously).
4. Close the superior again and allowed this to mix sit for a little bit.
5. The millet has to be well cooked (it ought to be yellow).

6. Stir, add the parsley and chives mix and serve in a very bowl. Squeeze some lemon juice and add salt by taste.

BAKED BEANS
Nutrition: Cal 230;Fat 6 g; Carb 40 g;Protein 2 g
Serving 8; Cook time 1 hour

Ingredients
- Beans (1 bag)
- Onion (half cup, chopped)
- Garlic (1 clove, chopped)
- Green bell pepper (half cup, chopped)
- Bacon (4 slices, cut in squares)
- Water (8 cups)
- Barbecue sauce (2 cups)
- Olive oil (1 tbsp)
- Mustard (optional, 2 tbsp)
- Salt and pepper to taste

Instructions
1. Pour water inside pressure cooker and adding the beans. Close and secure the lead, place it to "Manual" or "High Pressure" for 25 minutes.
2. Let the pressure out naturally.
3. Open the lid and strain the beans; wash it with cold water and hang up it aside in another pot or bowl.
4. Clean and dry pressure to succeed cooker then add the organic olive oil and the bacon. Add salt and pepper and sauté for 5 minutes (the bacon should be well fried.
5. Add the bell pepper and onion, stir and cook until the onion caramelizes.
6. Pour within the beans, mustard, garlic and barbecue sauce.
7. Close the cover and set to "High pressure" and cook for an additional fifteen minutes.
8. Release the pressure naturally. Open it, stir after which serve.

BLACK BEANS AND RICE
Nutrition: Cal 270;Fat 9 g; Carb 39 g;Protein 10 g
Serving 8; Cook time 70 min

Ingredients
- Black beans (1 along with a half cup)
- Rice (white or brown, 1 plus a half cup)
- Water (3 cups)
- Vegetable broth (3 cups)
- Onion (half, chopped)
- Garlic (4 cloves, chopped)
- Olive oil (2 teaspoons)
- Paprika (1 as well as a half teaspoons)
- Cumin (2 teaspoons)
- Oregano (1 as well as a half teaspoons)
- Chili powder (optional, 2 teaspoons)
- Lime juice

Instructions
1. Set pressure to succeed cooker to "Sauté"; add the essential olive oil and once it's hot enough add the onion and cook it till it's tender.

2. Add the paprika, cumin, garlic, oregano, salt, and chili powder and cook for half one minute, then shut off pressure cooker.
3. Pour inside water, vegetable broth, rice, and beans, stir and after that close and secure the cover, set to "High pressure" and cook for half an hour. Once you hear the timer, release pressure naturally for 10-fifteen minutes.
4. Open the lid, squeeze the juice of half lime, season with salt and pepper by taste, stir and serve. You will add avocado slices if you need, as well.

No-Cook Falafel
Nutrition: Cal 106;Fat 9 g; Carb 2,5 g;Protein 5,5 g
Serving 10; Cook time 10 min

Ingredients
- ¾ cup (120g) hulled hemp seeds
- 1 tablespoon dried parsley leaves
- 1½ teaspoons ground cumin
- 1 teaspoon granulated onion
- ½ teaspoon granulated garlic
- ¼ teaspoon cracked black pepper
- Grated zest of 1 lemon
- ¼ cup (64g) tahini, room temperature

Instructions
1. Line a rimmed baking sheet with parchment paper.
2. Using a food processor or blender, grind the hemp seeds until a coarse meal forms.
3. Transfer the hemp meal to a medium-sized mixing bowl, then add the rest of ingredients except the tahini and whisk together until combined.
4. Stir in the tahini and continue to mix until the ingredients are well combined and a somewhat crumbly dough forms. It will have the texture of pie dough and should hold together when pinched.
5. Using your hands, roll the mixture into 10 balls, about 1 tablespoon each. Place the balls on the lined baking sheet.
6. Chill in the freezer for at least 30 minutes or in the refrigerator for 2 hours so the falafel balls hold together.

Lupini Hummus
Nutrition: Cal 162;Fat 15 g; Carb 4 g;Protein 5 g
Serving 2; Cook time 5 min.

Ingredients
- 1½ cups (250g) jarred lupini beans (packed in brine), drained
- ½ cup (120 ml) extra-virgin olive oil
- ½ cup (120 ml) water
- ¼ cup (64g) tahini, room temperature
- Juice of 1 lemon
- 1 teaspoon crushed garlic
- 1 teaspoon ground cumin
- Paprika, for sprinkling

Instructions

1. Put the lupini beans, olive oil, water, tahini, lemon juice, garlic, and cumin in a food processor or high-powered blender and blend until smooth, 2 to 3 minutes. Transfer to a serving bowl and sprinkle with paprika.

Cucumber Avocado Pinwheels
Nutrition: Cal 201;Fat 16 g; Carb 10 g;Protein 7 g
Serving 2; Cook time 10 min.

Ingredients
- 1 medium Hass avocado (7½ ounces/212g)
- 2 sheets sushi nori
- 2 tablespoons (20g) sesame seeds
- ½ cup (50g) thinly sliced cucumbers
- ½ cup (30g) broccoli sprouts

DIPPING SAUCE SUGGESTIONS:
- Low-sodium tamari or coconut aminos with sliced scallions (green parts only)
- Tangy Avocado Mayo (here) or vegan mayo of choice

Instructions
1. Cut the avocado in half and remove the pit. Scoop the flesh into a small dish and mash with a fork.
2. Lay each sheet of nori on a flat surface and spread half of the mashed avocado on each sheet, leaving 1 inch (2.5 cm) of space at the far end of each sheet.
3. Sprinkle a tablespoon of the sesame seeds over the avocado on each sheet.
4. Lay out half of the cucumber slices on each sheet and top each with half of the broccoli sprouts.
5. Wet the far edge of each nori sheet with a little water. Starting at the edge closest to you, roll up the sheet into a roll. Press gently along the seam to make sure the wet edge of nori is sealed up against the roll.
6. Slice each roll into 6 to 8 pieces (depending on your preference), running the knife under water before each cut.
7. Serve with the dipping sauce of your choice.

Curry Tofu Salad Bites
Nutrition: Cal 148;Fat 10 g; Carb 6.5 g;Protein 11 g
Serving 8; Cook time 10 min.

Ingredients
- 1 (14-ounce/397-g) package extra-firm tofu, drained
- ¼ cup (60 ml) Tangy Avocado Mayo (here) or vegan mayo of choice
- ¼ cup (25g) diced celery
- 2 teaspoons curry powder or chili powder
- ¼ teaspoon salt
- 32 thin slices cucumber (about 1 cup/100g)
- Cracked black pepper
- 2 scallions (green parts only), sliced

Instructions
1. In a large mixing bowl, mash together the tofu, mayo, celery, curry powder, and salt until uniformly mixed.
2. Scoop about 1 tablespoon of the tofu mixture on top of each cucumber slice.
3. Top with freshly ground pepper and sliced scallions and serve.

Carrot Ginger Soup
Nutrition: Cal 234;Fat 20 g; Carb 7.7 g;Protein 20 g
Serving 4; Cook time 30 min.

Ingredients
- 2 tablespoons (30 ml) extra-virgin olive oil
- 1½ cups (190g) sliced carrots
- 1 tablespoon grated fresh ginger
- 1½ cups (360 ml) vegetable broth
- 1 (13.5-ounce/400-ml) can full-fat coconut milk
- Grated zest of 1 lemon
- ¼ teaspoon freshly ground black pepper

Instructions
1. Heat the oil in a large saucepan over medium heat. Add the carrots and ginger and cook for about 5 minutes, stirring occasionally, until the carrots begin to soften.
2. Add the broth and coconut milk to the pan and cover. Continue to cook for 20 minutes, until the carrots are tender and can easily be pierced with a knife.
3. Pour the soup into a blender and blend until smooth, about 2 minutes.
4. To serve, divide the soup among 4 bowls and top with the lemon zest and freshly ground black pepper

Spicy Coconut Soup
Nutrition: Cal 162;Fat 15 g; Carb 5 g;Protein 7 g
Serving 4; Cook time 30 min.

Ingredients
- 1 (14-ounce/397-g) block extra-firm tofu
- ½ cup (50g) sliced red bell peppers, plus extra for garnish
- ½ cup (30g) shredded red cabbage, plus extra for garnish

FOR GARNISH (OPTIONAL):
- Microgreens
- 1 stalk lemongrass, sliced
- Grated lime zest

Instructions
1. Heat the coconut milk, broth, tamari, chili paste, garlic, ginger, and lime juice in a large saucepan over medium heat, stirring just to mix the ingredients, about 5 minutes.
2. Drain, press, and cut the tofu into 1-inch (2.5-cm) cubes and add to the soup. Add the sliced peppers and shredded cabbage, cover, and continue to simmer for 15 minutes, until the peppers and cabbage are soft.
3. Remove from the heat and portion into bowls to serve. Garnish as desired.
4. To store: Refrigerate in a tightly sealed container for up to 4 days or freeze for up to a month.
5. To reheat: Warm in a covered saucepan over medium-low heat until the desired temperature is reached.

Creamy Cauliflower Soup
Nutrition: Cal 289;Fat 20 g; Carb 10.5 g;Protein 16 g
Serving 4; Cook time 25 min.

Ingredients
- 2 tablespoons (30 ml) extra-virgin olive oil

- 4 cups (400g) cauliflower pieces
- 3 cups (720 ml) vegetable broth
- ¾ cup (120g) hulled hemp seeds
- ¼ cup (20g) nutritional yeast
- 1 tablespoon chopped fresh chives

TOPPING SUGGESTIONS:
- Additional chopped fresh chives or sliced scallions (green parts only)
- Sauerkraut
- Freshly ground black pepper

Instructions
1. Heat the oil in a large saucepan over medium heat. Add the cauliflower and cook for about 5 minutes, stirring occasionally, until the pieces begin to soften.
2. Add the broth and continue to cook until the cauliflower is tender and can easily be pierced with a knife.
3. Carefully pour the soup into a heat-safe high-powered blender and add the hemp seeds, nutritional yeast, and chives. Blend until smooth, 2 to 3 minutes.
4. To serve, divide the soup among serving bowls and top as desired.

DESSERTS

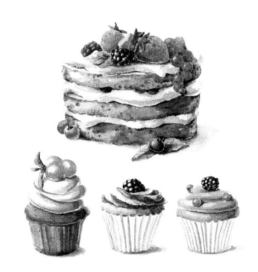

Samoa Bars
Nutrition: Cal 216;Fat 20 g; Carb 7 g;Protein 3 g
Serving 16; Cook time 30 min.

Ingredients
Crust
- 1 1/4 cups almond flour (125 g)
- 1/4 cup Swerve Sweetener
- 1/4 tsp salt
- 1/4 cup butter, melted

Chocolate Filling and Drizzle
- 4 oz sugar-free dark chocolate, chopped
- 2 TBSP coconut oil or butter

Coconut Caramel Filling
- 1 1/2 cups shredded coconut
- 3 TBSP butter
- 1/4 cup Swerve Brown
- 1/4 cup Bocha Sweet or additional Swerve Brown
- 3/4 cup heavy whipping cream
- 1/2 tsp vanilla extract
- 1/4 tsp salt

Instructions
Crust
1. Preheat the oven to 325°F. In a medium bowl, whisk together the almond flour, sweetener, and salt. Stir in the melted butter until the mixture begins to come together.
2. Turn out the mixture into an 8x8 baking pan and press firmly into the
bottom. Bake about 15 to 18 minutes, until just golden-brown. Remove and let cool while preparing the filling.

Chocolate Filling/Drizzle
3. In a small microwave-safe bowl, melt the chocolate and coconut oil in 30 second increments, stirring in between, until melted and smooth. Alternatively, you can melt it double boiler style over a pan of barely simmering water.
4. Spread about 2/3 of the chocolate mixture over the cooled crust.

Coconut Filling
5. In a medium skillet over medium heat, spread the coconut. Stir in frequently, toast until light golden-brown. Set aside.
6. In a large saucepan over medium heat, combine the butter and sweeteners. Cook until melted and then bring to a boil. Boil 3 to 5 minutes, until golden.
7. Remove from heat and add the cream, vanilla, and salt. The mixture will bubble vigorously—this is normal. Stir in the toasted coconut. Spread the mixture over the chocolate-covered
crust. Let cool completely (about 1 hour), then cut into squares. Gently reheat remaining chocolate mixture and drizzle over the bars.

LEMON BARS
Nutrition: Cal 190;Fat 19 g; Carb 2 g;Protein 4 g
Serving 16; Cook time 20 min.

Ingredients
Crust
- 6 TBSP butter

- 2 cups superfine blanched almond flour
- 1/3 cup granulated sugar substitute (I used Swerve)
- 1 TBSP freshly-grated lemon zest

Filling
- 1/2 cup butter
- 1/2 cup granulated sugar substitute (I used Swerve)
- 1/2 cup fresh lemon juice
- 1/4 cup grated lemon zest
- 6 egg yolks
- 1/2 tsp xanthan gum
- 2 TBSP unflavored collagen powder (or 1 tsp unflavored gelatin)

Instructions
Crust
1. Preheat the oven to 350°F.
2. Melt the butter in the microwave or a small saucepan.
3. Add the almond flour, sweetener, and lemon zest, stirring until fully combined.
4. Press the dough evenly along the bottom and 1/2 inch up the sides of an 8 x 8 inch square pan. For best results line the pan with parchment paper or foil first, then you can simply lift out the completed lemon bars.
5. Bake for 10 minutes.
6. Remove and cool while you make the filling.

Filling
7. Melt the butter in a small saucepan on low heat.
8. Remove from heat and whisk in sweetener, lemon juice, and lemon zest until dissolved.
9. Whisk in the egg yolks and return to the stove over low heat.
10. Whisk continually until the curd starts to thicken.
11. Remove from the heat and strain into a small bowl.
12. Whisk in the the xanthan gum and collagen (or gelatin) until dissolved and smooth.
13. Pour the filling over the pre-baked crust and spread out evenly to the edges of the pan.
14. Bake the bars at 350°F for 15 minutes.
15. Remove and cool.
16. Sprinkle with Powdered Swerve before serving, if desired.
17. Cut into sixteen 2 x 2 squares.

Almond Pecan Shortbread Cookies
Nutrition: Cal 190;Fat 19 g; Carb 2 g;Protein 3 g
Serving 20; Cook time 2 hours 20 min.

Ingredients
- 2 cups pecans
- 1 cup almonds
- 1 cup pastured butter, melted
- 3 TBSP Swerve
- 1 tsp vanilla extract

Instructions
Crust
1. Preheat oven to 350°F.
2. In a large food processor mix almond and pecans until they turn into a coarse flour.
3. Add butter and rest of ingredients to the food processor and blend until a dough is formed.

4. Now remove the dough from the food processor and with the aid of parchment paper shape it into a roll.

5. Put in the refrigerator for 2 hrs min, until dough hardens.

6. Now slice in to 1 inch-thick rounds.

7. Place on a cookie sheet on top of parchment paper.

8. Bake at 325°F for 10 minutes.

9. Be careful not to overbake or bottom will burn! Let cool before moving from the cookie sheet. If too crumbly, refrigerate before eating!

Lemon Poppyseed Cookies
Nutrition: Cal 190;Fat 15 g; Carb 8 g;Protein 5 g
Serving 8; Cook time 30 min.

Ingredients
Cookies
- 1 cup almond flour
- 1/4 cup coconut flour
- 3 TBSP poppyseeds
- 1 tsp baking powder
- 1/8 tsp salt
- 6 oz cream cheese, softened
- 1/2 cup Swerve Sweetener (granulated or confectioners)
- 1 large egg, room temperature
- Zest of one lemon
- 2 TBSP lemon juice
- 1/4 tsp liquid stevia extract

Glaze (optional)
- 1/4 cup confectioner's Swerve Sweetener
- 2 to 3 TBSP lemon juice

Instructions
Cookies
1. Preheat oven to 325°F and line a large baking sheet with parchment
paper.

2. In a medium bowl, whisk together the almond flour, coconut flour,
poppy seeds, baking powder, and salt.

3. In a large bowl, beat cream cheese, sweetener, egg, lemon zest, lemon

4. juice, and stevia extract. Beat in almond flour mixture until well combined.

5. Form by hand 8 to 10 even balls. Flatten with the palm of your hand to
about 1/2 inch-thick circles.

6. Bake about 20 minutes, until set and just barely brown around the edges. Remove and let cool on pan.

Glaze
7. In a small bowl, whisk together sweetener and enough lemon juice to make a thin glaze. Drizzle over cooled cookies.

Thin Mint Macaroon Cookies
Nutrition: Cal 56;Fat 5 g; Carb 4 g;Protein 7 g
Serving 24; Cook time 20 min.

Ingredients
- 2 cups desiccated unsweetened coconut

- 1/2 cup unsweetened almond milk
- 1 1/2 tsp peppermint extract
- 1/2 cup granulated sweetener
- 3 egg whites
- 1/4 tsp xanthan gum
- 1 oz 90% or greater cacao dark chocolate

Instructions
1. Combine the coconut, almond milk, peppermint extract, and sweetener in a medium bowl and stir well.

2. In a separate large bowl whisk the egg whites and xanthan gumtogether until soft peaks form.

3. Fold the egg mixture into the coconut mixture until fully combined.

4. Drop the dough mixture by scoop or tablespoon into 24 mounds onto a parchment-lined cookie sheet. Flatten into disks with your hand or aflat spatula.

5. Bake in a preheated 325°F oven for 16 minutes or until slightly firm.

6. Remove and cool.

7. Place the chocolate in a ziplock bag and melt in the microwave for 30seconds at a time until just liquid. Snip a tiny corner off of the bag and squeeze the chocolate out onto the cookies in a circular (or any) pattern. Cool and serve.

Chocolate Chunk Cookies
Nutrition: Cal 140;Fat 12 g; Carb 6 g;Protein 4 g
Serving 18; Cook time 50 min.

Ingredients
- 2 cups / 6.3 oz / 190 g blanched almond flour/meal
- ¼ tsp fine grain sea salt
- ½ tsp baking soda
- ¼ cup / 2 oz / 55 g coconut oil, melted
- 2 TBSP honey (or maple syrup)
- 1 TBSP vanilla extract
- ¾ cup / 3.5 oz / 100 g coarsely chopped +70% dark chocolate

Instructions
1. Preheat oven at 350°F (175°C), place a rack in the middle. Line a baking sheet with parchment paper and set aside.

2. In the bowl of a food processor combine almond flour, salt, and baking soda. Pulse in coconut oil, honey (or maple syrup) and vanilla extract until dough forms.

3. Remove the blade from the food processor and stir in chocolate chunks by hand. The dough will be very moist and oily—don't worry, that's how it's supposed to be.

4. Let the dough rest in the refrigerator for 30 minutes. The resting time will make the dough easier to handle.

5. Take the dough out of the fridge and scoop one level tablespoon at a time onto the prepared baking sheet.

6. With your hands, press balls of dough down gently and give them a look-alike cookie shape.

7. Bake in the oven for about 7 minutes (8 minutes for darker cookies).

8. Let cookies cool on the baking sheet (without touching) for 15 minutes, then with the help of a spatula place cookies onto a rack and let cool completely.

Iced Lemon Sugar Cookies

Nutrition: Cal 96;Fat 8 g; Carb 4 g;Protein 7 g
Serving 40; Cook time 30 min.

Ingredients
Sanding "Sugar"
- 2 TBSP Swerve Sweetener or other granulated erythritol or xylitol
- 1 drop yellow gel food coloring

Dough
- 1 1/2 cups almond flour
- 1/4 cup coconut flour
- 1 tsp baking powder
- 1/2 tsp xanthan gum
- 1/4 tsp salt
- 6 TBSP butter, softened
- 1/2 cup Swerve Sweetener (or other erythritol sweetener)
- 1 large egg, room temperature
- 3 TBSP fresh lemon juice
- Zest of one lemon

Glaze
- 6 TBSP powdered Swerve sweetener (or other powdered erythritol)
- 3 TBSP fresh lemon juice

Instructions
1. For the sanding "sugar," combine granulated sweetener and gel food coloring in a small bowl. Use the back of a spoon to work food coloring into sweetener granules. Set aside.
2. For the dough, whisk together almond flour, coconut flour, baking powder, xanthan gum, and salt in a medium bowl.
3. In a large bowl, beat butter with sweetener until well combined. Beat in egg, lemon juice, and lemon zest.
4. Add almond flour mixture and beat until dough comes together. Turn out dough onto a large piece of parchment paper. Pat into a rough circle and then top with another piece of parchment. Roll out to about 1/4-inch thickness. Place on a cookie sheet and chill in refrigerator for 30 minutes.
5. Preheat oven to 325°F and line another baking sheet with parchment. Cut out cookies into desired shape and lift carefully with a small, offset spatula or knife. Place cookies at least 1/2 inch apart on prepared baking sheet. Reroll your dough and cut out more cookies (if your dough gets too soft to work with, you can put it in the freezer for a bit to harden up).
6. Bake 12 to 14 minutes, or until just golden-brown and firm to the touch.
7. Let cool on pan 10 minutes, then transfer to a wire rack to cool completely.
8. For the glaze, stir powdered sweetener and lemon juice in a small bowl until smooth.
9. Spread a thin layer of glaze over each cookie and sprinkle with sanding sugar.

Rasberry Almond Thumbprint Cookies

Nutrition: Cal 180;Fat 16 g; Carb 4 g;Protein 4 g
Serving 24; Cook time 35 min.

Ingredients
Cookies
- 1 3/4 cup almond flour
- 1 TBSP coconut flour
- 1/2 tsp baking powder
- 1/2 cup butter, softened
- 1/2 cup confectioner's Swerve Sweetener
- 1 egg yolk
- 1 tsp almond extract
- 1/4 cup Raspberry Chia Seed Jam

Glaze
- 3 TBSP confectioner's Swerve Sweetener
- 1/4 tsp almond extract
- 1 to 2 TBSP water

Instructions
Cookies
1. Preheat oven to 325°F and line a baking sheet with parchment or a silicone liner.
2. In a medium bowl, whisk together almond flour, coconut flour, and baking powder.
3. In a large bowl, beat butter with sweetener until well combined and fluffy. Beat in egg yolk and almond extract. Beat in almond flour mixture until well incorporated.
4. Form dough into scant 1 inch balls and place two inches apart on prepared baking sheet. Press each ball down to about 1/2 inch high. Using your thumb, press an indentation into the center of each cookie.
5. Spoon about 1/2 teaspoon of jam into each and bake until just barely browning around the edges, 10 to 12 minutes. Cool on pan. The cookies will not seem set but will continue to firm up as they cool.

Glaze
6. In a small bowl, whisk together sweetener, almond extract, and water until a pourable consistency is achieved. Drizzle over cooled cookies.

Gingerbread Cookies

Nutrition: Cal 130;Fat 11 g; Carb 4 g;Protein 3 g
Serving 20; Cook time 35 min.

Ingredients
- 1/2 cup butter, softened
- 2 eggs
- 1 tsp vanilla extract
- 1 tsp cinnamon liquid stevia
- 1/4 cup heavy cream
- 1 TBSP molasses
- 2 cups sunflower seeds ground, or almond flour
- 1/2 cup coconut flour
- 1/4 cup Swerve or erythritol
- 1 tsp baking powder
- 1 tsp cinnamon
- 1 tsp ground ginger
- 1/4 tsp ground nutmeg
- 1/4 tsp ground cloves
- 1/4 tsp salt

Instructions
1. Preheat oven to 350°F.

2.Place the first 6 ingredients into a stand mixer and blend on high until incorporated.

3.Whisk the rest of the ingredients together in a bowl.

4.Slowly pour the dry ingredients into the wet in the stand mixer.

5.Blend until combined. It will be sticky so place dough in plastic wrap and refrigerate for at least one hour.

6.Flour surface of counter with gluten-free flour and your hands with flour then pat down dough or use a rolling pin until it's 1/2 inch in thickness.

7.Use cookie cutouts for gingerbread men and place on a silpat-lined baking sheet.

8.Add chocolate chip eyes and buttons, if desired.

9.Bake for 12 minutes.

10.Allow to cool for 10 minutes before removing gently from pan.

Almond Butter Chocolate Chip Cookies
Nutrition: Cal 130;Fat 9 g; Carb 12 g;Protein 4 g
Serving 10; Cook time 35 min.

Ingredients
- 1 large egg
- 1 cup almond butter
- 1/2 cup light brown sugar, lightly packed
- 1 tsp baking soda
- 1 cup dark chocolate chips

Instructions
1.Set oven to 350°F

2.Crack the egg into a medium bowl and beat it lightly. Add in the almond butter, baking soda, and sugar and mix everything together well.

3.Fold in the chocolate chips.

4.Scoop the dough onto a parchment or silpat-lined baking sheet. I use a (1 3/4 inch) scoop, but you can use a tablespoon. Space the cookies well apart, and flatten them slightly with the back of a spoon.

5.Bake for 8 to 10 minutes. Don't overbake these; the cookies will look underdone, but they will firm up as they cool.

6.Let them cool for a couple of minutes on the baking sheet, then transfer them carefully to a cooling rack.

Almond Crescent Cookies
Nutrition: Cal 185;Fat 11 g; Carb 6 g;Protein 5 g
Serving 15; Cook time 35 min.

Ingredients
- 1 stick salted butter, softened (1/2 cup)
- Pinch of kosher salt
- 1/2 cup granulated erythritol sweetener
- 1/2 tsp vanilla extract
- 1 tsp almond extract
- 2 cups superfine almond flour
- 1/3 cup sliced almonds

Instructions
1.Beat the butter, salt, and sweetener until fluffy. Add the vanilla and almond extracts and blend well.

2.Add the almond flour and beat until just blended to a stiff dough.

3.Divide the dough into 12 balls.

4.Roll each ball into a 3 inch log.

5.Spread the sliced almonds onto a clean surface and crush slightly into smaller pieces with the heel of your hand.

6.Roll the logs in the almond pieces and then bend the two ends in and pinch slightly to create a crescent shape.

7.Place the almond crescents on a parchment-lined cookie sheet and bake in apreheated 350°F oven for 15 minutes. Remove and cool before serving.

Maple Cream Sandwich Cookies
Nutrition: Cal 215;Fat 17 g; Carb 6 g;Protein 8 g
Serving 24; Cook time 40 min.

Ingredients
Cookies
- 2 cups almond flour
- 1/3 cup Swerve Sweetener
- 1 tsp baking powder
- 1/4 tsp salt
- 1 large egg
- 2 1/2 TBSP butter, melted
- 1 tsp maple extract
- 1/8 tsp stevia extract

Filling
- 1/4 cup butter, softened
- 1 cup powdered Swerve Sweetener
- 2 TBSP cream, room temperature
- 3/4 tsp maple extract

Instructions
Cookies
1.Preheat oven to 275°F and line two baking sheets with parchment paper.

2.Whisk almond flour, sweetener, baking powder, and salt together in a large bowl. Stir in egg, butter, maple extract, and stevia extract until dough comes together.

3.Turn dough out onto a large piece of parchment paper and pat into a rough rectangle. Top with another piece of parchment.

4.Roll dough out to about 1/8 inch thickness. Using a 2-inch maple leaf cookie cutter (or whatever shape you prefer) to cut out as many shapes as possible. Dough can be re-rolled multiple times to get more cookies.

5.Place half the cookies face up and half face down on the prepared baking sheet (if your cookie cutter is slightly irregular, this allows you to match them up properly after they are baked).

6.Bake about 20 minutes, until light golden-brown and firm to the touch. Watch them carefully, they can easily get too dark.

7.Remove from oven and let cool completely.

Filling
8.Beat butter and powdered sweetener together in a medium bowl until smooth. Beat in cream and maple extract to achieve a spreadable consistency.

9. To assemble, take one cookie and spread the backside with about a teaspoon of filling. Top with another cookie, backside towards the filling.

Matcha Fudge Fat Bombs
Nutrition: Cal 194;Fat 19 g; Carb 1 g;Protein 1 g
Serving 20; Cook time 15 min.

Ingredients
- 3.5 oz cocoa butter
- 1/2 cup coconut butter
- 1/2 cup sugar-free maple syrup
- 1/3 cup heavy cream
- 3 TBSP coconut oil
- 2 scoops matcha mct powder
- 2 tsp vanilla essence

Instructions
1. Place all the ingredients in a small saucepan and place over low heat.
2. Heat until the cocoa butter has melted, stir to combine all ingredients.
3. Pour the mixture into an 8x8 inch square cake pan, lined with parchment paper.
4. Set in the fridge for 3 hours, or until firm.
5. Cut into 24 pieces and serve.

Strawberry & Cream Fat Bombs
Nutrition: Cal 160;Fat 17 g; Carb 1 g;Protein 3 g
Serving 10; Cook time 15 min.

Ingredients
- 6 oz cream cheese, softened
- 5 fl.oz double cream
- 1 oz vanilla collagen protein powder
- 3 TBSP coconut oil, plus extra 2 tsp for rolling
- 1 tsp strawberry essence

Instructions
2. Mix all ingredients with a hand mixer for 5 minutes, until well combined.
3. Set the mixture in the fridge for 1 hour.
4. When the mixture is set, rub your hands with a little coconut oil and shape the mix into 10 evenly-sized fat bombs. The coconut oil will stop the mix from sticking to your hands.
5. Store the fat bombs in an airtight container in the fridge or freezer.

Zesty Lemon Fat Bombs
Nutrition: Cal 140;Fat 13 g; Carb 3 g;Protein 1 g
Serving 10; Cook time 15 min.

Ingredients
- 1 oz coconut butter
- 1 oz coconut oil
- 1 oz unsalted butter
- 1 TBSP sukrin melis
- 1 lemon zest & juice

Instructions

1. Place all the ingredients into a small saucepan over low heat. Heat until just melted, then remove from the heat.
2. Pour into silicone molds.
3. Place in the fridge and chill for 1 hour, until set.

Vanilla Strawberry Fudge Fat Bombs
Nutrition: Cal 150;Fat 16 g; Carb 1 g;Protein 1 g
Serving 25; Cook time 15 min.

Ingredients
Vanilla Layer
- 8 oz cream cheese, softened
- 8 oz butter, softened
- 2 tsp vanilla extract
- 3 TBSP erythritol

Strawberry Layer
- 8 oz cream cheese, softened
- 8 oz butter, softened
- 1 oz strawberry protein powder (low or no carb)

Instructions
Vanilla Layer
1. Line a baking tray with parchment paper and set aside.
2. Place the softened cream cheese, softened butter, vanilla extract, and erythritol in a bowl and mix with a hand mixer on low speed, slowly building up to medium/high speed until all ingredients are really well combined.
3. Pour the vanilla layer into the lined tray and smooth out as evenly as possible, set in the fridge for at least 30 minutes.

Strawberry Layer
4. As you did with the vanilla layer, place the softened cream cheese, butter, and strawberry protein powder in a bowl. Mix on low speed with a hand mixer and slowly increase the speed to medium/high until all ingredients are really well combined.
5. Pour the strawberry layer on top of the vanilla layer, smooth it out and set in the fridge for 1 hour.
6. Cut your fudge into bite-sized pieces and keep it cool, as it will soften very quickly in warm temperatures.

Chocolate Cheesecake Kisses Fat Bombs
Nutrition: Cal 97;Fat 9 g; Carb 1 g;Protein 1 g
Serving 25; Cook time 25 min.

Ingredients
- 8 oz cream cheese, softened
- 2 oz natvia icing mix
- 1 tsp vanilla essence
- 7 oz heavy cream
- 5 oz sugar-free chocolate

Instructions
1. Add the chocolate to a small heatproof bowl and place over a small saucepan of simmering water, ensuring that the bowl doesn't touch the water.
2. Melt the chocolate completely and remove from the heat. Set aside.

3. Place the softened cream cheese in a bowl, using your hand mixer, mix on medium speed until smooth.
4. Add the Natvia Icing Mix and vanilla essence and mix on low speed until combined.
5. Add the heavy cream and mix on medium speed until smooth and beginning to thicken.
6. Pour in the melted chocolate and mix on medium speed, until all ingredients are completely combined and the mixture is firm enough to pipe.
7. Add the mixture into a piping bag with a star nozzle. Pipe evenly into mini cupcake paper. We filled 24 cupcake papers, depending on your piping skills, you may get more or less.
8. Cover the kisses and set in the fridge for at least 3 hours, or overnight for best results.

Lemon & Poppyseed Fat Bomb
Nutrition: Cal 160;Fat 12 g; Carb 1 g;Protein 1 g
Serving 18; Cook time 25 min.

Ingredients
- 8 oz cream cheese, softened
- 3 TBSP erythritol
- 1 TBSP poppy seeds
- 1 lemon zest only
- 4 TBSP sour cream
- 2 TBSP lemon juice

Instructions
1. Place all ingredients in a bowl and using a hand mixer, mix on low speed; when ingredients are combined, mix on medium/high speed for 3 minutes.
2. Gently spoon mixture into mini cupcake cases or place into a piping bag and pipe into mini cupcakes cases. Refrigerate for at least 1 hour.
3. These cups will soften quickly in warm weather, we recommend to keep them refrigerated.

Pina Colada Fat Bombs
Nutrition: Cal 120;Fat 8 g; Carb 1 g;Protein 2 g
Serving 16; Cook time 25 min.

Ingredients
- 2 tsp pineapple essence
- 3 tsp erythritol
- 2 TBSP gelatin
- 1/2 cup boiling water
- 1/2 cup coconut cream
- 1 tsp rum extract
- 2 scoops MCT Powder (Optional)

Instructions
1. Dissolve the gelatin and erythritol in the boiling water in a heat-proof jug and add the pineapple essence.
2. Allow to cool for 5 minutes.
3. Add the coconut cream and rum extract and continue stirring for 2 minutes.
4. Pour into silicon molds and set for at least 1 hour, depending on the size of your mold.
5. Gently remove from the mold and enjoy. Store in the fridge.

6. Optional: If you want to get a real kick out of your fat bombs recipe try adding a scoop or two of MCT Powder, but be sure to mix it well in the hot water first (that may require a stick blender).

Red Velvet Fat Bombs
Nutrition: Cal 160;Fat 8 g; Carb 1 g;Protein 2 g
Serving 24; Cook time 40 min.

Ingredients
- 100 g 90% dark chocolate
- 125 g cream cheese, softened
- 100 g butter, softened
- 3 TBSP natvia
- 1 tsp vanilla extract
- 4 drops red food coloring
- 1/3 cup heavy cream, whipped

Instructions
1. Melt the chocolate in a heat-proof bowl over a small pot of simmering water. Make sure that the bowl isn't touching the water, as this will cause the chocolate to burn.
2. While the chocolate is melting, mix together the remaining ingredients with a hand mixer on medium speed for 3 minutes. Ensure the mix is fully combined.
3. With the hand mixer on low speed, slowly add the chocolate mixture to the other ingredients. Mix on medium speed for 2 minutes.
4. Add the mixture to a piping bag and pipe the fat bomb mixture onto a lined tray. Set in the fridge for 40 minutes.
5. Add the heavy cream to whipping canister and apply whipped cream to the fat bombs.

Raspberry Cream Fat Bombs
Nutrition: Cal 160;Fat 8 g; Carb 1 g;Protein 2 g
Serving 24; Cook time 40 min.

Ingredients
- 1 (9 g packet) raspberry sugar-free jello
- 15 g gelatin powder
- 1/2 cup water, boiling
- 1/2 cup heavy cream

Instructions
1. Dissolve gelatin and jello in boiling water.
2. Add the cream slowly while stirring and continue to stir for 1 minute. If you add the cold cream in all at once and don't thoroughly mix, the jellies will split, creating a layered affect.
3. Pour the mixture into candy molds and set in the fridge for at least 30 minutes.

Maple Pecan Fat Bombs
Nutrition: Cal 147;Fat 15 g; Carb 1 g;Protein 3 g
Serving 9; Cook time 25 min.

Ingredients
- 4 oz unsalted butter
- 2 oz pecan butter

- •1 scoop vanilla collagen powder
- •2 TBSP sugar-free maple syrup
- •9 pecan nuts

Instructions
1. Place all ingredients (except the pecans) into a small saucepan over low heat.
2. Whisk together until combined, then remove from heat. Allow to cool for 5 minutes.
3. Pour into a small heat-proof dish lined with parchment paper.
4. Sprinkle over the pecans then put in the fridge to chill.
5. Cool for 1-2 hours until set firm.
6. Cut into squares and enjoy.

Chocolate Zucchini Bread
Nutrition: Cal 185;Fat 17 g; Carb 6 g;Protein 5 g
Serving 12; Cook time 50 min.

Ingredients
Dry Ingredients
- •1 1/2 cup almond flour (170 g)
- •1/4 cup unsweetened cocoa powder (25 g)
- •1 1/2 tsp baking soda
- •2 tsp ground cinnamon
- •1/4 tsp sea salt
- •1/2 cup sugar-free crystal sweetener (Monk fruit or erythritol) (100 g) or coconut sugar if refined sugar-free

Wet Ingredients
- •1 cup zucchini, finely grated measure packed, discard
- •juice/liquid if there is some - about 2 small zucchini
- •1 large egg
- •1/4 cup + 2 TBSP canned coconut cream (100 ml)
- •1/4 cup extra virgin coconut oil, melted (60ml)
- •1 tsp vanilla extract
- •1 tsp apple cider vinegar

Filling (optional)
- •1/2 cup sugar-free chocolate chips
- •1/2 cup chopped walnuts (or nuts you like)

Instructions
1. Preheat oven to 180°C (375°F). Line a baking loaf pan (9 inches x 5 inches) with parchment paper. Set aside.
2. Remove both extremity of the zucchinis, keep skin on.
3. Finely grate the zucchini using a vegetable grater. Measure the amount needed in a measurement cup. Make sure you press/pack them firmly for a precise measure and to squeeze out any liquid from the grated zucchini, I usually don't have any! If you do, discard the liquid or keep for another recipe.
4. In a large mixing bowl, stir all the dry ingredients together: almond flour, unsweetened cocoa powder, sugar   free crystal sweetener, cinnamon, sea salt, and baking soda. Set aside.
5. Add all the wet ingredients into the dry ingredients: grated zucchini, coconut oil, coconut cream, vanilla, egg, apple cider vinegar.
6. Stir to combine all the ingredients together.
7. Stir in the chopped nuts and sugar-free chocolate chips.

8. Transfer the chocolate bread batter into the prepared loaf pan.
9. Bake 50 - 55 minutes—you may want to cover the bread loaf with a piece of foil after 40 minutes to avoid the top to darken too much, up to you.
10. The bread will stay slightly moist in the middle and firm up after fully cooled down.
11. Transfer pan to a wire rack; let bread cool 15 minutes before removing from pan.

Cinnamon Almond Flour Bread
Nutrition: Cal 221;Fat 15 g; Carb 10 g;Protein 9 g
Serving 8; Cook time 30 min.

Ingredients
- •2 cups fine blanched almond flour (I use Bob's Red Mill)
- •2 TBSP coconut flour
- •1/2 tsp sea salt
- •1 tsp baking soda
- •1/4 cup flaxseed meal or chia meal (ground chia or flaxseed, see notes for how to make your own)
- •5 eggs and 1 egg white whisked together
- •tsp apple cider vinegar or lemon juice
- •2 TBSP maple syrup or honey
- •2–3 TBSP of clarified butter (melted) or coconut oil (divided). Vegan butter also works.
- •1 TBSP cinnamon, plus extra for topping
- •Optional: Chia seeds to sprinkle on top before baking

Instructions
1. Preheat oven to 350°F. Line an 8×4 bread pan with parchment paper at the bottom and grease the sides.
2. In a large bowl, mix together your almond flour, coconut flour, salt, baking soda, flaxseed meal or chia meal, and 1/2 tablespoon of cinnamon.
3. In another small bowl, whisk together your eggs and egg white. Then add in your maple syrup (or honey), apple cider vinegar, and melted butter (1.5 to 2 tablespoons).
4. Mix wet ingredients into dry. Be sure to remove any clumps that might have occurred from the almond flour or coconut flour.
5. Pour batter into a your greased loaf pan.
6. Bake at 350°F for 30-35 minutes, until a toothpick inserted into center of loaf comes out clean. Mine came to around 35 minutes, but I am at altitude.
7. Remove from the oven.
8. Next, whisk together the other 1 to 2 tablespoons of melted butter (or oil) and mix it with 1/2 tablespoon of cinnamon. Brush this on top of your cinnamon almond flour bread.
9. Cool and serve, or store for later.
10. Transfer pan to a wire rack; let bread cool 15 minutes before removing from pan.

Blueberry English Muffin Bread
Nutrition: Cal 156;Fat 13 g; Carb 4 g;Protein 5 g
Serving 12; Cook time 45 min.

Ingredients

- 1/2 cup almond butter, cashew, or peanut butter
- 1/4 cup butter ghee or coconut oil
- 1/2 cup almond flour
- 1/2 tsp salt
- 2 tsp baking powder
- 1/2 cup almond milk, unsweetened
- 5 eggs, beaten
- 1/2 cup blueberries

Instructions

1. Preheat oven to 350°F.
2. In a microwavable bowl melt nut butter and butter together for 30 seconds, stir until combined well.
3. In a large bowl, whisk almond flour, salt, and baking powder together. Pour the nut butter mixture into the large bowl and stir to combine.
4. Whisk the almond milk and eggs together then pour into the bowl and stir well.
5. Drop in fresh blueberries or break apart frozen blueberries and gently stir into the batter.
6. Line a loaf pan with parchment paper and lightly grease the parchment paper as well.
7. Pour the batter into the loaf pan and bake 45 minutes or until a toothpick in center comes out clean.
8. Cool for about 30 minutes then remove from pan.
9. Slice and toast each slice before serving.1/2 cup chopped walnuts (or nuts you like)

Zucchini Bread with Walnuts
Nutrition: Cal 200;Fat 18 g; Carb 3 g;Protein 5 g
Serving 16; Cook time 60 min.

Ingredients
- 3 large eggs
- ½ cup olive oil
- 1 tsp vanilla extract
- 2 1/2 cups almond flour
- 1 1/2 cups erythritol
- ½ tsp salt
- 1 1/2 tsp baking powder
- ½ tsp nutmeg
- 1 tsp ground cinnamon
- ¼ tsp ground ginger
- 1 cup grated zucchini
- ½ cup chopped walnuts

Instructions
1. Preheat oven to 350°F. Whisk together the eggs, oil, and vanilla extract. Set to the side.
2. In another bowl, mix together the almond flour, erythritol, salt, baking powder, nutmeg, cinnamon, and ginger. Set to the side.
3. Using a cheesecloth or paper towel, take the zucchini and squeeze out the excess water.
4. Then, whisk the zucchini into the bowl with the eggs.
5. Slowly add the dry ingredients into the egg mixture using a hand mixer until fully blended.
6. Lightly spray a 9x5 loaf pan, and spoon in the zucchini bread mixture.

7. Then, spoon in the chopped walnuts on top of the zucchini bread. Press walnuts into the batter using a spatula.
8. Bake for 60-70 minutes at 350°F or until the walnuts on top look browned.

Keto Bagel
Nutrition: Cal 168;Fat 17 g; Carb 8 g;Protein 5 g
Serving 4; Cook time 45 min.

Ingredients
- 1 cup (120 g) of almond flour
- 1/4 cup (28 g) of coconut flour
- 1 TBSP (7 g) of psyllium husk powder
- 1 tsp (2 g) of baking powder
- 1 tsp (3 g) of garlic powder
- Pinch of salt
- 2 medium eggs (88 g)
- 2 tsp (10 ml) of white wine vinegar
- 2 1/2 TBSP (38 ml) of ghee, melted
- 1 TBSP (15 ml) of olive oil
- 1 tsp (5 g) of sesame seeds

Instructions
1. Preheat the oven to 320°F (160°C).
2. Combine the almond flour, coconut flour, psyllium husk powder, baking powder, garlic powder, and salt in a bowl.
3. In a separate bowl, whisk the eggs and vinegar together. Slowly drizzle in the melted ghee (which should not be piping hot) and whisk in well.
4. Add the wet mixture to the dry mixture and use a wooden spoon to combine well. Leave to sit for 2-3 minutes.
5. Divide the mixture into 4 equal-sized portions. Using your hands, shape the mixture into a round shape and place onto a tray lined with parchment paper. Use a small spoon or apple corer to make the center hole.
6. Brush the tops with olive oil and scatter over the sesame seeds. Bake in the oven for 20-25 minutes until cooked through. Allow to cool slightly before enjoying!

Chocolate Coconut Mounds Pie
Nutrition: Cal 242;Fat 21 g; Carb 12 g;Protein 5 g
Serving 8; Cook time 60 min.

Ingredients
- 2 cups unsweetened coconut milk
- 4 eggs
- 1 tsp vanilla extract
- 1-1/2 tsp coconut stevia
- 2 cups unsweetened shredded coconut
- 1/2 cup unsweetened cocoa powder
- 1/4 cup coconut flour
- 1/2 tsp salt

Coconut Cream Topping
- 1 can (15 oz) coconut milk (opened, overnight in fridge)
- Optional: 2 ounces Lily's sugar-free coconut chocolate Bar

Instructions
1. In a stand mixer with a whisk attachment blend the first 4 ingredients together.
2. Change to the paddle attachment and add the rest of the ingredients on low speed.
3. Pour mixture into a pie plate and bake for 40 minutes.
4. Allow to cool before adding coconut cream topping.
5. Keep refrigerated.

5. Pour batter into crust and bake 30 minutes, covering with foil about halfway through. Remove and let cool 10 minutes, then refrigerate half an hour until cool.

Topping
6. Combine cream, sweetener, and vanilla extract in a large bowl. Beat until cream holds stiff peaks. Spread over cooled filling. Shave dark chocolate over top. Chill another hour or two until completely set.

Brownie Truffle Pie
Nutrition: Cal 370;Fat 33 g; Carb 6 g;Protein 8 g
Serving 4; Cook time 60 min.

Ingredients
Crust
- 1 1/4 cup almond flour
- 3 TBSP coconut flour
- 1 TBSP granulated Swerve Sweetener
- 1/4 tsp salt
- 5 TBSP butter chilled and cut into small pieces
- 2-4 TBSP ice water

Filling
- 1/2 cup almond flour
- 6 TBSP cocoa powder
- 6 TBSP Swerve Sweetener
- 1 tsp baking powder
- 2 large eggs
- 5 TBSP water
- 1/4 cup melted butter
- 1 TBSP Sukrin Fiber Syrup (optional, but helps create a more gooey center)
- 1/2 tsp vanilla extract
- 3 TBSP sugar-free chocolate chips

Topping
- 1 cup whipping cream
- 2 TBSP confectioner's Swerve Sweetener
- 1/4 tsp vanilla extract
- 1/2 oz sugar-free dark chocolate

Instructions
Crust
1. Preheat oven to 325°F and grease a glass or ceramic pie pan.
2. In a large bowl, combine almond flour, coconut flour, sweetener, and salt. Cut in butter using a pastry cutter or two sharp knives until mixture resembles coarse crumbs. Add two tablespoons water and mix until dough comes together. Add more water only if necessary to get dough to come together.
3. Press evenly into the bottom and up the sides of prepared pie pan, crimp edges, and prick bottom all over with a fork. Bake 12 minutes.

Filling
4. In a large bowl, whisk together the almond flour, cocoa powder, sweetener, and baking powder. Stir in eggs, water, melted butter, and vanilla extract until well combined. Stir in chocolate chips.

Coconut Key Lime Pie
Nutrition: Cal 460;Fat 42 g; Carb 6 g;Protein 11 g
Serving 9; Cook time 50 min.

Ingredients
Crust
- 2 cups raw hazelnuts
- 1 egg
- 4 TBSP chia seeds
- 4 TBSP organic butter, melted
- 1 TBSP coconut oil
- 1 TBSP Swerve

Filling
cup coconut cream
- 1.5 cup sour cream
- 3 large eggs
- 1 cup fresh key lime juice
- 3 TBSP Swerve
- 1 TBSP key lime zest
- ½ cup unsweetened coconut shavings

Instructions
1. Pre heat oven to 375°F.
2. In a food processor grind the hazelnuts until they turn in to a flour, then add the chia seeds, Swerve, egg, and melted butter. Mix everything together until a dough is formed.
3. Now grease a 6 by 9 inch pyrex with coconut oil.
4. Press the crust flat into the pyrex.
5. Bake for 20 min at 375°F.
6. In the meantime, prepare the filling.
7. In a large bowl mix all the filling ingredients and blend with an immersion blender until smooth and frothy.
8. Remove the crust from the oven once done.
9. Pour filling onto crust and put back in the oven at 350°F.
10. Bake for 45 minutes.
11. Remove from the oven, and let cool, then sprinkle evenly with the coconut flakes. Then refrigerate overnight.

Sweet Ricotta Cheese Pie
Nutrition: Cal 270;Fat 12 g; Carb 4 g;Protein 14 g
Serving 8; Cook time 50 min.

Ingredients
- 1 1/2 cups almond flour, sifted
- 3 TBSP low carb sugar substitute (I used Swerve)
- 1/4 tsp salt
- 1/4 cup butter, melted

- 1 egg
- 1 tsp vanilla extract
- 4 eggs, beaten
- 1 tsp vanilla extract
- 15 oz ricotta cheese
- 1 TBSP coconut flour
- 3/4 cup Swerve (add more if desired; up to 1 cup)
- 2 TBSP low carb sugar substitute or 24 drops liquid stevia to help round out sweetness

Instructions

1. In deep dish pie plate, mix together almond flour, 3 tablespoons equivalent sugar substitute and 1/4 teaspoon salt.
2. Pour in butter, 1 egg and 1 teaspoon vanilla.
3. Mix until dough forms.
4. Press into pie plate. Bake at 350 degrees F for 10 minutes.
5. Set on rack to cool slightly.
6. In a large bowl mix 4 beaten eggs, 1 teaspoon vanilla, ricotta cheese, coconut flour, 1 cup equivalent sugar substitute and 2 tablespoons other sweetener.
7. Beat until smooth.
8. Pour into crust and bake at 350°F for 45 minutes or until lightly browned and firm.

Chayote Squash Mock Apple Pie
Nutrition: Cal 190;Fat 16 g; Carb 6 g;Protein 2 g
Serving 16; Cook time 45 min.

Ingredients
Crust
- 1/2 cup butter, melted
- 1 1/2 cup almond flour
- 3/4 cup coconut flour
- 4 eggs
- 1 TBSP whole psyllium husks
- 1/2 tsp salt

Filling
- 5 medium chayote squash
- 3/4 cup low carb sugar substitute
- 1 1/2 tsp cinnamon
- 1/4 tsp ginger
- 1/8 tsp nutmeg
- 1 TBSP xanthan gum
- 1 TBSP lemon juice
- 2 tsp apple extract (optional)
- 1/3 cup butter cut in small pieces

Topping
- 1 egg
- Low carb sugar substitute

Instructions
Crust
1. Mix crust ingredients to form dough.
2. Separate into two dough balls.
3. Roll each crust ball out into pie crust.
4. Transfer one crust to 9 inch pie dish. Smooth out any cracks.
5. Reserve remaining crust for pie top.

Filling
6. Filling
7. Peel chayote and cut into slices.
8. Boil sliced chayote until fork tender. Drain. Return to pot.
9. Add sweetener, xanthan gum, lemon juice, and apple extract to cooked chayote squash.
10. Pour chayote mixture into prepared pie crust. Dot filling with butter.

Topping
11. Cover filling with reserved pie crust.
12. Flute edges of pie crust together and cut slits on pie top.
13. Brush egg on top crust and sprinkle with additional sweetener, if desired.
14. Bake at 375°F for 30-35 minutes (I took mine out after 30 minutes).

Lemon Meringue Pie
Nutrition: Cal 218;Fat 17 g; Carb 7 g;Protein 6 g
Serving 12; Cook time 60 min.

Ingredients
Pastry Crust
- 1 1/4 cup almond flour
- 2 TBSP coconut flour
- 2 TBSP arrowroot starch OR 2 TBSP oat fiber for THM
- 1 TBSP granulated Swerve Sweetener
- 1 tsp xanthan gum
- 1/4 tsp salt
- 5 TBSP butter, chilled and cut into small pieces
- 2-4 TBSP ice water

Filling
- 1 cup plus 2 TBSP water, divided
- 1 cup granulated Swerve Sweetener
- 2 tsp lemon zest
- 1/4 tsp salt
- 4 large egg yolks
- 1/3 cup lemon juice
- 3 TBSP butter
- 1/2 tsp xanthan gum
- 1 TBSP grassfed gelatin (can use 1 envelope Knox gelatin)

Meringue Topping
- 4 large egg whites at room temperature
- 1/4 tsp cream of tartar
- Pinch of salt
- 1/4 cup powdered Swerve Sweetener
- 1/4 cup granulated Swerve Sweetener
- 1/2 tsp vanilla extract

Instructions
Crust
1. Preheat oven to 325°F.
2. Combine almond flour, coconut flour, arrowroot starch, sweetener, xanthan gum, and salt in the bowl of a food processor. Pulse to combine.
3. Sprinkle surface with butter pieces and pulse until mixture resembles coarse crumbs.

4. With processor running on low, add ice water, one tablespoon at a time until dough begins to clump together.
5. Place a large piece of parchment on work surface and dust liberally with additional almond flour. Turn out dough and pat into a circle. Sprinkle with more almond flour and over with another large piece of parchment.
6. Roll out carefully into an 11-inch circle. Remove top layer of parchment. Place a 9-inch pie pan upside down on crust and then carefully flip both over so crust is lying in the pie pan. Remove parchment. (Alternatively, you can skip rolling out the pastry and simply press the crust into the bottom and up the sides of the pan).
7. You may get some cracking and tears. Simply use small pieces of pastry from the overhang to patch them up. Crimp the edges of the crust and prick all over with a fork.
8. Bake crust 12 minutes, then remove and let cool.

Lemon Filling

9. In a medium saucepan over medium heat, combine 1 cup of the water, sweetener, lemon zest, and salt. Bring to just a boil, whisking frequently, until sweetener dissolves.
10. In a medium bowl, whisk egg yolks until smooth. Slowly add about 1/2 cup of the water to the egg yolks, whisking constantly. Then gradually whisk the egg yolks back into the pan and lower the heat to low. Cook for 1 minute more, stirring continuously.
11. Stir in lemon juice and butter and whisk until smooth. Sprinkle surface with xanthan gum and whisk vigorously to combine.
12. In a small bowl, stir together the remaining two tablespoons of water and the gelatin. Let sit 2 minutes until gelled, then stir into hot lemon mixture, whisking until well combined. Cover and set aside while making the meringue.

Meringue Topping

13. In a large bowl, beat egg whites with cream of tartar and salt until frothy. With beaters going, slowly add sweeteners and vanilla extract and continue to beat until stiff peaks form.

To Assemble

14. Preheat oven to 300°F.
15. Pour warm filling into crust. Dollop with meringue and spread right to the edges so that the meringue meets the crust. Swirl the top with the back of a spoon.
16. Bake 20 minutes or until meringue topping is golden andьjust barely firm to the touch. Remove and let pie cool 20 minutes, then refrigerate at least 3 hours to set

Grasshopper Mousse Pie
Nutrition: Cal 261;Fat 26 g; Carb 5 g;Protein 3 g
Serving 12; Cook time 45 min.

Ingredients
No-bake Chocolate Pie Crust
• 3/4 cup unsweetened shredded coconut

• 1/4 cup unsweetened cocoa powder
• 1/2 cup sunflower seeds raw, unsalted
• 4 TBSP butter, softened
• 1/4 tsp salt
• 1/4 cup Swerve confectioners

Filling
• 1/2 cup water
• 1 tsp gelatin
• 5 oz avocado, mashed
• 8 oz cream cheese, softened
• 1 tsp peppermint extract
• 1 tsp peppermint liquid stevia
• Pinch of salt
• 1 cup heavy cream

Instructions
Crust
1. Combine all ingredients into a food processor and blend just enough to combine. Don't over blend or you will have the texture of peanut butter.
2. Taste crust to see if you need more salt or sweetness.
3. Using your fingers spread and mold crust onto bottom and sides of pie plate. Set aside.

Filling
1. Pour the water into a small saucepan and sprinkle the gelatin on top.
2. Turn on low heat, stirring constantly until gelatin is dissolved. Let cool.
3. Place the avocado, cream cheese, peppermint extract, stevia, and salt into a stand mixer and blend on high until smooth.
4. Taste and adjust sweetness if needed.
5. Pour in heavy cream in another bowl and use an electric mixer to blend on high until soft peaks form. Fold into the cream cheese mixture.
6. Gradually pour in the cooled gelatin and stir until combined.
7. Pour filling into pie crust.
8. Refrigerate at least 2 hours, loosely covered or up to 1 day.
9. When ready to serve add optional chocolate drizzle if desired.

Coconut Flour Chocolate Cupcakes
Nutrition: Cal 270;Fat 22 g; Carb 6 g;Protein 6 g
Serving 12; Cook time 40 min.

Ingredients
Cupcakes
• 1/2 cup butter, melted
• 7 TBSP cocoa powder
• 1 tsp instant coffee granules (optional, enhances chocolate flavor)
• 7 eggs room temperature
• 1 tsp vanilla extract
• 2/3 cup coconut flour
• 2 tsp baking powder
• 2/3 cup Swerve Sweetener
• 1/2 tsp salt

- 1/2 cup unsweetened almond milk (more if your batter is too thick)

Espresso Butter cream
- 2 TBSP hot water
- 2 tsp instant espresso powder or instant coffee
- 1/2 cup whipping cream
- 6 TBSP butter, softened
- 4 oz cream cheese, softened
- 1/2 cup powdered Swerve Sweetener

Instructions
Cupcakes
1. Preheat oven to 350°F and line a muffin tin with parchment or silicone liners
2. In a large bowl, whisk together the melted butter, cocoa powder, and espresso powder.
3. Add the eggs and vanilla and beat until well combined. Then add the coconut flour, sweetener, baking powder and salt and beat until smooth.
4. Beat in the almond milk. If that batter is still very thick, beat in more almond milk 1 tablespoon at a time until it thins out a bit (batter will still be thick, but should be of scoopable consistency; it will not be pourable).
5. Divide batter among prepared muffin tins and bake in center of oven for 20 to 25 minutes. Cupcakes are done when the top is set and a tester inserted into the middle comes out clean. Cool in pan for 5-10 minutes and then transfer to a wire rack to cool completely.

Butter cream
1. In a small bowl, stir together hot water and espresso until coffee dissolves. Set aside.
2. With an electric mixer, whip cream until it forms stiff peaks. Set aside.
3. In a medium bowl, beat butter, cream cheese, and sweetener together until creamy. Add coffee mixture and beat until combined. With a rubber spatula, fold in whipped cream carefully until well combined.
4. Spread frosting on cooled cupcakes with a knife or offset spatula, or pipe on with a decorating bag.

Pumpkin Pie Cupcakes
Nutrition: Cal 170;Fat 12 g; Carb 5 g;Protein 3 g
Serving 6; Cook time 45 min.

Ingredients
- 3 TBSP coconut flour
- 1 tsp pumpkin pie spice
- 1/4 tsp baking powder
- 1/4 tsp baking soda
- Pinch of salt
- 3/4 cup pumpkin puree
- 1/3 cup Swerve Brown or Swerve Granular
- 1/4 cup heavy whipping cream
- 1 large egg
- 1/2 tsp vanilla

Instructions
1. Preheat oven to 350°F and line 6 muffin cups with silicone or parchment liners.
2. In a small bowl, whisk together the coconut flour, pumpkin pie spice, baking powder, baking soda, and salt.
3. In a large bowl, whisk pumpkin puree, sweetener, cream, egg, and vanilla until well combined. Whisk in dry ingredients. If your batter seems very thin, whisk in an additional tbsp of coconut flour.
4. Divide among prepared muffin cups and bake 25 to 30 minutes, until just puffed and barely set. Remove from oven and let cool in pan (they will sink...that's okay, all the better for plopping your whipped cream on top!).
5. Refrigerate for at least one hour before serving. Dollop whipped cream generously on top.

Peanut Butter Molten Lava Cakes
Nutrition: Cal 270;Fat 22 g; Carb 6 g;Protein 10 g
Serving 4; Cook time 40 min.

Ingredients
- 1/4 cup butter
- 1/4 cup peanut butter
- 2 TBSP coconut oil
- 6 TBSP powdered Swerve Sweetener
- 2 large eggs2 large egg yolks
- 1/2 tsp vanilla extract
- 6 TBSP almond flour
- Low carb chocolate sauce

Instructions
1. Preheat oven to 350°F and grease 4 small (about 1/2 cup capacity each) ramekins very well. I used both butter and coconut oil spray.
2. In a medium-sized microwave safe bowl, combine butter, peanut butter, and coconut oil. Cook on high in 30 second increments until melted. Stir together until smooth.
3. Whisk in powdered sweetener until smooth. Whisk in eggs, egg yolks, and vanilla extract. Then whisk in almond flour until smooth.
4. Divide batter among prepared ramekins and bake 12 to 15 minutes, until sides are set but the center still jiggles a bit. Remove and let cool a few minutes.
5. Run a sharp knife around the inside of the ramekin to loosen the cakes. Cover each with an upside-down plate and flip over to turn the cake out onto the plate (you may need to give it one good shake, holding the plate and ramekin together tightly).
6. Drizzle with low carb chocolate sauce and serve immediately.

Texas Sheet Cake
Nutrition: Cal 230;Fat 20 g; Carb 6 g;Protein 6 g
Serving 12; Cook time 40 min.

Ingredients
Cake
- 2 cups almond flour
- 3/4 cup Swerve Sweetener
- 1/3 cup coconut flour

- 1/3 cup unflavoured whey protein powder
- 1 TBSP baking powder
- 1/2 tsp salt
- 1/2 cup butter
- 1/2 cup water
- 1/4 cup cocoa powder
- 3 large eggs
- 1 tsp vanilla extract
- 1/4 cup heavy cream
- 1/4 cup water

Frosting
- 1/2 cup butter
- 1/4 cup cocoa powder
- 1/4 cup cream
- 1/4 cup water
- 1 tsp vanilla extract
- 1 1/2 cups powdered Swerve Sweetener
- 1/4 tsp xanthan gum
- 3/4 cup chopped pecans

Instructions
Cake
1. Preheat oven to 325°F and grease a 10x15 inch rimmed sheet pan very well.
2. In a large bowl, whisk together the almond flour, sweetener, coconut flour, protein powder, baking powder, and salt. Break up any clumps with the back of a fork.
3. In a medium saucepan over medium heat, combine the butter, water, and cocoa powder, stirring until melted. Bring to a boil and then remove from heat. Add to the bowl.
4. Add eggs, vanilla extract, cream and water and stir until well combined. Spread in prepared baking pan.
5. Bake 15 to 20 minutes, until cake is set and a tester inserted in the center comes out clean.

Frosting
6. In another medium saucepan, combine butter, cocoa powder, cream, and water. Bring to a simmer, stirring until smooth. Stir in vanilla extract. Add powdered sweetener 1/2 a cup at a time, whisking vigorously to dissolve any clumps. Whisk in xanthan gum.
7. Pour over warm cake and sprinkle with pecans. Let cool until frosting is set, about 1 hour.

Gingerbread Cake Roll
Nutrition: Cal 206;Fat 18 g; Carb 4 g;Protein 6 g
Serving 12; Cook time 40 min.

Ingredients
Cake
- 1 cup almond flour
- 1/4 cup powdered Swerve Sweetener
- 2 TBSP cocoa powder
- 1 TBSP grassfed gelatin
- 2 tsp ground ginger
- 1 tsp ground cinnamon
- 1/4 tsp ground cloves
- 4 large eggs room temperature, separated

- 1/4 cup granulated Swerve Sweetener, divided
- 1 tsp vanilla extract
- 1/4 tsp salt, divided
- 1/4 tsp cream of tartar

Vanilla Cream Filling
- 2 oz cream cheese, softened
- 1 1/2 cups whipping cream, divided
- 1/4 cup powdered Swerve Sweetener
- 1/2 tsp vanilla extract

Instructions
Cake
1. Preheat oven to 350°F and line an 11x17 inch rimmed baking sheet with parchment paper. Grease the parchment paper and pan sides very well.
2. In a medium bowl, whisk together the almond flour, powdered sweetener, cocoa powder, gelatin, ginger, cinnamon, and cloves.
3. In another medium bowl, beat the egg yolks with 2 tablespoons of the granulated sweetener until lighter yellow and thickened. Beat in the vanilla extract
4. Using clean beaters and a large clean bowl, beat the egg whites with the salt and cream of tartar until frothy. Beat in the remaining two tablespoons sweetener until stiff peaks form.
5. Gently fold the egg yolk mixture into the whites. Then gently fold in the almond flour mixture, taking care not to deflate them, until no streaks remain.
6. Spread the batter evenly into the prepared baking pan and bake 10 to 12 minutes, until the top springs back when touched.
7. Remove from the oven and let let cool a few minutes, then run a knife around the edges to loosen. Cover with another large piece of parchment paper and then a kitchen towel. Place another large baking sheet overtop and flip over.
8. Gently peel the parchment from what is now the top of the cake. While still warm, gently roll up inside the kitchen towel, starting from one of the shorter ends. Don't roll too tightly or it will crack. Let cool while preparing the filling.

Vanilla Cream Filling
9. In a small bowl, beat the cream cheese with 1/4 cup whipping cream until smooth.
10. In a large bowl, beat the remaining whipping cream with the sweetener and vanilla extract until it holds soft peaks. Then add the cream cheese mixture and continue to beat until stiff peaks form. Do not overbeat. Remove ½ cup and set aside for decorating.
11. Gently and carefully unroll the cake. Do not try to lay it completely flat, let it curl up on the ends. Spread with the remaining filling to within 1/2 inch of the edges. Gently roll back up without the kitchen towel. Place seam side down on a serving platter.
12. Sprinkle with some more powdered sweetener, if desired. Pipe remaining vanilla cream mixture in stars or other shapes down the center of the top of the cake.
13. Refrigerate 1 hour before slicing. Store in the refrigerator.

Mini Cinnamon Roll Cheesecakes

Nutrition: Cal 240;Fat 20 g; Carb 5 g;Protein 5 g
Serving 6; Cook time 40 min.

Ingredients
Crust
- 1/2 cup almond flour
- 2 TBSP Swerve Sweetener
- 1/2 tsp cinnamon
- 2 TBSP melted butter
- Cheesecake Filling
- 6 oz cream cheese, softened
- 5 TBSP Swerve Sweetener, divided
- 1/4 cup sour cream
- 1/2 tsp vanilla extract
- 1 large egg
- 2 tsp cinnamon

Frosting
- 1 TBSP butter, softened
- 3 TBSP confectioners Swerve Sweetener
- 1/4 tsp vanilla extract
- 2 tsp heavy cream

Instructions
Crust
1. Preheat the oven to 325°F and line a muffin pan with 6 parchment or silicone liners.
2. In a medium bowl, whisk together the almond flour, sweetener and cinnamon. Stir in the melted butter until the mixture begins to clump together.
3. Divide among the prepared muffin cups and press firmly into the bottom. Bake 7 minutes, then remove and let cool while preparing the filling.

Cheesecake Filling
4. Reduce oven temperature to 300°F. In a large bowl, beat the cream cheese and 3 tablespoons of the sweetener together until smooth. Beat in the sour cream, vanilla and egg until well combined.
5. In a small bowl, whisk together the remaining 2 tablespoons sweetener and the cinnamon.
6. Dollop about 3/4 tablespoon of the cream cheese mixture into each of the muffin cups and sprinkle with a little of the cinnamon mixture. Repeat 2 more times. If you have any leftover cinnamon "sugar," reserve to sprinkle on after the cheesecakes are baked.
7. Bake 15 to 17 minutes, until mostly set but centres jiggle slightly. Turn off the oven and let them remain inside for 5 more minutes, then remove and let cool 30 minutes. Refrigerate at least 2 hours until set.

Frosting
8. In a medium bowl, beat butter with powdered sweetener until well combined. Beat in vanilla extract and heavy cream.
9. Transfer to a small ziplock bag and snip the corner. Drizzle decoratively over the chilled cheesecakes.

Chocolate Peanut Butter Lava Cakes

Nutrition: Cal 345;Fat 30 g; Carb 7 g;Protein 8 g
Serving 3; Cook time 35 min.

Ingredients
- 1/4 cup butter
- 1 oz unsweetened chocolate chopped
- 3 TBSP Swerve Sweetener
- 1 large egg
- 1 large egg yolk
- 3 TBSP almond flour
- 1/4 tsp vanilla extract
- Pinch of salt
- 2 TBSP peanut butter

Instructions
1. Preheat oven to 375°F and grease 3 small ramekins. Dust the ramekins with cocoa powder and shake out the excess.
2. In a microwave safe bowl, melt butter and chocolate together, whisking until smooth. Alternatively, you can melt it carefully over low heat.
3. Add the sweetener and whisk until combined. Then add the egg and egg yolk and whisk until smooth.
4. Whisk in the almond flour, vanilla extract, and salt until well combined.
5. Divide about 2/3 of the batter between the three ramekins, making sure to cover the bottom.
6. Divide peanut butter between the ramekins, placing in center of the batter. Cover with remaining batter. Bake 10 to 12 minutes, or until the edges of the cakes are set but the center still jiggles slightly.
7. Remove and let cool 5 to 10 minutes. Then run a sharp knife around the edges and flip out onto platesIn a medium-sized microwave safe bowl, combine butter, peanut butter, and coconut oil. Cook on high in 30 second increments until melted. Stir together until smooth.

Pecan Pie Cheesecake

Nutrition: Cal 340;Fat 30 g; Carb 5 g;Protein 6 g
Serving 10; Cook time 35 min.

Ingredients
Crust
- 3/4 cup almond flour
- 2 TBSP powdered Swerve Sweetener
- Pinch of salt
- 2 TBSP melted butter

Pecan Pie Filling
- 1/4 cup butter
- 1/3 cup powdered Swerve Sweetener
- 1 tsp Yacon syrup or molasses optional, for color and flavor
- 1 tsp caramel extract or vanilla extract
- 2 TBSP heavy whipping cream
- 1 large egg
- 1/4 tsp salt
- 1/2 cup chopped pecans

Cheesecake Filling

- 12 oz cream cheese, softened
- 5 TBSP powdered Swerve Sweetener
- 1 large egg
- 1/4 cup heavy whipping cream
- 1/2 tsp vanilla extract

Topping
- 2 TBSP butter
- 2 1/2 tbsp powdered Swerve Sweetener
- 1/2 tsp Yacon syrup or molasses
- 1/2 tsp caramel extract or vanilla extract
- 1 TBSP heavy whipping cream
- Whole toasted pecans for garnish

Instructions
Crust
1. In a medium bowl, whisk together the almond flour, sweetener, and salt. Stir in the melted butter until the mixture begins to clump together.
2. Press into the bottom and partway up the sides of a 7-inch springform pan. Place in the freezer while making the pecan pie filling.

Pecan Pie Filling
3. In a small saucepan over low heat, melt the butter. Add the sweetener and Yacon syrup and whisk until combined, then stir in the extract and heavy whipping cream.
4. Add the egg and continue to cook over low heat until the mixture thickens (this should only take a minute or so). Immediately remove from heat and stir in the pecans and salt.
5. Spread mixture over the bottom of the crust.

Cheesecake Filling
6. Beat the cream cheese until smooth, then beat in the sweetener. Beat in the egg, whipping cream, and vanilla a extract.
7. Pour this mixture over the pecan pie filling and spread to the edges.

To Bake
8. Wrap the bottom of the springform pan tightly in a large piece of foil. Place a piece of paper towel over the top of the springform pan (not touching the cheesecake) and then wrap foil around the top as well. Your whole pan should be mostly covered in foil to keep out excess moisture.
9. Place the rack that came with your Instant Pot or pressure cooker into the bottom. Pour a cup of water into the bottom.
10. Carefully lower the wrapped cheesecake pan onto the rack (there are ways to do this with a sling made out of tin foil but I didn't bother with that).
11. Close the lid and set the Instant Pot to manual mode for 30 minutes on high. Once the cooking time is complete, let the pressure to release naturally (do not vent it).
12. Lift out the cheesecake and let it cool to room temperature, and then refrigerate for 3 or 4 hours, or even overnight.

Topping
13. In a small saucepan over low heat, melt the butter. Add the sweetener and Yacon syrup and whisk until combined, then stir in the extract and heavy whipping cream. Drizzle over the chilled cheesecake and garnish with toasted pecans.

Peanut Butter Mug Cakes
Nutrition: Cal 210;Fat 20 g; Carb 6 g;Protein 7 g
Serving 6; Cook time 10 min.

Ingredients
- 1/3 cup peanut butter
- 1/4 cup butter
- 2/3 cup almond flour
- 1/3 cup Swerve Sweetener
- 2 tsp baking powder
- 2 large eggs
- 1/2 tsp vanilla extract
- 1/4 cup water
- 3 TBSP sugar-free chocolate chips

Instructions
1. In a microwave-safe bowl, melt peanut butter and butter together until smooth.
2. In a medium bowl, whisk together the almond flour, sweetener, and baking powder. Stir in the eggs, vanilla extract, melted peanut butter mixture and water until well combined. Stir in chocolate chips.
3. Divide among 6 ramekins or mugs and microwave each for 1 minute, until puffed and set. Serve warm.

Kentucky Butter Cake
Nutrition: Cal 310;Fat 27 g; Carb 6 g;Protein 7 g
Serving 16; Cook time 60 min.

Ingredients
Cake
- 2 1/2 cups almond flour
- 1/4 cup coconut flour
- 1/4 cup unflavored whey protein powder
- 1 TBSP baking powder
- 1/2 tsp salt
- 1 cup butter, softened
- 1 cup Swerve Granular
- 5 large eggs room temperature.
- 2 tsp vanilla extract
- 1/2 cup whipping cream
- 1/2 cup water

Butter Glaze
- 5 TBSP butter
- 1/3 cup Swerve Granular
- 2 TBSP water
- 1 tsp vanilla extract

Garnish
- 1 to 2 TBSP Confectioner's Swerve

Instructions
1. Preheat oven to 325°F. Grease a bundt cake pan VERY well and then dust with a few tbsp of almond flour.

2. In a medium bowl, whisk together the almond flour, coconut flour, whey protein, baking powder, and salt.
3. In a large bowl, beat the butter and the sweetener together until light and creamy. Beat in the eggs and vanilla extract.
4. Beat in the almond flour mixture and then beat in the whipping cream and water until well combined.
5. Transfer the batter to the prepared baking pan and smooth the top. Bake 50 to 60 minutes, until golden brown and the cake is firm to the touch. A tester inserted in the center should come out clean.
6. Butter Glaze:In a small saucepan over low heat, melt the butter and sweetener together. Whisk until well combined. Whisk in the water and vanilla extract.
7. While the cake is still warm and in the pan, poke holes all over with a skewer. Pour the glaze over and let cool completely in the pan.
8. Gently loosen the sides with a knife or thin rubber spatula, then flip out onto a serving platter. Dust with powdered sweetener.
9. Serve with lightly sweetened whipped cream and fresh berries.

Chocolate Walnut Torte
Nutrition: Cal 343;Fat 31 g; Carb 9 g;Protein 9 g
Serving 1; Cook time 45 min.

Ingredients
Torte
- 1 1/2 cup walnuts
- 3/4 cup Swerve Sweetener
- 1/4 cup cocoa powder
- 1 tsp espresso powder (optional, enhances chocolate flavor)
- 1/2 tsp baking powder
- 1/4 tsp salt
- 1/2 cup butter
- 4 oz unsweetened chocolate
- 5 large eggs
- 1/2 tsp vanilla extract
- 1/2 cup almond milk
Glaze
- 1/2 cup whipping cream
- 2 1/2 oz sugar-free dark chocolate chopped
- 1/3 cup walnut pieces
Instructions
Torte
1. Preheat oven to 325°F and grease a 9-inch round baking pan. Line the bottom with parchment paper and grease the paper.
2. In a food processor, process walnuts until finely ground. Add sweetener, cocoa powder, espresso powder, baking powder, and salt and pulse a few times to combine.
3. In a large saucepan set over low heat, melt butter and chocolate together until smooth. Remove from heat and whisk in eggs and vanilla extract. Add almond milk and whisk until mixture smooths out. Stir in walnut mixture until well combined.

4. Spread batter in prepared baking pan and bake about 30 minutes, until edges are set but center still looks slightly wet. Let cool 15 minutes in pan, then invert onto a wire rack to cool completely. Remove parchment paper.
Glaze
5. In a small saucepan over medium heat, bring cream to just a simmer. Remove from heat and add chopped chocolate. Let sit to melt 5 minutes, then whisk until smooth.
6. Cool another 10 minutes, then pour the glaze over the cake, smoothing the sides. Sprinkle top with walnut pieces and chill until chocolate is firm, about 30 minutes.

Cinnamon Roll Coffee Cake
Nutrition: Cal 222;Fat 20 g; Carb 5 g;Protein 7 g
Serving 8; Cook time 45 min.

Ingredients
- Cinnamon Filling
- 3 TBSP Swerve Sweetener
- 2 tsp ground cinnamon
- Cake
- 3 cups almond flour
- 3/4 cup Swerve Sweetener
- 1/4 cup unflavored whey protein powder
- 2 tsp baking powder
- 1/2 tsp salt
- 3 large eggs
- 1/2 cup butter, melted
- 1/2 tsp vanilla extract
- 1/2 cup almond milk
- 1 TBSP melted butter
- Cream Cheese Frosting
- 3 TBSP cream cheese, softened
- 2 TBSP powdered Swerve Sweetener
- 1 TBSP heavy whipping cream
- 1/2 tsp vanilla extract
Instructions
1. Preheat oven to 325°F and grease an 8x8 inch baking pan.
2. For the filling, combine the Swerve and cinnamon in a small bowl and mix well. Set aside.
3. For the cake, whisk together almond flour, sweetener, protein powder, baking powder, and salt in a medium bowl.
4. Stir in the eggs, melted butter and vanilla extract. Add the almond milk and continue to stir until well combined.
5. Spread half of the batter in the prepared pan, then sprinkle with about two thirds of the cinnamon filling mixture. Spread the remaining batter over top and smooth with a knife or an offset spatula.
6. Bake 35 minutes, or until top is golden brown and a tester inserted in the center comes out with a few crumbs attached.
7. Brush with melted butter and sprinkle with remaining cinnamon filling mixture. Let cool in pan.

8. For the frosting, beat cream cheese, powdered erythritol, cream and vanilla extract together in a small bowl until smooth. Pipe or drizzle over cooled cake.

Butter Cake
Nutrition: Cal 269;Fat 24 g; Carb 5 g;Protein 6 g
Serving 15; Cook time 40 min

Ingredients
Cake
- 2 cups almond flour
- 1/2 cup Swerve Sweetener
- 2 TBSP unflavored whey protein powder
- 2 tsp baking powder
- 1/4 tsp salt
- 1/2 cup butter, melted
- 1 large egg
- 1/2 tsp vanilla extract

Filling
- 8 oz cream cheese, softened
- 1/2 cup butter, softened
- 3/4 cup powdered Swerve
- 2 large eggs
- 1/2 tsp vanilla extract
- Powdered Swerve for dusting

Instructions
1. Preheat the oven to 325°F and lightly grease a 9x13 baking pan.
2. In a large bowl, combine the almond flour, sweetener, protein powder, baking powder, and salt. Add the butter, egg, and vanilla extract and stir to combine well. Press into the bottom and partway up the sides of the prepared baking pan.
3. In another large bowl, beat the cream cheese and butter together until smooth. Beat in the sweetener until well combined, then beat in the eggs and vanilla until smooth.
4. Pour the filling over the crust. Bake 35 to 45 minutes, until the filling is mostly set, but the center still jiggles, and the edges are just golden-brown.
5. Remove and let cool, then dust with powdered Swerve and cut into bars.

Classic New York Keto Cheesecake
Nutrition: Cal 284;Fat 24 g; Carb 3 g;Protein 7 g
Serving 8; Cook time 1 hour 30 min.

Ingredients
- 24 oz cream cheese, softened
- 5 TBSP unsalted butter, softened
- 1 cup powdered Swerve Sweetener
- 3 large eggs, room temperature
- 3/4 cup sour cream, room temperature
- 2 tsp grated lemon zest
- 1 1/2 tsp vanilla extract

Instructions

1. Preheat the oven to 300°F and generously grease a 9-inch springform pan. Cut a circle of parchment to fit the bottom the pan and grease the paper. Wrap 2 pieces of aluminum foil around the outside of the pan to cover the bottom and most of the way up the sides.
2. In a large bowl, beat the cream cheese and butter until smooth, then beat in the sweetener until well combined. Add the eggs, once at a time, beating after each addition. Clean the beaters and scrape down the sides of the bowl as needed.
3. Add the sour cream, lemon zest, and vanilla extract and beat until the batter is smooth and well combined. Pour into the prepared springform pan and smooth the top.
4. Set the pan inside a roasting pan large enough to prevent the sides from touching. Place the roasting pan in the oven and carefully pour boiling water into the roasting pan until it reaches halfway up the sides of the springform pan.
5. Bake 70 to 90 minutes, until the cheesecake is mostly set but still jiggles just a little in the center when shaken. Remove the roasting pan from the one, then carefully remove the springform pan from the water bath. Let cool to room temperature.
6. Run a sharp knife around the edges of the cake to loosen, the release the sides of the pan. Refrigerate for at least 4 hours before serving.

Italian Cream Cake
Nutrition: Cal 335;Fat 30 g; Carb 6 g;Protein 6 g
Serving 12; Cook time 45 min.

Ingredients
Cake
- 1/2 cup butter, softened
- 1 cup Swerve Sweetener
- 4 large eggs, room temperature, separated
- 1/2 cup heavy cream room temperature
- 1 tsp vanilla extract
- 1 1/2 cups almond flour
- 1/2 cup shredded coconut
- 1/2 cup chopped pecans
- 1/4 cup coconut flour
- 2 tsp baking powder
- 1/2 tsp salt
- 1/4 tsp cream of tartar

Frosting
- 8 oz cream cheese, softened
- 1/2 cup butter, softened
- 1 cup powdered Swerve Sweetener
- 1 tsp vanilla extract
- 1/2 cup heavy whipping cream, room temperature

Garnish
- 2 TBSP shredded coconut, lightly toasted
- 2 TBSP chopped pecans, lightly toasted

Instructions
Cake

1. Preheat the oven to 325°F and grease two 8 inch or 9 inch round cake pans very well (the 8 inch pans will take a little longer to cook but the layers will be higher and I think they will look better). Line the pans with parchment paper and grease the paper.
2. In a large bowl, beat the butter with the sweetener until well combined. Beat in the egg yolks one at a time, mixing well after each addition. Beat in the heavy cream and vanilla extract.
3. In another bowl, whisk together the almond flour, shredded coconut, chopped pecans, coconut flour, baking powder, and salt. Beat into the butter mixture until just combined.
4. In another large bowl, beat the egg whites with the cream of tartar until they hold stiff peaks. Gently fold into the cake batter.
5. Divide the batter evenly among the prepared pans and spread to the edges. Bake 35 to 45 minutes (or longer, depending on your pans), until the cakes are golden on the edges and firm to the touch in the middle.
6. Remove and let cool completely in the pans, then flip out onto a wire rack to cool completely. Remove the parchment from the layers if it comes out with them.

Frosting
7. In a large bowl, beat the cream cheese and butter together until smooth. Beat in the sweetener and vanilla extract until well combined.
8. Slowly add the heavy whipping cream until a spreadable consistency is achieved.

To Assemble
9. Place the bottom layer on a serving plate and cover the top with about 1/3 of the frosting. Add the next layer and frost the top and the sides.
10. Sprinkle the top with the toasted coconut and pecans. Refrigerate at least half an hour to let set.

COCONUT-ALMOND CAKE
Nutrition: Cal 231;Fat 19 g; Carb 12 g;Protein 3 g
Serving 8; Cook time 50 min.

Ingredients
- nonstick cooking spray
- 1 cup almond flour
- ½ cup unsweetened shredded coconut
- ⅓ cup Swerve
- 1 teaspoon apple pie spice
- 2 eggs, lightly whisked
- ¼ cup unsalted butter, melted
- ½ cup heavy (whipping) cream

Instructions
1. Grease a 6-inch round cake pan while using cooking spray.
2. In a medium bowl, mix together the almond flour, coconut, Swerve, and apple pie spice. Add the eggs, then the butter, and then your cream, mixing well after each addition.

3. Pour the batter in to the pan and cover with aluminum foil. Pour 2 glasses of water to the inner cooking pot, then place a trivet inside pot. Place the pan around the trivet.
4. Latch the lid. Select "Pressure Cook" or "Manual" and hang pressure to high and cook for 40 minutes. After enough time finishes, allow ten mins to naturally release pressure to succeed. For any remaining pressure, just quick-release it. Open the lid.
5. Carefully get the pan and allow it to cool for 15 to twenty minutes. Invert the dessert onto a plate. Sprinkle with shredded coconut, almond slices, or powdered sweetener, if desired, and serve.

DARK CHOCOLATE CAKE
Nutrition: Cal 225;Fat 20 g; Carb 4 g;Protein 5 g
Serving 6; Cook time 30 min.

Ingredients
- 1 cup almond flour
- ⅔ cup Swerve
- ¼ cup unsweetened powered cocoa
- ¼ cup chopped walnuts
- 1 teaspoon baking powder
- 3 eggs
- ⅓ cup heavy (whipping) cream
- ¼ cup coconut oil
- nonstick cooking spray

Instructions
1. Put the flour, Swerve, cocoa powder, walnuts, baking powder, eggs, cream, and coconut oil inside a large bowl. Using a hand mixer on very fast, combine the
2. Ingredients until the mix is well incorporated and appearance fluffy. This step will keep your cake from being too dense.
3. With the cooking spray, grease a heatproof pan, such like a 3-cup Bundt pan, that fits with your Instant Pot. Pour the dessert batter in the pan and cover with aluminum foil.
4. Pour 2 servings of water to the inner cooking pot, then place a trivet within the pot. Place the pan for the trivet.
5. Latch the lid. Select "Pressure Cook" or "Manual" and hang pressure to high and cook for 20 mins. After time finishes, allow 10 minutes to naturally release pressure to succeed. For any remaining pressure, just quick-release it. Carefully remove the pan and allow it to go cool for 15 to 20 mins. Invert the wedding cake onto a plate. It can be served hot or at room temperature. Serve having a dollop of whipped cream, if desired.

VANILLA CREAM WITH RASPBERRIES
Nutrition: Cal 302;Fat 30 g; Carb 4 g;Protein 4 g
Serving 4; Cook time 50 min.

Ingredients
- 1 ½ cup coconut milk, full-fat
- 1 tbsp. almond flour

- 2 tbsps. butter
- ¼ cup raspberries
- 3 egg yolks
- 3 tbsps. Swerve
- 1 tbsp. agar powder
- 1 vanilla bean
- 2 tsps. vanilla flavoring

Instructions

1. Using a sharp paring knife, slice the vanilla bean lengthwise and take away the seeds, schedule.
2. Plug inside instant pot and press the "Sauté" button.
3. Grease the inner pot with butter and add coconut milk. Warm up, stirring constantly, and adding egg yolks, swerve, and vanilla flavor.
4. Cook for 3 - 4 minutes, stirring constantly.
5. Finally, add agar powder, and vanilla seeds. Give it a good stir and then cook for an additional little bit, or until the mixture thickens.
6. Press the "Cancel" button and remove the cream in the pot. Divide between serving bowls and optionally top with a few whipped cream or fresh strawberries.
7. Plug inside instant pot and pour in the milk. Press the "Sauté" button and warm up. Add Swerve, cocoa powder, coconut cream, and vanilla extract.
8. Bring it to a boil, stirring constantly, and adding agar powder. Continue in order to smoke for 1 - 2 minutes.
9. Press the "Cancel" button and stir in finely chopped almonds.
10. Transfer the mix to a large mixing bowl and pour in the whipping cream. Beat well on high-speed for two main - 3 minutes.
11. Finally, divide the amalgamation between serving bowls and top each with raspberries. Serve cold.

KETO CHOCOLATE CAKE
Nutrition: Cal 300;Fat 12 g; Carb 7 g;Protein 8 g
Serving 6; Cook time 40 min.

Ingredients

- Almond flour (1 cup)
- Cocoa powder (unsweetened, ¼ cup)
- Coconut oil (1/4 cup)
- Eggs (3)
- Artificial sweetener by choice (2/3 cups)
- Walnuts (1/4 cups, chopped)
- Baking soda (1 teaspoon)

Instructions

1. All with the ingredients go in a very bowl and must be mixed which has a hand mixture (till everything gets to be a fluffy homogeny texture).
2. Pick a pan which will fit in the pressure cooker, grease it and pour the batter inside.
3. Pour water (2 cups) inside the pressure cooker, adding the steamer rack and ahead of it place the pot with the amalgamation.
4. Close and secure the lid, set to "High pressure" for 20 minutes; when cooking is completed, release the pressure naturally for 10 mins.
5. Cut it in pieces and serve.

PECAN PIE CHEESECAKE
Nutrition: Cal 340;Fat 31 g; Carb 5 g;Protein 6 g
Serving 10; Cook time 30 min.

Ingredients
FOR PECAN PIE FILLING

- Egg (1)
- Butter (1/4 cup)
- Artificial sweetener by choice (1/3 cup)
- Vanilla extract (1 teaspoon)
- Pecans (chopped)
- Heavy cream (2 tbsp)
- Salt (1/4 teaspoon)
- For cheesecake filling
- Cream cheese (12 oz.)
- Egg (1)
- Artificial sweetener by choice (5 tbsp)
- Heavy cream (1/4 cup)
- Vanilla extract (1/2 teaspoon)

FOR THE CRUST

- Almond flour (3/4 cups)
- Butter (2 tablespoons)
- Artificial sweetener by choice (2 tablespoons)
- Salt

Topping

- Toasted pecans
- Butter (2 tablespoons)
- Molasses (half tablespoon)
- Vanilla extract (half teaspoon)
- Heavy cream (1 tablespoon)

Instructions
Pecan pie filling

1. Melt the butter and adding the artificial sweetener, stir and adding the heavy cream.
2. Add the egg and cook on low heat (it should thicken). Remove it after a minute and atart exercising . the pecans and salt and stir.
3. This mixture goes on the crust.
4. Cheesecake filling
5. Add the artificial sweetener to the cheese cream and beat well. Then add the egg, vanilla flavor and whipping cream and beat well.
6. Add this mix within the pecan pie mix and spread well (over the crust).

For baking

1. The entire pan (crust, pecan pie, and cheesecake spreading) must be covered with foil.
2. Make sure the container will fit inside pressure to succeed cooker.
3. Pour water in the cooker after which put the rack inside; place the pan on the top from the rack.
4. Close the cover and hang the cooker to "Manual" for 30 minutes.
5. Release pressure naturally.
6. Take out the cheesecake, cool it to room temperature and after that input it in the fridge for 3-4 hours.

Topping:

1. Melt the butter and add the artificial sweetener, you can add the Molasses; whisk well and after that pour inside heavy cream.
2. Pour it over the cheesecake and top by incorporating more pecans (previously toasted). Serve and get!

CARROT CAKE
Nutrition: Cal 268;Fat 25 g; Carb 6 g;Protein 6 g
Serving 8; Cook time 60 min.

Ingredients
- Eggs (3)
- Carrots (1 cup, chopped)
- Artificial sweetener by choice (2/3 cups)
- Baking powder (1 teaspoon)
- Almond flour (1 cup)
- Coconut oil (1/4 cup)
- Cinnamon (1.5 teaspoons)
- Walnuts (half cup, chopped)
- Heavy cream (half cup)

Instructions
1. Use the coconut oil to grease a pan (be sure it's sufficient to suit within the pressure cooker).
2. Mix all of the Ingredients by using a hand mixer (the batter ought to be fluffy).
3. Pour the dough inside pan and place aluminum foil over it.
4. Pour two cups of water, add the steamer rack and put the pan while using batter into it.
5. Set pressure to succeed cooker to "Cake" and hang the timer for 40 minutes.
6. Release the stress naturally for ten minutes.
7. Let it cool well.
8. Serve with some extra heavy cream or any other toppings by choice.

CHOLATE MINT CAKE
Nutrition: Cal 214;Fat 19 g; Carb 8 g;Protein 6 g
Serving 8; Cook time 3 hours.

Ingredients
- Chocolate chips (make sure they may be reduced carbohydrate, 1/3 cup)
- Almond flour (1 cup)
- Almond milk (unsweetened, 2/3 cup)
- Artificial sweetener by choice (half cup)
- Cocoa powder (unsweetened, 1/3 cup)
- Butter (unsalted, 6 tablespoons)
- Eggs (3)
- Baking powder (1 ½ cup)
- Peppermint extract (half teaspoon)
- Salt (a pinch)

Instructions
1. Mix the powered cocoa, almond flour, artificial sweetener, salt, and baking powder.
2. Add the beaten eggs for this dry mix, almond milk, peppermint extract, chocolate chips, and melted butter.
3. The batter goes inside a previously greased pan or bowl that fits in the pressure cooker.
4. Set it to "Low" and let it bake for two-3 hours.

5. Let it cool for around 30 minutes (inside pressure cooker) and serve it while it's still warm.

MINI CHOCO CAKE
Nutrition: Cal 156;Fat 11 g; Carb 10 g;Protein 7 g
Serving 2; Cook time 15 min

Ingredients
- Eggs (2, beat them previously)
- Artificial sweetener by choice (2 tbsp)
- Baking cocoa (1/4 cup)
- Baking powder (half teaspoon)
- Vanilla extract (1 teaspoon)
- Heavy cream (2 tbsp)

Instructions
1. Mix the dry
2. Ingredients in the bowl and atart exercising . the wet
3. Ingredients and whisk well and soon you have a smooth batter.
4. Get bowls (ensure they can fit inside pressure cooker) and grease them.
5. Pour the dough inside the bowls (up on the half).
6. Add a cup full of water in the pressure cooker, put within the trivet and place the bowls inside.
7. Close and secure the lid; set to "High pressure" for 9 minutes.
8. Quick-release pressure to succeed then obtain the bowls out.
9. Serve with heavy cream.

COCONUT CUSTARD
Nutrition: Cal 174;Fat 14 g; Carb 6 g;Protein 6 g
Serving 4; Cook time 30 min.

Ingredients
- Eggs (3)
- Coconut milk (unsweetened, 1 cup)
- Vanilla extract (3 drops)
- Artificial sweetener by choice (1/3 cup)

Instructions
1. Mix well the milk, artificial sweetener, vanilla flavor, and eggs; work with a heatproof bowl and cover it with aluminum foil.
2. Put two cups inside the pressure cooker, put inside trivet and place the bowl over it.
3. Set to "High pressure" for 30 minutes once it's cooked release pressure naturally.
4. Cool the custard inside the fridge (until it's well set).
5. Serve in bowls and eat cooled.

AVOCADO PUDDING
Nutrition: Cal 251;Fat 21 g; Carb 3.7 g;Protein 6 g
Serving 2; Cook time 10 min.

Ingredients
- ½ ripe avocado, cut into cubes
- 1 tsp. agar powder
- 1 cup whole milk
- ¼ cup coconut cream
- 2 tsps. Stevia powder

•1 tsp. vanilla extract
Instructions
1. Combine avocado and coconut cream in a food processor or a high-speed blender. Pulse until smooth and creamy. Then put aside.
2. In a large mixing bowl, combine milk, agar powder, Stevia, and vanilla flavor. Mix until well combined and then add avocado mixture. Stir all well and pour into an oven-safe bowl.
3. Pour 1 cup of water inside the metal insert of your Instant Pot. Set the trivet around the bottom make the bowl on the top.
4. Securely lock the lid as well as set the steam release handle by moving the valve on the "Sealing" position. Set the timer for 3 minutes for the "Manual" mode.
5. When you hear the cooker's end signal, perform a quick pressure release and open the pot.
6. Transfer the bowl to a wire rack and allow it to cool completely.
7. Refrigerate for 30 minutes before serving

Salted Caramel Peanut Delight Milkshake
Nutrition: Cal 220;Fat 16 g; Carb 3 g;Protein 6 g
Serving 1; Cook time 10 min.

Ingredients
•1 cup Coconut Milk
•7 Ice Cubes
•2 tbsp. Peanut Butter
•2 tbsp. SF Torani Salted Caramel
•1 tbsp. MCT Oil
•1/4 tsp. Xanthan Gum
Instructions
1. Add all ingredients to a blender.
2. Blend 1-2 minutes.

Nutty Cookie Butter
Nutrition: Cal 174;Fat 14 g; Carb 6 g;Protein 6 g
Serving 1; Cook time 20 min.

Ingredients
•1 cup Raw Macadamias
•3/4 cup Raw Cashews
•1 tsp. Vanilla
•1/4 tsp. Cinnamon
•1/4 tsp. Ginger
•1/8 tsp. Nutmeg
•1/8 tsp. Cloves
•2 tbsp. Butter
•2 tbsp. Heavy Cream
•2 tbsp. Swerve, powdered
•Pinch Salt
Instructions
1. In a food processor, blend together macadamia nuts and cashews until smooth.
2. In a saucepan, begin to brown butter along with the Swerve.
3. Once browned, mix in heavy cream.
4. Remove from heat.

5. To nut mixture, add vanilla and spices, cream and butter.
6. Process again, ensuring no lumps.
7. Add in caramel sauce and process until desired consistency is reached.

Chocolate Chia Raspberry Pudding
Nutrition: Cal 246;Fat 12 g; Carb 7 g;Protein 23 g
Serving 1; Cook time 40 min.

Ingredients
•3 tablespoons Chia Seeds
•1 cup Unsweetened Almond Milk
•1 scoop Chocolate Protein Powder
•1/4 cup Raspberries fresh or frozen
•1 teaspoon Optional : Honey
Instructions
1. Mix together almond milk and protein powder.
2. Mix in chia seeds.
3. Let rest 5 minutes before stirring.
4. Refrigerate 30 minutes.
5. Top with raspberries.

Lemon Coconut Vanilla Bean
Nutrition: Cal 246;Fat 16 g; Carb 7 g;Protein 20 g
Serving 1; Cook time 40 min.

Ingredients
•½ cup extra virgin coconut oil, softened
•½ cup coconut butter, softened
•zest and juice of one lemon
•seeds from ½ a vanilla bean
Instructions
1. Whisk ingredients in an easy to pour cup.
2. Pour into lined cupcake or loaf pan.
3. Refrigerate 30 minutes.
4. Top with lemon zest.

Caramel Chocolate Brownies
Nutrition: Cal 320;Fat 7 g; Carb 12 g;Protein 10 g
Serving 8; Cook time 30 min.

Ingredients
•2 cups Almond Flour
•1/2 cup Unsweetened Cocoa Powder
•1/3 cup Erythritol
•1/4 cup Coconut Oil
•1/4 cup Maple Syrup
•2 large Eggs
•1 tbsp. Psyllium Husk Powder
•2 tbsp. Torani Salted Caramel
•1 tsp. Baking Powder
•1/2 tsp. Salt
Instructions
1. Preheat oven to 350 degrees.
2. In a bowl, beat together wet ingredients.
3. To the wet ingredients, slowly beat in dry ingredients.
4. Bake in an 11x7 well-greased brownie pan for 20 minutes.

White Chocolate Summer Berry Cheesecake
Nutrition: Cal 280;Fat 14 g; Carb 6 g;Protein 14 g
Serving 2; Cook time 15 min.

Ingredients
- 8 oz. cream cheese, softened
- 2 oz. heavy cream
- 1 teaspoon Stevia Glycerite
- 1 teaspoon low sugar raspberry preserves
- 1 tablespoon Da Vinci Sugar Free Syrup, White Chocolate flavor

Instructions
1. Whip together ingredients to a pudding consistency.
2. Put in cups.
3. Refrigerate.

Autumn Spice Scone Cookies
Nutrition: Cal 240;Fat 8 g; Carb 12 g;Protein 8 g
Serving 12; Cook time 60 min.

Ingredients
- 1 Sweet Lightning Winter Squash (or 1 1/4 cup Pumpkin Puree, strained)
- 2 tsp. Cinnamon
- 2 tsp. Garam Masala
- 1 tbsp. Coconut Oil Cooking Spray
- 2 large Eggs
- 1 tsp. Vanilla Extract
- 1 tsp. Baking Powder
- 1 cup Almond Flour
- 1/4 cup Butter
- 1/4 cup Pumpkin Pie Spice

Instructions
1. Preheat oven to 400 degrees.
2. Remove flesh from squash.
3. Slice squash.
4. Spray with coconut oil.
5. Place on parchment paper
6. Season with cinnamon and garam marsala.
7. Bake until tender 30-35 minutes.
8. Remove and place in food processor and process along with other ingredients.
9. Bake at 350 degrees.

Decadent Coconut Macaroons
Nutrition: Cal 320;Fat 7 g; Carb 12 g;Protein 10 g
Serving 8; Cook time 30 min.

Ingredients
- 4 large egg whites
- 1 tsp. vanilla
- 1/4 tsp. cream of tartar
- 1/8 tsp. salt
- 1 cup erythritol
- 16 ounces finely shredded, unsweetened dried coconut
- 8 ounces cream cheese, softened
- 2 ounces heavy cream
- 2 ounces Da Vinci Sugar Free White Chocolate Syrup
- 2 ounces Enjoy Life Semi-Sweet Mini Chocolate Chips

Instructions
1. Preheat oven to 325 degrees.
2. Line 2 large baking sheets with parchment paper.
3. In a large mixing bowl, on low, beat together egg whites, vanilla, cream of tartar and salt until soft peaks form.
4. Add erythritol a tablespoon at a time.
5. Beat until stiff peaks form.
6. Fold in coconut.
7. Beat together cream cheese and cream until smooth.
8. Mix in syrup.
9. Add in coconut mixture, a little at a time.
10. Fold in chocolate chips.
11. Using a small ice cream scoop, place mixture on baking sheet.
12. Bake 20-25 minutes.
13. Turn off oven leaving cookies in for 30 minutes.
14. Move to wire rack.

Raspberry Coconut Pancakes
Nutrition: Cal 280;Fat 14 g; Carb 6 g;Protein 14 g
Serving 2; Cook time 15 min.

Ingredients
Pancakes:
- 2 large eggs
- 1 tbsp. fine coconut flour
- 2 tbsp. desiccated coconut (unsweetened)
- ¼ tsp. baking soda
- 3 tbsp. coconut milk
- ½ tsp. pure vanilla bean extract
- 1 tbsp. extra virgin coconut oil
- 3-6 drops liquid Stevia extract

Topping:
- ½ cup plain organic yogurt
- ½ tsp. pure vanilla bean extract
- ⅓ cup fresh raspberries
- 1 tsp. desiccated coconut (unsweetened)

Instructions
1. Beat eggs.
2. In a separate bowl, combine coconut flour, coconut, vanilla bean extract and baking soda.
3. Add to eggs.
4. Add coconut a little at a time.
5. Mix well.
6. Add sweetener.
7. In a separate bowl, mix the yogurt.
8. Grease a pan with coconut oil and turn heat to low.
9. Pour half a ladle of batter into the pan.
10. Flip when bubbles form.
11. Cook for 1 minute.
12. Top with coconut.

No Crust Chocolate Cheesecake
Nutrition: Cal 310;Fat 18 g; Carb 3 g;Protein 14 g
Serving 2; Cook time 15 min.

Ingredients
- 8 oz. cream cheese, softened
- 2 oz. heavy cream

- 1 teaspoon Stevia Glycerite
- 1 teaspoon (packet) Splenda or other powdered or liquid low carb sweetener
- 1 ounce Enjoy Life Mini chocolate chips

Instructions
1. Whip together all ingredients except chocolate until a pudding consistency.
2. Fold in chocolate chips.
3. Refrigerate in serving cups.

Peanutty Frozen Dessert
Nutrition: Cal 340;Fat 22 g; Carb 7 g;Protein 20 g
Serving 1; Cook time 40 min.

Ingredients
- 1 Cup Cottage Cheese
- 1 Scoop Protein Powder
- 2 Tbsp. Peanut Butter
- 2 Tbsp. Heavy Cream
- 6 Drops Splenda
- 1 Hand blender or food processor

Instructions
1. In a food processor, blend together ingredients except protein powder.
2. When smooth mix in protein powder, blend to remove chunks.
3. Freeze for 40 minutes.

Chocolate Caramel Chip Muffins
Nutrition: Cal 250;Fat 7 g; Carb 12 g;Protein 8 g
Serving 1; Cook time 40 min.

Ingredients
- 2 cups Almond Flour
- 1/8 cup erythritol
- 1/2 tsp. baking soda
- 1/2 tsp. salt
- 1/2 tsp. xanthan gum
- 2 large eggs, lightly beaten
- 1 cup sour cream
- 2 T butter, melted, and slightly cooled
- 1 tsp. stevia glycerite
- ½ cup of Walden Farms SF Caramel Dip
- ¾ cup Enjoy Life Semi-Sweet Chocolate Chips

Instructions
1. Preheat oven to 350 degrees.
2. Using paper liners, line 45 muffin cups.
3. In a medium sized bowl, whisk almond flour, erythritol, baking soda, salt and xanthan gum.
4. In a separate bowl, lightly beat eggs.
5. Add sour cream, cooled butter and stevia
6. Stir liquid into flour and mix well.
7. Fill each muffin cup 3/4 full.
8. Bake 20-25 minutes until tops are light brown and springs to touch.

Cream Cheese Filled Chocolate Roll Cake
Nutrition: Cal 280;Fat 12 g; Carb 10 g;Protein 12 g
Serving 1; Cook time 40 min.

Ingredients
- 1 cup Almond Flour
- 4 tbsp. Butter, melted
- 3 large Eggs
- 1/4 cup Psyllium Husk Powder
- 1/4 cup Cocoa Powder
- 1/4 cup Coconut Milk
- 1/4 cup Sour Cream
- 1/4 cup Erythritol
- 1 tsp. Vanilla
- 1 tsp. Baking Powder
- Cream Cheese Filling:
- 8 oz. Cream Cheese
- 8 tbsp. Butter
- 1/4 cup Sour Cream
- 1/4 cup Erythritol
- 1/4 tsp. Stevia
- 1 tsp. Vanilla

Instructions
1. Preheat oven to 350 degrees.
2. Stir together dry ingredients.
3. Slowly mix in wet ingredients.
4. Spread dough on a baking sheet.
5. Bake 12-15 minutes.
6. Mix together cream cheese filling.
7. Spread cream cheese filling over cake.
8. Roll tightly.

ChocoCherry No Bake Cheesecake
Nutrition: Cal 340;Fat 22 g; Carb 7 g;Protein 20 g
Serving 1; Cook time 40 min.

Ingredients
1. 8 oz. cream cheese, softened
2. 2 oz. heavy cream
3. 1 teaspoon Stevia Glycerite
4. 1 tablespoon Dutch process cocoa powder
5. 1 tablespoon Da Vinci Sugar Free Syrup, Cherry flavor
6. 3-5 drops EZSweet liquid Splenda

Instructions
7. Whip together all ingredients except Ezsweet until a pudding consistency.
8. Sweeten to taste with Ezsweet.
9. Refrigerate in small cups.

Brown Butter Blackberry Cake
Nutrition: Cal 240;Fat 16 g; Carb 7 g;Protein 20 g
Serving 1; Cook time 40 min.

The Cake
- 1 1/2 cups Almond Flour
- 1/4 cup Erythritol, powdered
- 2 tbsp. Psyllium Husk Powder
- 1/2 cup Sour Cream
- 1/3 cup Salted Butter

- •2 large Eggs
- •1 1/2 tsp. Baking Powder
- •2 tbsp. Poppy Seeds
- •Zest of 1 Lemon
- •1 tsp. Vanilla Extract
- •1/4 tsp. Liquid Stevia

The Icing

- •2 tbsp. Lemon Juice
- •1/2 cup Erythritol, powdered
- •1/2 cup Blackberries, strained
- •1/4 cup Heavy Cream
- •6 tbsp. Butter

Instructions

1. Preheat oven to 350 degrees.
2. Over medium low heat, brown butter.
3. Mix together all dry ingredients.
4. In separate bowl, mix together all wet ingredients.
5. Add brown butter to wet ingredients.
6. Slowly mix in dry ingredients to wet ingredients
7. Mix until dough forms.
8. Put dough into greased round cake pan.
9. Bake 20-25 minutes.
10. Let cool on cooling rack.
11. In a food processor, purée blackberries.
12. Mix with lemon and erythritol.
13. Cream together, butter and heavy cream.
14. Mix into blackberry purée.
15. Ice the cake and refrigerate 20-30 minutes.

Dark Chocolate Peppermint Frozen Cream
Nutrition: Cal 290;Fat 16 g; Carb 3 g;Protein 20 g
Serving 2; Cook time 30 min.

Ingredients

- •1 Cup Heavy Cream
- •½ Cup Light Cream
- •½ tsp. Liquid Stevia Extract
- •½ tsp. Vanilla (Optional)
- •Several Drops Peppermint Extract (Optional)
- •1 Square Dark Chocolate (Optional)
- •Several Drops Green food coloring (Optional)

Instructions

1. Whisk together all ingredients except chocolate.
2. Freeze for 5 minutes.
3. Add to ice-cream maker.
4. Add shavings before ice cream has set.

Keto Chocolate Chunk Avocado Ice Cream
Nutrition: Cal 310;Fat 18 g; Carb 3 g;Protein 20 g
Serving 2; Cook time 30 min.

Ingredients

- •2 ripe Hass Avocados
- •1 cup Coconut Milk (from carton)
- •1/2 cup Heavy Cream
- •1/2 cup Cocoa Powder
- •2 tsp. Vanilla Extract
- •1/2 cup Erythritol, Powdered

- •25 drops Liquid Stevia
- •6 squares Unsweetened Baker's Chocolate

Instructions

1. Scoop avocado into a bowl.
2. Add coconut milk, cream, and vanilla extract.
3. With an immersion blender, proceed to cream together.
4. Add Erythritol, stevia, and cocoa powder to the avocado mixture and mix well.
5. Add chop bakers chocolate.
6. Chill 6-12 hours, then about 20 minutes before you're ready to serve, add mixture to ice cream machine as per manufacturer's instructions.

Keto Blackberry Pudding Delight
Nutrition: Cal 310;Fat 18 g; Carb 3 g;Protein 20 g
Serving 2; Cook time 40 min.

Ingredients

- •1/4 cup Coconut Flour
- •1/4 tsp. Baking Powder
- •5 large Egg Yolks
- •2 tbsp. Coconut Oil
- •2 tbsp. Butter
- •2 tbsp. Heavy Cream
- •2 tsp. Lemon Juice
- •Zest 1 Lemon
- •1/4 cup Blackberries
- •2 tbsp. Erythritol
- •10 drops Liquid Stevia

Instructions

1. Preheat oven to 350 degrees.
2. Mix together dry ingredients.
3. Add butter and coconut oil to a bowl
4. Beat egg yolks until pale and add erythritol and Stevia.
5. Beat until well mixed.
6. Add heavy cream, lemon juice, lemon zest, coconut oil and butter and beat until fully mixed.
7. Sift dry ingredients into wet and mix well.
8. Put batter into two ramekins.
9. Push in 2 tbsp. blackberries.
10. Bake for 20-25 minutes.

Coconut Macaroons Bites
Nutrition: Cal 240;Fat 3 g; Carb 6 g;Protein 15 g
Serving 2; Cook time 25 min.

Ingredients

- •4 Egg Whites (1/2 Cup)
- •1 tsp. Vanilla
- •½ tsp. EZ-Sweet (Or equivalent of 1 cup artificial sweetener)
- •4½ tsp. Water
- •2 Cups Unsweetened Coconut

Instructions

1. Pre-heat to 375 degrees.
2. Mix together egg whites and liquids
3. Mix in coconut.
4. Put into whoopee pie pan.
5. Put in oven and reduce to 325 degrees.

6. Bake 14 minutes.

Baked Keto Strawberry Cheesecake
Nutrition: Cal 280;Fat 18 g; Carb 6 g;Protein 15 g
Serving 2; Cook time 120 min.

Ingredients
Crust:
- ¾ Cup Pecans (84g)
- ¾ Cup Almond Flour
- 4 Tbsp. Butter
- 2 Tbsp. Splenda

Filling:
- 1½ lbs. Cream Cheese
- 4 Eggs
- ½ Tbsp. Liquid Vanilla
- ½ Tbsp. Lemon Juice
- ½ tsp. EZ-Sweetz (Equivalent to 1 cup sugar, if Splenda, use 1 cup)
- ¼ Cup Sour Cream
- 9 Strawberries

Instructions
1. Preheat to oven to 400 degrees.
2. Crush the pecans.
3. In a saucepan, melt butter and add pecans, Splenda and flour.
4. Mix for several minutes.
5. Grease a 9" spring form pan and add the dough.
6. Cook for 7 minutes until it starts to brown.
7. Combine all ingredients at room temperature
8. Mix well.
9. Slice and Place strawberries along the sides of the crust and fill with filling.
10. Place in oven and lower heat to 250 degrees.
11. Bake 60-90 minutes.

Creamy Chocoberry Fudge Sauce
Nutrition: Cal 320;Fat 20 g; Carb 3 g;Protein 17 g
Serving 2; Cook time 15 min

Ingredients
- 4 ounces cream cheese, softened
- 1-3.5 ounce bar Lindt 90% chocolate, chopped
- 1/4 cup powdered erythritol
- 1/4 cup of heavy cream
- 2 tbsp. Monin sugar free Raspberry Syrup

Instructions
1. Melt together cream cheese and chocolate.
2. Once melted, stir in sweetener.
3. Remove from heat and let cool.
4. Once cool, mix in cream and syrup.
5. Mix well.

Easy Choco-Coconut Pudding
Nutrition: Cal 246;Fat 16 g; Carb 7 g;Protein 15 g
Serving 1; Cook time 50 min.

Ingredients
- 1 cup coconut milk (full fat, canned)

- 2 tbsp. cacao powder or organic cocoa
- 1/2 tsp. stevia powder extract
- Or 2 Tbsp. honey or maple syrup
- 1 Tbsp. quality gelatin
- 2 Tbsp. water

Instructions
1. Over medium heat whisk together coconut milk, cocoa, and sweetener.
2. In a separate bowl, mix the gelatin and water.
3. Add to pan and stir until fully dissolved.
4. Pour into small dishes and refrigerate 30-45 minutes.

Microwave Tiramisu
Nutrition: Cal 270;Fat 16 g; Carb 9 g;Protein 17 g
Serving 1; Cook time 15 min.

Ingredients
- 1 tbsp. eryithol or any sweetener of choice
- 1/2 tsp. of LC sweet brown sugar without the carbs, you can omit this if you want
- 1 tbsp. of unsalted soften butter
- 3 tbsp. of almond flour (honeyville brand)
- 2 tbsp. of vanilla whey protein powder
- 1/4 tsp. of baking powder
- 1 tbsp. of almond milk
- 2 tbsp. of beaten egg or egg whites

Coffee Mixture:
- 1 tbsp. of instant coffee
- 2 tbsp. of water

Filling:
- 2 oz. cream cheese or if you have mascarpone cheese use it
- 2 tbsp. whipped cream or heavy cream
- 1 tsp. of eyrithol

Garnish:
- 1 tsp. unsweetened cocoa powder
- 1 tsp. of unsweetened grated chocolate

Instructions
1. First, mix together the sweetener and the softened butter.
2. Next, mix in the rest of the ingredients.
3. Divide into 2 ramekins.
4. Wait 1 minute for baking powder to activate.
5. Microwave for 1 minute.
6. Melt cream cheese in microwave for 30 seconds and mix in cream and sweetener.
7. Cut cake in half.
8. Dip 2 pieces of cake into coffee.
9. Layer the cake with the filling and sprinkle with cocoa and grated chocolate.

Hazelnut Cheesecake Balls
Nutrition: Cal 315;Fat 20 g; Carb 4 g;Protein 20 g
Serving 4; Cook time 30 min.

Ingredients
- 8 oz. package cream cheese
- 1/4 cup cocoa powder
- Stevia to taste

- 1 or 2 tbsp. Sugar Free Hazelnut syrup
- 1/4 cup ground hazelnuts

Instructions
1. Mix together all ingredients at room temperature except for the hazelnuts.
2. Roll into 16 balls.
3. Cover in hazelnuts.

Berry Layer Cake
Nutrition: Cal 246;Fat 16 g; Carb 7 g;Protein 15 g
Serving 1; Cook time 15 min.

Ingredients15
- 1/4 of the lemon pound cake
- 1/4 cup of whipping cream
- 1/2t Truvia
- 1/8t orange flavor
- Mixed berries

Instructions
1. Cut lemon cake into small cubes.
2. Cut strawberries into small pieces.
3. Whip together whipping cream, Truvia, and orange flavor.
4. Layer fruit, cake and cream in a clear cup.

Coconut Cream Macaroons
Nutrition: Cal 246;Fat 12 g; Carb 5 g;Protein 17 g
Serving 2; Cook time 35 min.

Ingredients
- 1 teaspoon vanilla
- 4 or 5 egg whites
- 1/4 teaspoon cream of tartar
- 9 ounces cream cheese
- 1 cup erythritol
- 3 ounces heavy cream
- 1/8 teaspoon salt
- 18 ounces dried coconut

Instructions
1. Preheat oven to 325 degrees.
2. Whisk together egg whites, cream of tartar, vanilla and salt.
3. Occasionally add erythritol.
4. Add coconut.
5. Whisk together cream cheese, heavy cream and chocolate syrup.
6. Mix in egg mixture.
7. Mix in chocolate.
8. Scoop into baking sheet.
9. Bake 25 minutes.

Rich Brownie Cheesecake
Nutrition: Cal 320;Fat 10 g; Carb 12 g;Protein 15 g
Serving 2; Cook time 35 min.

Ingredients
Brownie:
- 1/2 cup Kerry Gold Butter
- 2 oz. chopped unsweetened chocolate
- 1/2 cup almond flour
- 1/4 cup cocoa powder
- 1/8 tsp. salt
- 2 eggs
- 3/4 cup sweetner equivalent to sugar (we used liquid Splenda)
- 1/4 tsp. vanilla
- 1/4 cup chopped Pecans

Cheesecake:
- 1 lb. softened Cream Cheese
- 2 large Eggs
- 1/2 cup sweetener equivalent to sugar (again we used liquid Splenda)
- 1/4 cup Organic Heavy Cream
- 1/2 tsp. Organic Vanilla Extract

Instructions
1. Preheat oven to 325 degrees.
2. Butter a pie pan.
3. Melt butter and chocolate together in the microwave.
4. In a bowl, mix almond flour, cocoa powder and salt.
5. In separate bowl, mix eggs, sweetener and organic vanilla extract.
6. Add in almond flour mix.
7. Mix in melted butter and chocolate and pecans.
8. Pour into pie pan.
9. Spread out evenly.
10. Bake 15 minutes.
11. Cool 15 minutes.
12. Reduce heat to 300.
13. Beat softened cream cheese
14. Add eggs, sweetener, cream, and vanilla extract.
15. Mix well.
16. Pour over brownie crust.
17. Bake around 40 minutes until center hardly jiggles.
18. Drizzle chocolate sauce on top.

Creamy Banana Fat Bombs
Nutrition: Cal 134;Fat 12 g; Carb 1 g;Protein 3 g
Serving 12; Cook time 70 min.

Ingredients
- 1&1/4 cups cream cheese, at room temperature
- 3/4 cup heavy (whipping) cream
- 1 tablespoon pure banana extract
- 6 drops liquid stevia

Instructions
1. Line a baking sheet with parchment paper and set aside.
2. In a medium bowl, beat together the cream cheese, heavy cream, banana extract, and stevia until smooth and very thick, about 5 minutes.
3. Gently spoon the mixture onto the baking sheet in mounds, leaving some space between each mound, and place the baking sheet in the refrigerator until firm, about 1 hour.
4. Store the fat bombs in an airtight container in the refrigerator for up to 1 week.

BlueberRy Fat Bombs

Nutrition: Cal 115;Fat 12 g; Carb 1 g;Protein 1 g
Serving 12; Cook time 3 hours 10 min.

Ingredients
- ½ cup coconut oil, at room temperature
- ½ cup cream cheese, at room temperature
- ½ cup blueberries, mashed with a fork
- 6 drops liquid stevia
- Pinch ground nutmeg

Instructions
1. Line a mini mufn tin with paper liners and set aside.
2. In a medium bowl, stir together the coconut oil and cream cheese until well blended.
3. Stir in the blueberries, stevia, and nutmeg until combined.
4. Divide the blueberry mixture into the mufn cups and place the tray in the freezer until set, about 3 hours.
5. Place the fat bombs in an airtight container and store in the freezer until you wish to eat them

Spiced-Chocolate Fat Bombs

Nutrition: Cal 117;Fat 12 g; Carb 2 g;Protein 2 g
Serving 12; Cook time 15 min.

Ingredients
- ¾ cup coconut oil
- ¼ cup cocoa powder
- ¼ cup almond butter
- ⅛ teaspoon chili powder
- 3 drops liquid stevia

Instructions
1. Line a mini mufn tin with paper liners and set aside.
2. Put a small saucepan over low heat and add the coconut oil, cocoa powder, almond buter, chili powder, and stevia.
3. Heat until the coconut oil is melted, then whisk to blend.
4. Spoon the mixture into the mufn cups and place the tin in the refrigerator until the bombs are firm, about 15 minutes.
5. Transfer the cups to an airtight container and store the fat bombs in the freezer until you want to serve them.

Chocolate-Coconut Treats

Nutrition: Cal 43;Fat 5 g; Carb 1 g;Protein 1 g
Serving 16; Cook time 35 min.

Ingredients
- ⅓ cup coconut oil
- ¼ cup unsweetened cocoa powder
- 4 drops liquid stevia
- Pinch sea salt
- ¼ cup shredded unsweetened Coconut

Instructions
1. Line a 6-by-6-inch baking dish with parchment paper and set aside.
2. In a small saucepan over low heat, stir together the coconut oil, cocoa, stevia, and salt for about 3 minutes.

3. Stir in the coconut and press the mixture into the baking dish.
4. Place the baking dish in the refrigerator until the mixture is hard, about 30 minutes.
5. Cut into 16 pieces and store the treats in an airtight container in a cool place.

Almond ButTer Fudge

Nutrition: Cal 204;Fat 22 g; Carb 3 g;Protein 3 g
Serving 36; Cook time 2 hours 10 min.

Ingredients
- 1 cup coconut oil, at room temperature
- 1 cup almond butter
- ¼ cup heavy (whipping) cream
- 10 drops liquid stevia
- Pinch sea salt

Instructions
1. Line a 6-by-6-inch baking dish with parchment paper and set aside.
2. In a medium bowl, whisk together the coconut oil, almond buter, heavy cream, stevia, and salt until very smooth.
3. Spoon the mixture into the baking dish and smooth the top with a spatula.
4. Place the dish in the refrigerator until the fudge is firm, about 2 hours.
5. Cut into 36 pieces and store the fudge in an airtight container in the freezer for up to 2 weeks

NutTy Shortbread CoOkies

Nutrition: Cal 105;Fat 10 g; Carb 2 g;Protein 3 g
Serving 18; Cook time 50 min.

Ingredients
- ½ cup butter, at room temperature, plus additional for greasing the baking sheet
- ½ cup granulated sweetener
- 1 teaspoon alcohol-free pure
- vanilla extract
- 1&½ cups almond flour
- ½ cup ground hazelnuts
- Pinch sea salt

Instructions
1. In a medium bowl, cream together the buter, sweetener, and vanilla until well blended.
2. Stir in the almond four, ground hazelnuts, and salt until a firm dough is formed.
3. Roll the dough into a 2-inch cylinder and wrap it in plastic wrap. Place the dough in the refrigerator for at least 30 minutes until firm.
4. Preheat the oven to 350°F. Line a baking sheet with parchment paper and lightly grease the paper with buter; set aside.
5. Unwrap the chilled cylinder, slice the dough into 18 cookies, and place the cookies on the baking sheet.
6. Bake the cookies until firm and lightly browned, about 10 minutes.

7. Allow the cookies to cool on the baking sheet for 5 minutes and then transfer them to a wire rack to cool completely.

VanilLa-Almond Ice Pops
Nutrition: Cal 166;Fat 15 g; Carb 4 g;Protein 3 g
Serving 8; Cook time 4 hours 10 min.

Ingredients
- 2 cups almond milk
- 1 cup heavy (whipping) cream
- 1 vanilla bean, halved lengthwise
- 1 cup shredded unsweetened Coconut

Instructions
1. Place a medium saucepan over medium heat and add the almond milk, heavy cream, and vanilla bean.
2. Bring the liquid to a simmer and reduce the heat to low. Continue to simmer for 5 minutes.
3. Remove the saucepan from the heat and let the liquid cool.
4. Take the vanilla bean out of the liquid and use a knife to scrape the seeds out of the bean into the liquid.
5. Stir in the coconut and divide the liquid between the ice pop molds.
6. Freeze until solid, about 4 hours, and enjoy.

RaspberRy CheEsecake
Nutrition: Cal 176;Fat 18 g; Carb 3 g;Protein 6 g
Serving 12; Cook time 1 hours 10 min.

Ingredients
- ⅔ cup coconut oil, melted
- ½ cup cream cheese, at room temperature
- 6 eggs
- 3 tablespoons granulated sweetener
- 1 teaspoon alcohol-free pure vanilla extract
- ½ teaspoon baking powder
- ¾ cup raspberries

Instructions
1. Preheat the oven to 350°F. Line an 8-by-8-inch baking dish with parchment paper and set aside.
2. In a large bowl, beat together the coconut oil and cream cheese until smooth.
3. Beat in the eggs, scraping down the sides of the bowl at least once.
4. Beat in the sweetener, vanilla, and baking powder until smooth.
5. Spoon the bater into the baking dish and use a spatula to smooth out the top. Scater the raspberries on top.
6. Bake until the center is firm, about 25 to 30 minutes.
7. Allow the cheesecake to cool completely before cuting into 12 squares.

Peanut ButTer MousSe
Nutrition: Cal 280;Fat 28 g; Carb 4 g;Protein 6 g
Serving 4; Cook time 40 min.

Ingredients
- 1 cup heavy (whipping) cream
- ¼ cup natural peanut butter
- 1 teaspoon alcohol-free pure
- vanilla extract
- 4 drops liquid stevia

Instructions
1. In a medium bowl, beat together the heavy cream, peanut buter, vanilla, and stevia until firm peaks form, about 5 minutes.
2. Spoon the mousse into 4 bowls and place in the refrigerator to chill for 30 minutes.

Cauliflower Chaffle
Nutrition: Cal 246;Fat 16 g; Carb 7 g;Protein 20 g
Serving 2; Cook time 30 min.

Ingredients
- 2 cups cauliflower florets, grated
- ½ teaspoon garlic powder
- ½ teaspoon salt
- ½ teaspoon ground black pepper
- 1 teaspoon Italian seasoning
- 2 eggs, pasteurized, at room temperature
- 1 cup mozzarella cheese, full-fat, shredded
- 1 cup parmesan cheese, full-fat, shredded

Instructions
5. Switch on the waffle maker and set it to preheat according to the manufacturer's instructions.
6. Meanwhile, prepare the batter and for this, take a medium-sized bowl, add all the ingredients to it, and whisk well by using an electric mixer at medium speed until incorporated and smooth batter comes together.
7. Grease the waffle maker with avocado oil spray, sprinkle 2 tablespoons of parmesan cheese on waffle trays until covered, and ladle the prepared batter on top.
8. Shut the waffle maker with its lid and let cook for 5–8 minutes until waffle turns firm and golden-brown.
9. When done, remove waffles by using a tong or a fork and repeat with the remaining batter.
10. Let waffles cool slightly and serve.

Parmesan and Garlic Chaffles
Nutrition: Cal 352;Fat 24 g; Carb 2 g;Protein 18 g
Serving 4; Cook time 30 min.

Ingredients
- 1 teaspoon garlic powder
- 2 cups mozzarella cheese, full-fat, shredded
- 4 teaspoons Italian seasoning
- 4 eggs, pasteurized, at room temperature
- 1 cup parmesan cheese, full-fat, grated

Instructions
1. Switch on the waffle maker and set it to preheat according to the manufacturer's instructions.
2. Meanwhile, prepare the batter and for this, take a medium-sized bowl, add all the ingredients (except for cheese), whisk until incorporated, and fold in cheese until mixed.
3. Grease the waffle maker with avocado oil spray and ladle the prepared batter on waffle trays.

4. Shut the waffle maker with its lid and let cook for 5–8 minutes until waffle turns firm and golden-brown.
5. When done, remove waffles by using a tong or a fork and repeat with the remaining batter.
6. Let waffles cool slightly and serve.

Pizza Chaffle
Nutrition: Cal 337;Fat 24 g; Carb 7 g;Protein 25 g
Serving 4; Cook time 30 min.

Ingredients
- 4 eggs, pasteurized, at room temperature
- 2 cups mozzarella cheese, full-fat, shredded
- ¼ teaspoon Italian seasoning
- 4 tablespoons pizza sauce, sugar-free
- ½ cup parmesan cheese, grated
- Pepperoni slices, as needed for topping

Instructions
1. Switch on the waffle maker and set it to preheat according to the manufacturer's instructions.
2. Meanwhile, prepare the batter and for this, take a medium-sized bowl, crack eggs in it, add Italian seasoning and mozzarella cheese, and whisk well by using an electric mixer at medium speed until incorporated and smooth batter comes together.
3. Grease the waffle maker with avocado oil spray, sprinkle 1 tablespoon of parmesan cheese on waffle trays until covered, and ladle the prepared batter on top.
4. Shut the waffle maker with its lid and let cook for 5–8 minutes until waffle turns firm and golden-brown.
5. When done, remove waffles by using a tong or a fork and repeat with the remaining batter.
6. Let waffles cool slightly, spread pizza sauce over each waffle, and top with pepperoni and some more mozzarella cheese.
7. Microwave each waffle for 20 seconds at a high heat setting and then serve.

Buffalo Chicken Chaffle
Nutrition: Cal 465;Fat 24 g; Carb 8 g;Protein 35 g
Serving 4; Cook time 30 min.

Ingredients
- ½ cup celery, diced
- ½ cup almond flour
- 1 cup chicken, pasteurized, shredded
- 2 teaspoons baking powder
- ½ cup Frank red hot sauce and more for topping
- 4 eggs, pasteurized, at room temperature
- ½ cup mozzarella cheese, full-fat, shredded
- ½ cup feta cheese, full-fat, crumbled
- 1 ½ cup cheddar cheese, full-fat, shredded

Instructions
1. Take a small bowl, place flour in it, and stir in the baking powder until mixed, set aside until required.
2. Switch on the waffle maker and set it to preheat according to the manufacturer's instructions.

3. Meanwhile, prepare the batter and for this, take a medium-sized bowl, crack eggs in it, and whisk until blended.
4. Beat in red hot sauce, beat in flour mixture until incorporated, beat in all the cheeses until well combined, and then fold in chicken.
5. Grease the waffle maker with avocado oil spray and ladle the prepared batter on waffle trays.
6. Shut the waffle maker with its lid and let cook for 5–8 minutes until waffle turns firm and golden-brown.
7. When done, remove waffles by using a tong or a fork and repeat with the remaining batter.
8. Let waffles cool slightly, top with some more hot sauce and feta cheese, and serve.

Cheddar Chaffles
Nutrition: Cal 240 Fat 14 g; Carb 4 g;Protein 14 g
Serving 4; Cook time 30 min.

Ingredients
- 4 tablespoons almond flour
- 2 cups cheddar cheese, full-fat, shredded
- 4 eggs, pasteurized, at room temperature

Instructions
1. Switch on the waffle maker and set it to preheat according to the manufacturer's instructions.
2. Meanwhile, prepare the batter and for this, take a medium-sized bowl, add all the ingredients, and whisk well by using an electric mixer at medium speed until incorporated and smooth batter comes together.
3. Grease the waffle maker with avocado oil spray and ladle the prepared batter on waffle trays.
4. Shut the waffle maker with its lid and let cook for 5–8 minutes until waffle turns firm and golden-brown.
5. When done, remove waffles by using a tong or a fork and repeat with the remaining batter.
6. Let waffles cool slightly and serve.

Egg and Mozzarella Chaffle
Nutrition: Cal 258 Fat 19 g; Carb 2 g;Protein 20 g
Serving 4; Cook time 30 min.

Ingredients
- 4 eggs, pasteurized, at room temperature
- 2 cups mozzarella cheese, full-fat, shredded

Instructions
1. Switch on the waffle maker and set it to preheat according to the manufacturer's instructions.
2. Meanwhile, prepare the batter and for this, take a medium-sized bowl, crack eggs in it, add cheese, and whisk well until incorporated and smooth batter comes together.
3. Grease the waffle maker with avocado oil spray and ladle the prepared batter on waffle trays.
4. Shut the waffle maker with its lid and let cook for 5–8 minutes until waffle turns firm and golden-brown.
5. When done, remove waffles by using a tong or a fork and repeat with the remaining batter.
6. Let waffles cool slightly and serve.

Jalapeno and Cheddar Chaffle

Nutrition: Cal 258 Fat 19 g; Carb 2 g;Protein 20 g
Serving 4; Cook time 30 min.

Ingredients
- 4 tablespoons jalapenos, chopped
- 4 tablespoons almond flour
- 4 eggs, pasteurized, at room temperature
- 2 cups cheddar cheese, full-fat, shredded

Instructions
1. Switch on the waffle maker and set it to preheat according to the manufacturer's instructions.
2. Meanwhile, prepare the batter and for this, take a medium-sized bowl, crack eggs in it, add remaining ingredients, and whisk well by using an electric mixer at medium speed until incorporated and smooth batter comes together.
3. Grease the waffle maker with avocado oil spray and ladle the prepared batter on waffle trays.
4. Shut the waffle maker with its lid and let cook for 5–8 minutes until waffle turns firm and golden-brown.
5. When done, remove waffles by using a tong or a fork and repeat with the remaining batter.
6. Let waffles cool slightly and serve.

Beef and Onion Bun Chaffle

Nutrition: Cal 593 Fat 40 g; Carb 2 g;Protein 55 g
Serving 4; Cook time 30 min.

Ingredients
Sauce
- 8 tablespoons horseradish
- 8 teaspoons erythritol sweetener
- 1 teaspoon salt
- 2 cups mayonnaise, full-fat

Chaffle
- 4 tablespoons white onion, minced
- ½ teaspoon salt
- 2 cups mozzarella cheese, full-fat, grated
- 4 eggs, pasteurized, at room temperature
- 16 ounces deli roast beef

Instructions
1. Prepare the sauce and for this, take a medium-sized bowl, place all of its ingredients in it, and whisk until combined. Set aside until needed.
2. Switch on the waffle maker and set it to preheat according to the manufacturer's instructions.
3. Meanwhile, prepare the batter and for this, take a medium-sized bowl, crack eggs in it, add onion, salt, and cheese, and whisk well by using an electric mixer at medium speed until incorporated and smooth batter comes together.
4. Grease the waffle maker with avocado oil spray and ladle the prepared batter on waffle trays.
5. Shut the waffle maker with its lid and let cook for 5–8 minutes until waffle turns firm and golden-brown.
6. When done, remove waffles by using a tong or a fork and repeat with the remaining batter.

7. Let waffles cool slightly, drizzle 2 tablespoons of the horseradish sauce over two waffles, top with beef, and cover the other waffles.
8. Serve chaffle buns with the remaining horseradish sauce and then serve.

Belgian Chaffles

Nutrition: Cal 400 Fat 28.5 g; Carb 3 g;Protein 28 g
Serving 4; Cook time 30 min.

Ingredients
- 3 cups cheddar and jack cheese blend, full-fat, shredded
- 4 eggs, pasteurized, at room temperature

Instructions
1. Switch on the waffle maker and set it to preheat according to the manufacturer's instructions.
2. Meanwhile, prepare the batter and for this, take a medium-sized bowl, crack eggs in it, and whisk until blended.
3. Add cheese blend into the eggs and stir until combined.
4. Grease the waffle maker with avocado oil spray and ladle the prepared batter on waffle trays.
5. Shut the waffle maker with its lid and let cook for 5–8 minutes until waffle turns firm and golden-brown.
6. When done, remove waffles by using a tong or a fork and repeat with the remaining batter.
7. Let waffles cool slightly and serve.

Broccoli and Cheese Chaffle

Nutrition: Cal 340 Fat 26 g; Carb 4 g;Protein 24 g
Serving 4; Cook time 30 min.

Ingredients
- 4 tablespoons almond flour
- 1 cup broccoli florets, chopped
- 1 teaspoon garlic powder
- 4 eggs, pasteurized, at room temperature
- 2 cups cheddar cheese, full-fat, shredded

Instructions
1. Switch on the waffle maker and set it to preheat according to the manufacturer's instructions.
2. Meanwhile, prepare the batter and for this, take a medium-sized bowl, crack eggs in it, add flour, cheese, and garlic powder, and then whisk well by using an electric mixer at medium speed until incorporated and smooth batter comes together.
3. Grease the waffle maker with avocado oil spray, spread half the broccoli into the waffle tray, and ladle the prepared batter on top.
4. Shut the waffle maker with its lid and let cook for 5–8 minutes until waffle turns firm and golden-brown.
5. When done, remove waffles by using a tong or a fork and repeat with the remaining batter and broccoli.
6. Let waffles cool slightly and serve.

Bacon Chaffles
Nutrition: Cal 380 Fat 29 g; Carb 4 g;Protein 24 g
Serving 4; Cook time 30 min.

Ingredients
- 4 tablespoons green onion, chopped
- 1 tablespoon almond flour
- ½ cup bacon, pasteurized, chopped
- ½ teaspoon baking powder
- 4 eggs, pasteurized, at room temperature
- 1 cup cheddar cheese, full-fat, shredded
- 1 cup mozzarella cheese, full-fat

Instructions
1. Switch on the waffle maker and set it to preheat according to the manufacturer's instructions.
2. Meanwhile, prepare the batter and for this, take a medium-sized bowl, crack eggs in it, add flour, baking powder, and both kinds of cheese, and whisk well until incorporated.
3. Add bacon and onion, and stir until mixed and smooth batter comes together.
4. Grease the waffle maker with avocado oil spray and ladle the prepared batter on waffle trays.
5. Shut the waffle maker with its lid and let cook for 5–8 minutes until waffle turns firm and golden-brown.
6. When done, remove waffles by using a tong or a fork and repeat with the remaining batter.
7. Let waffles cool slightly and serve.

Cannabis Chaffles
Nutrition: Cal 422 Fat 37 g; Carb 4 g;Protein 17 g
Serving 4; Cook time 30 min.

Ingredients
- 2 tablespoons melted cannabutter
- 1 cup mozzarella cheese, full-fat, shredded
- 1 cup cream cheese, full-fat, softened
- 4 eggs, pasteurized, at room temperature

Instructions
1. Switch on the waffle maker and set it to preheat according to the manufacturer's instructions.
2. Meanwhile, prepare the batter and for this, take a medium-sized bowl, crack eggs in it, add remaining ingredients, and whisk well by using an electric mixer at medium speed until incorporated and smooth batter comes together.
3. Grease the waffle maker with avocado oil spray and ladle the prepared batter on waffle trays.
4. Shut the waffle maker with its lid and let cook for 5–8 minutes until waffle turns firm and golden-brown.
5. When done, remove waffles by using a tong or a fork and repeat with the remaining batter.
6. Let waffles cool slightly and serve.

Conclusion

I hope this book helps those women out there that are looking for a diet that will help them change their entire lifestyle. The ketogenic diet has helped me in so many ways to recover from the diseases that I had to face due to the growing age. Females, unlike males, have to go through a lot in a lifetime. Menopause is one of the biggest changing factors that is the start of the decline in our health. Just like how we first encounter our first period, stopping the menstrual cycle can have a huge impact on our body. With that comes a lot of issues such as obesity, joint problems (arthritis), fatigue, hormonal imbalances, mood swings, insomnia, acne, and so much more that you have read about in this book. It doesn't only talk about the problems women over 50 faces but how the keto diet can help fight those problems more healthily. No diet only benefits, just like how trying out a new workout can be hard on your body and in the beginning, starting a new diet can have some problematic impact on your body as well. Some problems that come alongside the ketogenic diet have been discussed in this book as well. Like the keto flu (ugh! don't get me started on that one), keto rash, keto cramps, and more. But, unlike other books, you will find solutions alongside every problem enlisted in this book. And not only solutions but a handful of some delicious recipes for your beginner keto-friendly meal and all the ingredients you might need to start this diet. Hopefully, this will help you grasp the technicalities of the keto diet and help you make a healthier you.

Sandra Grant

2022

Printed in Great Britain
by Amazon

11840767R10106